The Developing Genome

CONTENTS

The Developing Genome

Genome

An Introduction to Behavioral Epigenetics

DAVID S. MOORE

OXFORD
UNIVERSITY PRESS

OXFORD

UNIVERSITY PRESS

Oxford University Press is a department of the University of
Oxford. It furthers the University's objective of excellence in research,
scholarship, and education by publishing worldwide.

Oxford   New York

Auckland   Cape Town   Dar es Salaam   Hong Kong   Karachi
Kuala Lumpur   Madrid   Melbourne   Mexico City   Nairobi
New Delhi   Shanghai   Taipei   Toronto

With offices in

Argentina   Austria   Brazil   Chile   Czech Republic   France   Greece
Guatemala   Hungary   Italy   Japan   Poland   Portugal   Singapore
South Korea   Switzerland   Thailand   Turkey   Ukraine   Vietnam

Oxford is a registered trademark of Oxford University Press
in the UK and certain other countries.

Published in the United States of America by
Oxford University Press
198 Madison Avenue, New York, NY 10016

A copy of this book's Cataloging-in-Publication Data is on file with the Library of Congress
ISBN 978-0-19-992234-5

1 3 5 7 9 8 6 4 2
Printed in the United States of America
on acid-free paper

The beginning of modern science can be dated from the time when such general questions as, "How was the universe created? What is matter made of? What is the essence of life?" were replaced by such limited questions as "How does a stone fall? How does water flow in a tube? How does blood circulate in vessels?" This substitution had an amazing result. While asking general questions led to limited answers, asking limited questions turned out to provide more and more general answers.

—François Jacob, 1977

The biology of the mind has now captured the imagination of the scientific community of the 21st century, much as the biology of the gene fascinated the scientists of the 20th century.

—Eric Kandel, in his speech to the Nobel Foundation, 2000

ACKNOWLEDGMENTS

It would have been completely impossible for me to write this book without the support and active help of numerous individuals and institutions. I am particularly grateful to Philip D. Zelazo for motivating me to learn about behavioral epigenetics; to Mark S. Blumberg for calling the attention of Oxford University Press to my nascent book on this topic; and to my agent, Miriam Altshuler, for her tireless and ongoing efforts on my behalf. In addition, I received feedback on earlier versions of my manuscript from several friends and colleagues to whom I am indebted; the final version is undoubtedly better than it would have been without the helpful comments of Dawn M. Moore, J. Steven Reznick, Daniel K. Feinberg, Mark S. Blumberg, Jerome Kagan, and one anonymous reviewer. From the earliest stages of my career through the final stages of this book project, I have been lucky enough to have a large number of colleagues and friends with whom I have been able to share ideas, books, and/or papers, and I greatly appreciate their intellectual generosity; they include Robert Lickliter, J. Steven Reznick, Jerome Kagan, Philip R. Zelazo, David J. Lewkowicz, Moshe Szyf, Patrick O. McGowan, Ziv Machnes, Janet F. Werker and the students and staff in her lab, and several members of the faculty at Pitzer College, notably Emily Wiley, Brian L. Keeley, and Alan P. Jones. Writing a book like this also required some very special locations where I could sit undisturbed for hours on end while remaining near outstanding libraries and exceptional caffeinated beverages; my efforts to get my thoughts on "paper" were greatly facilitated by the Whiteley Center at the University of Washington's Friday Harbor Laboratories, the University of British Columbia, the Claremont Colleges, Niall and Cathy Burnett, Cynthia Adams, and numerous cafés in Victoria and Vancouver, British Columbia. And although all of the members of my family were helpful and supportive as I worked on this project, I benefited in particular from conversations with Irwin B. Moore, Beryl Moore, and Michael B. Jones.

Special thanks are due to my beloved wife, Dawn M. Moore, who tolerated my struggles with this project, who sacrificed years without a proper vacation, who read each of my words with thoughtful consideration, who created all but four of the beautiful figures gracing the pages of this book, and who provided me with indispensable encouragement whenever I ran into obstacles while composing this treatise. She was absolutely the sine qua non for this project, and I cannot possibly thank her enough.

D. S. M.

Claremont, California 2014

PART I

WHAT'S THE BIG DEAL? GETTING UP TO SPEED

1

Context

The British Empire in North America got off to a rocky start. A metal plaque in St. John's, Newfoundland—the easternmost spot in Canada—commemorates the landing of Sir Humphrey Gilbert, who on August 5, 1583, took possession of "this new found land in the name of his sovereign Queen Elizabeth [and] thereby founded Britain's overseas empire." Looking at the plaque, it is easy to imagine Gilbert's sense of victory at his accomplishment and to imagine him returning to great fanfare in London, where he could live out the rest of his days amid an adoring public. What the plaque fails to record is that Gilbert was actually lost at sea 35 days later as he sailed home; he was never seen again.

Fortunately for the English, Gilbert's mother had another son, Gilbert's half-brother Walter. When his half-brother drowned, Walter was only 29 years old, but his youth didn't stop Queen Elizabeth from granting him a charter to carry out the transatlantic expeditions Gilbert had planned and financed before his death. Just 6 months after Gilbert disappeared at sea, the queen granted Walter the right "to discover, search, finde out, and view such remote, heathen and barbarous lands, countries, and territories, not actually possessed of any Christian Prince." Walter ultimately became such a favorite of the queen that she knighted him in the mid-1580s, which is why we have since known him as *Sir* Walter Raleigh.

Elizabeth's charge to Raleigh was to establish a colony—in her words, "to inhabite or remaine, there to build and fortifie, at the discretion of the said *Walter Ralegh*." Raleigh never traveled to North America himself, but an expedition he sent in 1587 did establish a colony in what is now North Carolina. But "remaine" it did not. The Roanoke Colony was founded as a collection of families with a combined population of more than 100 men, women, and children, but less than two years after the colonists were left to live off of the rich American land, ships returning to the location from England found not a soul in residence.[1] The site did not contain any signs of distress or struggle, and to this day, no one knows for sure what happened to the colonists, which is why Roanoke is now known as "the lost colony." Among the hypotheses that have been floated to explain the mysterious disappearance of the colonists are that they tried to sail back to England and died at sea or that they relocated to live among local Native American tribes. But there is little archaeological support for any of these claims.

In the late 1990s, a tantalizing new bit of evidence about the failure of the colony came to light. By looking at the rings in centuries-old cypress trees in southeastern Virginia, a team of scientists discovered that in the three-year period when the Roanoke Colony disappeared, the region was in the midst of the worst drought in 800 years.[2] The extreme lack of available water during this period would have made it very difficult for the colonists to survive. Armed with their data, the scientists concluded that although the "colonists have been criticized for poor planning, poor support, and a startling indifference to their own subsistence, . . . the tree-ring reconstruction indicates that even the best planned and supported colony would have been supremely challenged by the climatic conditions of 1587–1589."[3]

In the 1960s and 1970s, social psychologists learned from their experiments that observers often underestimate the power of situations to influence what people do. For instance, if an observer hears a person tell a lie, the observer will typically attribute the lie to the individual's personality, even if virtually everyone would lie *in the situation the person was in*; that is, the observer will judge the person's character and fail to understand that it was really the context that provoked the lie.[4] In evaluating what happened to the Roanoke Colony, this kind of error-of-attribution could explain why the colonists have traditionally been criticized for their own demise, even when the failure of the colony might best be understood as having been caused by a situational factor, the drought. It seems that for human beings, it is always easier to see the influences of a person—or any active party—than it is to see the influences of the person's *context*, even if the contextual factors might be just as important as the active party's characteristics.

Of course, it is a mistake to see the failure of the Roanoke Colony as being *completely* determined by the weather. After all, the colony at Jamestown was established not long after the Roanoke Colony, and although the residents at Jamestown also experienced a drought worse than any in that area for over 750 years,[5] their colony survived—if only by the skin of its teeth!—and went on to serve as the capital of the colony of Virginia for over 80 years. So rather than understanding these historical events as reflecting the characteristics of the colonists *or* the characteristics of their situations, a better way to think about these events is in terms of the *interactions* that occur between people and their contexts. When we try to understand why things unfold as they do, it's often helpful to recognize that multiple factors play a role in any outcome. For colonial America to emerge as it did, some vital *combination* of people and situations was required.

The End of Nature Versus Nurture

This book is about how individuals come to be as they are. For thousands of years, words in the Hebrew bible about sparing "the rod" have been understood to mean that we grow up to be the adults we are at least in part because of the experiences we have at the hands of our parents. In the 20th century, biologists discovered that we are also profoundly influenced by the molecules of DNA we inherit from our parents. These dual influences—experiences and DNA—are associated with nurture and nature, respectively, ideas theorists have been arguing about at least since 1582, the year before Gilbert claimed Newfoundland for the Crown; that year marked the publication of an influential book on education called *Elementarie*, written by one Richard Mulcaster—the headmaster of what was at the time the largest school in England—who used the words "nature" and "nurture" to describe the factors that influence how children develop.[6]

My earlier book *The Dependent Gene* is about how genes cannot be single-handedly responsible for our characteristics; that book is essentially an argument against *genetic determinism*, the idea that genes can determine the nature of our characteristics. Even though many nonscientists think there are genes that cause us to have the eye colors we have, genes that cause some of us to develop certain diseases, and genes that cause some of us to be smart or musical or funny, the truth is that genes are only half of the story. Just as we can't understand the fate of the Roanoke Colony by considering only its colonists (or the drought), we can't understand why some of us have brown eyes and some of us have blue eyes by considering genetic factors alone (even if your biology teachers in school told you we can). The fact is, people's characteristics—including both physical traits like facial structure or psychological traits like personality—result from interactions that occur between biological molecules and their contexts.[7] This will not be news to people who have read about this topic before, but to anyone new to the area, it might be surprising. The nature-versus-nurture debate is passé, because scientists now understand that genetic factors and situational factors both always play roles in the development of our traits. Consequently, as I explained in my earlier book, it is useful to adopt the perspective that neither factor is ever more important than the other.

In the late 1990s while I was working on *The Dependent Gene*, I had a conversation with my father about the nature of development. He was engaged by this question because he is a medical doctor, and he remains interested in the questions that drive contemporary scientists. But when I told him about my interest in a process called "epigenesis," he confessed to me a natural dislike of that term. As a physician, he was familiar with the prefix "epi," from the Greek root meaning "above," "on," or "on top of," but the whole notion of there being things "on top of" genes made no sense to him. I countered that the word really just captured the idea that there are factors that are *metaphorically* "above" genes, factors that influence genetic functioning and, as a result, development. When scientists talk about epigenesis like this, they have in mind all of the nongenetic factors that influence an organism's development, including factors like hormones or the social contexts in which some animals live their lives. But to my father-the-doctor, this metaphorical meaning was unsatisfying; for him, the word "epigenetic" should refer only to things physically "on top of" the genes. And in the 1990s, my understanding of such things was vague at best, and my father was not convinced that any such things even existed at all.

Now, less than two decades later, things are different. Epigenetics is a well established subbranch of biology, and the new discoveries of epigeneticists have generated an enormous amount of excitement in several different disciplines, including oncology, nutrition, psychology, philosophy, and others. In fact, there actually *are* things *on* (or, at any rate, attached to) our DNA—they are often referred to as "epigenetic marks"—and as it turns out, these things play critical roles in how DNA functions. For this reason, epigenetic processes influence virtually all of our characteristics. And although scientists have only just started learning what there is to know about epigenetic marks, the discoveries made so far have been truly groundbreaking. Because some epigenetic marks can be influenced by our experiences (and other aspects of the environments we occupy), such marks are being invoked to explain things as diverse as the differences between identical twins, the effects of our diets on our health, and the influence of mothers' behaviors on how stressed their offspring are as adults. This is why discoveries about epigenetics have helped undermine the nature-nurture debate; because epigenetic events happen at the interface between DNA and its environment, they can help us see how our features always arise from *both* nature and nurture, just as the success or failure of the first American colonies depended on *both* the colonists and their situations.

Psychology and Biology

As a developmental psychologist, I'm interested in how psychological traits develop. To get a grasp on those processes, I've found it useful to learn about biology. Biology is important for psychology because our personalities, behaviors, emotions, and thoughts all depend on the structures and functions of our brains, a biological organ. Other organs contribute to psychological characteristics as well; our guts, for instance, have long been known to play critical roles in influencing our emotions and motivating our behaviors. Of course, understanding someone's psychology will always require more than just understanding their organs, because what we think, feel, and do is affected by factors *outside* of our bodies. But because biology *contributes* to all psychological phenomena, trying to understand psychology with very little understanding of biology is a bad idea (even if some of my students are not happy to hear this news on the first day of my Introduction to Psychology courses)!

It is equally important, though, to remember that factors outside of our bodies affect our biological systems just as they affect our thoughts and behaviors. If you were trying to understand a normal person's heart rate changes over the course of a day, you would be hopelessly confused by the sudden spike in her pulse if you didn't realize that it was correlated with the unexpected sight of her latest flame. Just as we understand that our experiences influence our mental states, anyone who has studied, for example, how depression influences weight gain[8] or how psychological stress contributes to adverse cardiac events[9] understands that our experiences influence our bodily states as well. Once you start to think about it, it becomes clear that there is a fundamental similarity between what happens when your *organs* behave (e.g., your heart beats) and what happens when *you* behave (e.g., you smile at a friend). For this reason, biological and psychological characteristics really ought not be considered distinctly different things.

Scientists have been interested in how psychology is related to biology for well over 100 years,[10] but it is only recently that they have started to get a handle on how DNA, proteins, and the other molecules in our cells contribute to our psychological traits. The new understandings now coming into focus have their roots in biology, but recent research in a field known as behavioral epigenetics has started to show how our molecular biology influences our psychological states *and* how our psychological states influence our molecular biology. This book will focus on this two-way highway of influence.

The insights of behavioral epigenetics have the potential to change how we treat ourselves and other people, so they are too important to remain the property of biologists alone. These lessons must be made available to everyone. But while the conclusions we can draw from recent work in epigenetics are fascinating and potentially important, the real news here is in the molecular details. It is difficult to get a deep appreciation of the power of this emerging domain of knowledge just by hearing the takeaway message; getting a good feel for epigenetics requires looking under the hood. Unfortunately, what is under the hood can be a bit intimidating, because molecular biology is extremely complex. My hope is that my background as a nonbiologist will enable me to tell the story of epigenetics in a comprehensible, relatively jargon-free way.

Having said that, different readers will almost certainly be looking for different levels of detail from a book like this, so I will tell the story of behavioral epigenetics on two different levels. Six of the 23 chapters in this book will involve "Zooming in" on the topic of the preceding chapter. It is possible to skip these more detailed chapters and still have the experience of reading a seamless book, because the other seventeen chapters provide all of the information required to understand the principal messages that have emerged from research in this field.

The six "Zooming in" chapters provide a glimpse of the truly exciting molecular details emerging from the world's behavioral epigenetics labs, and although they should still be accessible to readers who have not previously studied biology, they provide a level of detail that only some readers will be seeking. But do note: The "Zooming in" chapters work together, so understanding the information in a later "Zooming in" chapter will likely require a reader to have read the earlier "Zooming in" chapters as well.

Our Focus and a Note of Caution

The growth in the field of epigenetics has been astonishing in the last few years. Although I used the word "epigenetic" nearly two dozen times when I was writing *The Dependent Gene* in 1999, a PubMed search for "epigenetics" yields only 46 references that used that word in the three dozen years between 1964 and 2000. The same search finds more than 40 times that number of references—1,922—published in just the first decade of the 21st century. And between 2010 and 2014, the same search finds nearly four times that number of references, 7,462. In 2013 alone, PubMed reports that 2,413 scientific papers mentioned epigenetics, 25% more than were published in the first *decade* of the 21st century. The recent proliferation of research in this area reflects the fact that epigenetic processes are helping to explain an enormous number of phenomena, including—fasten your seatbelts—psychosis, memory and learning, depression, cancer, circadian rhythms, obesity and diabetes, autism, trait inheritance, homosexuality,[11] addiction, aging, insects' body shapes, the effects of factors like exercise, nutrition, environmental toxins, and early-life experiences . . . the list goes on and on. Clearly, a book like this cannot consider all of the emerging work on epigenetics in a comprehensive way, so a word is needed here about what this book will and will not focus on.

My primary concentration will be on *behavioral* epigenetics, the branch of epigenetics that studies how epigenetic effects influence psychological processes like emotional reactivity, memory and learning, mental health, and behavior.[12] Because of this emphasis, I will not focus on topics like cancer or senescence (i.e., biological aging); in *The Epigenetics Revolution* (2011), Nessa Carey does an excellent job of introducing readers with a strong background in biology to these topics. Likewise, this book will not be *primarily* about the discovery that some epigenetic effects can be transmitted from ancestors to descendants (i.e., epigenetic inheritance). But because the inheritance of epigenetic states is one of the most interesting—and controversial[13]—aspects of some recent work in epigenetics, I will devote Part III of this book to this topic. Until then, I will emphasize how experience can influence our epigenetic states in our own lifetimes, because this phenomenon, independently of whether or not these states can be inherited, bears on how we think about human nature. Although the idea of epigenetic inheritance is exciting, it has the potential to distract us from other implications of epigenetics that are just as groundbreaking.

A note of caution is also warranted here. Excitement about behavioral epigenetics has been increasing so rapidly that several writers have begun to worry that "this hot new field [might be] getting ahead of itself."[14] There have been a few recent articles expressing concern about the so-called hype surrounding behavioral epigenetics,[15a–15b] and a group of eight well-respected scientists signed a letter—published in *Science* in 2010—that "expressed serious reservations about the scientific basis of the epigenome project."[16] It is perhaps no surprise that I think the excitement generated by research in this domain is justified. Nonetheless, science proceeds slowly, and it is clear that it will be some time before behavioral epigenetics is completely free from controversy, particularly with respect to epigenetic inheritance. But even if the skeptics are right and epigenetic inheritance (as some theorists define it) proves to be exceedingly rare, I am still confident that insights from research on epigenetics will help us understand how genetic and experiential factors work together in an interdependent way to build all of our psychological and biological characteristics. Because some authors continue to promote genetic determinism by writing as if there are genes that can single-handedly determine the nature of some of our characteristics—be they diseases, talents, or vices—we should value the ability of epigenetics to underscore how genetic and nongenetic factors always work *together* to produce our traits. In this way, recent discoveries about epigenetics really should be recognized as revolutionary.

2

Phenotypes

The Academy Award-winning actress Angelina Jolie was perfectly healthy when she made the decision to have both of her breasts surgically removed. As she explained in an essay published in the *New York Times*, her decision was motivated by the discovery that she has "a 'faulty' gene, *BRCA1*, which sharply increases [the] risk of developing breast cancer and ovarian cancer."[1] In the following days, the range of opinions I heard on her decision was startling, running the gamut from laudatory to critical. Maureen Dowd, a columnist for the *Times*, wrote that Jolie's "courage in going public with the graphic details of her mutilation and reconstruction . . . makes her a real-life action heroine."[2] In contrast, an author of multiple respected books on genetics commented that her decision seemed "pretty stupid." Conflicting reactions like this reflect the fact that our understanding of breast cancer remains so murky that different people can look at the same situation and see different things, as if Jolie were some sort of a medical Rorschach test.

To her credit, her writing revealed that she had established a relatively sophisticated understanding of her predicament before she made her decision. The gene in question—*BRCA1* (pronounced like "bracka-one")—is known by its acronym, but this nickname was derived from its more formal name: "Breast cancer 1." Given its name, most people would conclude that this is an abnormal gene that causes breast cancer. But this would be a mistake in two important ways. First, *BRCA1* is not abnormal; it is present in everyone's body, and thank goodness, because it performs the vital function of repairing damaged DNA, a task required quite frequently. Second, even the various mutated forms of *BRCA1* that *are* associated with cancer do not *cause* it in the kind of straightforward way implied by the gene's name. If a mutated *BRCA1* gene *caused* breast cancer, anyone with that mutated gene would develop breast cancer, but some people with mutated *BRCA1* genes remain cancer free throughout their lives.[3] Jolie telegraphed her understanding of these things by using quotation marks when she described the gene as "faulty" and when she noted that it merely imparted on her an increased risk, not a certain death sentence.

When doctors tell their patients about "risk," what they are doing is providing statistical information, based on past observations, about what seems likely to occur in the future. As it is with meteorology, so it is with biology: If your local weather forecaster tells you there is a 75% chance of precipitation tomorrow, you know she is just offering her best guess about what will happen. But when tomorrow comes, it may or may not rain. This is why Jolie's decision was a difficult one. To some observers, she decided to risk radical surgery even though there was a real chance she would never develop breast cancer. As three science-and-health writers for the *New York Times* subsequently pointed out, some physicians were worried that Jolie's "disclosure could be misinterpreted by other women, fueling the trend toward [breast-removal surgeries] that are not medically necessary."[4] Asked about the choices facing women in Jolie's position, the highly respected surgeon Susan Love observed, "When you have to cut off normal body parts to prevent a disease, that's really pretty barbaric."[5] Of course, how a person responds to the discovery that she has a *BRCA1* mutation is a personal decision that no one has a right to second-guess. But Jolie's choice to announce her decision publicly threw the issue of genetic contributions to diseases squarely into the public spotlight. The more we know about DNA and how it works, the more equipped we will be to make some of the important decisions we might face in the future.

DNA and Phenotypes: A Complex Relationship

There is a more general message to be gleaned from reading extensively about *BRCA1*. It turns out that there is a good reason why the DNA that is the *BRCA1* gene doesn't cause breast cancer: DNA cannot single-handedly cause diseases. In fact, DNA can't single-handedly cause *any* of our characteristics! This statement might be surprising, because most of us have been explicitly taught that the genes in our DNA *do* cause some of our phenotypes (to use the word biologists use when referring to traits or characteristics). Phenotypes can be physical or psychological, and they include everything from a person's eye color and head size, to their musical talent, attention span, and penchant for drunkenness (and everything in between). But even though genes do not *determine* phenotypes, many of the world's current biology textbooks still suggest that they do, thereby espousing a form of genetic determinism; eye color is a particularly noteworthy example, as many biology textbooks leave students with the impression that this phenotype is genetically determined in a simple way.[6a–6c] Likewise, the mass media often reinforces the idea that there can be genes "for" things like hair textures, personality traits, or tumors; in a perfectly mundane occurrence, the homepage of the *New York Times* on the day I was writing this chapter contained the headline "Overweight? Maybe Your Genes Really Are at Fault."[7] And some writers in the social sciences, humanities, and even the life sciences still write as if certain phenotypes are already inherent in us when we are just embryos, as if these characteristics are somehow unavoidably part of our destinies—*predestined*, or predetermined—regardless of the experiences we might have as we develop.

Despite these kinds of statements, DNA doesn't work like this. Instead, our traits—whether you're considering the characteristics of your bones, your brain, your eyes, or anything else[8a–8c]—emerge because of how genetic and nongenetic factors interact as we develop and live our lives.[9a–9n] Genes—that is, DNA segments—are always influenced by their contexts, so there is never a perfect relationship between the presence of a gene and the ultimate appearance of a phenotype. Genes do not determine who we become, because nongenetic factors play critical roles in trait development; genes do what they do at least in part *because* of their contexts. This is why doctors are unable to provide more than the *probability* that you will develop a disease based on your genetic constitution. Genes alone can't be used to accurately predict what will happen, because the contexts in which we live our lives always play a role in life's outcomes.[10a–10e] If this doesn't sound like a revelation to you, it's probably because you have read about this topic before; but to many people, this really is news.

A Little Information About Breast Cancer

Given this scenario, it should be no surprise that information about a given woman's *BRCA1* gene cannot be used to accurately predict if she will develop breast cancer. This fundamental ignorance is hard to reconcile with what sounds like relatively confident predictions coming from doctors, who in Angelina Jolie's case estimated her risk of developing breast cancer at a whopping 87%. Faced with a number like this, many women with financial resources might choose surgery despite currently being in excellent health. But such a large (and notably precise) number gives the impression that we understand more about breast cancer than we actually do.

To see just how wary we should be of these kinds of estimates, consider the following passage from the current factsheet on *BRCA* mutations, written by the world's foremost breast cancer experts at the National Institute of Health's Cancer Institute (I have italicized phrases that warrant special attention):

> It is important to note . . . that estimates of breast and ovarian cancer risk associated with *BRCA1* and *BRCA2* mutations have been calculated from studies of [large families with many individuals affected by cancer]. Because family members share a proportion of their genes and, often, their environment, *it is possible that the large number of cancer cases seen in these families may be due in part to other genetic or environmental factors.* Therefore, [these] risk estimates . . . *may not accurately reflect the levels of*

risk for *BRCA1* and *BRCA2* mutation carriers in the general population. In addition, no data are available from long-term studies of [cancer risk using the proper comparison groups in] the general population . . . [so] the percentages given above are estimates that may change as more data become available.[11]

This statement should clarify why some healthcare professionals were alarmed when Angelina Jolie became a potential role model for women with *BRCA1* gene mutations. Not to make an agonizing decision any more agonizing, but the truth is that we are still largely in the dark about breast cancer, and just because a person has a particular genetic variant does not mean we really know what the future holds for that person.

Nonetheless, some things are known. First, certain kinds of cancers—prostate and colon cancers, along with breast cancer, for example—sometimes run in families, and genetic factors play a role in these cases.[12] Second, certain behaviors (e.g., smoking cigarettes) severely increase the risk of developing cancer.[13] These two kinds of contributions to cancer represent nature and nurture, the poles of the age-old debate about what makes us who we are. But cancer researchers in the forefront of the field now recognize another factor that is critically important in cancer: epigenetics. As Andrew Feinberg, a professor of molecular medicine at Johns Hopkins University, wrote in 2006, "cancer seems to have both a genetic and epigenetic basis."[14] Likewise, Osamu Nakanishi, the cancer research division leader for Asia's largest pharmaceutical company, said in 2010, "Epigenetics controls so many things . . . and it has decisive power for inducing cancer."[15] The important role of epigenetics in cancer was underscored in 2004, when the Food and Drug Administration began approving new drugs that fight particular cancer types by influencing epigenetic factors in our bodies. But what does this terribly awkward word "epigenetics" mean?

Introducing Epigenetics: The Developing Genome

In the era of the 24-hour news cycle, information reaches us quickly. So if you suddenly start to hear a lot about a musician you've never heard of before, odds are it is because she has just released her first recordings and they're good enough to have garnered some new fans quickly. And if you've suddenly started to hear a lot about epigenetics, you might reasonably conclude there's a new discipline on the scene, which has been given this new, rather odd name. But there is actually quite a lot of history behind the word "epigenetics," going back hundreds of years.[16a–16c]

The word "epigenetics" has been defined in different ways in different eras, depending on what was known about biology at the time, and I will talk about a few of the more recent definitions in the next chapter. But throughout most of this book, I will use a definition that reflects how contemporary biologists use the word: *Epigenetics refers to how genetic material is activated or deactivated—that is, expressed—in different contexts or situations.* Think of it like this: DNA works like a light switch that can be turned on or off. Even better, DNA works like a *dimmer* switch; it can be turned on just a little bit, a moderate amount, a lot, full-blast, or any amount in between. How active a DNA segment is depends on its epigenetic state, which depends on factors like its context.

This definition represents a fairly radical change in perspective on genes and what they do. The traditional perspective holds that what really matters is the genes that you *have.* From this perspective, if you have genes associated with blue eyes, this is why you have blue eyes. If you have a gene associated with breast cancer, you have an increased risk of developing breast cancer. And so on. But the definition of epigenetics suggests that we should be thinking about these things in a very different way. Given that genetic activity levels change in different circumstances, what really matters is what your DNA is *doing.* It doesn't matter if you *have* a particular gene if that gene might be "turned off." From the perspective of epigenetics, having a gene is a little bit like having a key, which when you think about it, is completely useless in the absence of the right keyhole. To quote Benjamin Franklin out of context, such a gene would be like "silver in the mine"—of little consequence.

An excellent example of epigenetics in action could be called "the case of the skittish rats." In a remarkable program of research, scientists in Montreal have discovered that the behaviors of mother rats alter the activity of genes in their baby pups, genes that play a role in modulating stress reactions.[17] Specifically, mothers that spend a lot of time licking and grooming their babies effectively "turn on" specific genes in those pups, and as a result, the offspring grow up to be adult rats that respond well to stressful events. Mothers that don't treat their pups this way end up with offspring that respond to stress in much less healthy ways. Because people have nervous systems that respond to stress in much the same was as rats' nervous systems do, the implications of this discovery have been recognized as extremely important. (In fact, the work of these scientists is so important that I'll devote an entire chapter—titled "Experience"—to describing this research.)

Changing the focus from what genes you *have* to what your genes are *doing* might seem like a subtle shift, but it's actually game changing. The idea that we are as we are because of the genes we inherit implies that at least some of our phenotypes are predetermined when we are conceived. In contrast, the recognition that epigenetic processes influence the functioning of our genes means that our experiences *and* our DNA together make us as we are, so our characteristics cannot be predetermined. The contexts in which we live our lives—how we are nurtured—definitely matter. This is one reason cancer researchers believe the vast majority of cancer cases are associated with environmental or lifestyle factors.[18]

The genome of an individual—that is, the full complement of genetic material in that person's cells—is usually thought to remain unchanged across the person's life. Other than random mutations, the DNA sequence information you received at conception is identical to the DNA sequence information that will be in your body when you die. Now, keep in mind that the genome of the human *species* is undergoing changes because of the process of evolution, but evolutionary changes occur in a *population*'s genome across multiple generations, so these kinds of changes are decidedly different from any changes that could occur in an individual's genome in a single lifetime. For this reason, biologists have traditionally considered *development* to be a characteristic of an organism, not a genome; the thinking has been that although people change as they grow from infants into adults, their genomes don't.

However, once we understand that some of our DNA behaves differently at different times, we're forced to accept the fact that in very significant ways, our genomes are dynamic. And because we now know that the variations in how our genomes function reflect changes in the chemical structure of DNA, we can no longer ignore the fact that people's genomes effectively change as they live out their lives. So the traditional idea that the genetic material in an individual's body remains unchanged across the lifespan needs to be revised. We are all born with *a developing genome*, one that changes in response to its environmental context.

It is one thing to discover that our DNA can be affected by its context and that the environment in which we develop can affect that context in important ways. But it is something else to discover *how* DNA and its context work together—in a mechanical way—to make us who we are. By the mid-1960s, some developmental biologists already understood that genes are affected by factors present in their environments.[19] But nearly five decades later, we are still just beginning to get an inkling of *how* our environments affect the molecules inside us and thereby collaborate with our genes to build us from the ground up. In the following pages, I will provide several examples that illustrate how all of this works.

Why Everyone Needs to Know About Behavioral Epigenetics

Discoveries of previously unimagined epigenetic phenomena have provided compelling empirical evidence that DNA-context interactions are continuously present in development. Epigeneticists have already begun unraveling how it is that our experiences influence genetic activity and thereby contribute to our future phenotypes. As the American neurobiologist David Sweatt put it, "there is an emerging fascination with epigenetics, because it has been a hidden mechanistic layer operating at the environment–genome interface."[20] The conclusion that developmental circumstances—"nurture"—can influence how a person's genome functions does not mean that "nature" is any less important than we all previously thought. But it does mean that DNA cannot specify destiny. The implications of epigenetic research are enormous, because the belief that experiences matter is likely to affect how we live our lives and how we treat those around us.

For example, a teacher who believes some children are born with genes that produce insurmountable learning disabilities will be less inclined to invest time and energy teaching these children than will a teacher who believes all children can learn. An employer who believes people of a particular racial background are "naturally" competent will be more likely to hire someone with that background. And if you believe you are destined to be overweight because both of your parents are obese, you might be less likely to even try to control the number of calories you eat; why deny yourself the pleasures of chocolate cake when you are destined to be heavy anyway? But anyone who knows that genes alone cannot determine traits like body mass, competence in the workplace, or aptitude for learning is likely to behave very differently in these situations. Epigenetics also has important implications for doctors trying to understand how drugs work, for politicians deciding how to keep their constituents safe from environmental toxins, and for anyone considering whether they should bother starting on an exercise regime. This is big stuff, because in one way or another, it will ultimately touch all of us.

Most people have never heard of epigenetics, and it might seem as though they never will, because after all, most people aren't particularly interested in molecular biology. But a mere 50 years ago, most people had never heard of DNA, and in a single generation we have developed into a world where Verizon sells "DNA" phones and where car manufacturers are confident that consumers will understand what they mean when their ads refer to the DNA of their automobiles. Epigenetics, likewise, will be a household word in the future, for several reasons.

Some people will learn about epigenetics because they or someone they love will be afflicted by a medical condition caused by epigenetic abnormalities. Besides cancer, epigenetic phenomena have been implicated in some autoimmune diseases and in some lesser-known disorders like Prader-Willi syndrome and Angelman syndrome. Some psychological disorders, too, are associated with epigenetic abnormalities, for example schizophrenia and bipolar (i.e., manic-depressive) disorders. Other people will become aware of epigenetics because of its role in everyday psychological functioning. For example, epigenetic events are involved in learning and memory formation, and in generating the daily cycles that cause us to go to sleep each night and awaken each morning.

Still other people will find epigenetics to be important because of what epigenetic *inheritance* means for biologists' current theory of evolution, a theory known as the neo-Darwinian (or "modern") synthesis. The neo-Darwinian synthesis underlies virtually all of the work done in biology over the past 60 years; it holds that the traits we acquire during our lifetimes (i.e., as a result of our experiences) cannot possibly be inherited by our children.[21] Nonetheless, the discovery of epigenetic inheritance indicates otherwise, and will therefore force a rethinking of some of the basic tenets of biology. In the words of Evelyn Fox Keller, Professor Emerita of History and Philosophy of Science at MIT, "there is little doubt that its discovery and its integration into mainstream genetics is indeed rocking the foundations of that science."[22]

Perhaps the most important application of epigenetics will be the development of *treatments* for disorders, specifically dietary or drug treatments that target epigenetic marks. For example, current work in epigenetics appears poised to lead to "designer drugs" that effectively treat abnormal stress reactions related to traumatic events experienced in childhood. The discovery of these types of treatments will be groundbreaking and potentially monumental. I'll be considering these and other exciting implications of behavioral epigenetics in the coming chapters.

3

Development

In the late 1880s and early 1890s, a German biologist named Hans Driesch conducted experiments that changed everything about our conceptions of development. Building on his work, the scientists who followed have been able to treat spinal cord injuries using transplanted stem cells,[1] to clone mammals,[2] and to start thinking about engineering blood vessels for use in people with heart disease.[3] The importance of Driesch's foundational work can hardly be overestimated.

Like his late-Victorian peers, Driesch knew that shortly after fertilization, an egg divides into two cells, which then each divide as well, so that the number of cells in an embryo-to-be changes quickly from 1 to 2 to 4 to 8 to 16 . . . and so on, ultimately leaving people with about 50 trillion cells in their bodies. In the waning decades of the 19th century, a prevailing theory held that when a single fertilized egg divides in two, the parts of the egg that specify how to develop an animal's head region all move into one of the two cells, while the parts that specify how to develop its tail region all move into the other cell. This, they thought, is how the top halves of bodies wind up with heads, shoulders, and everything else in the top half of a body, while the bottom halves wind up with legs, genitalia, and everything else in the bottom half of a body.

Although most 19th-century biologists were not experimentally inclined, Driesch was ahead of his time, so he set about trying to see if he could *prove* that animals' bodies develop in accord with this theory. In the crucial test, he *separated* the two cells of a recently divided sea urchin embryo and then gave them some time to develop. Given the theory he was testing, he expected to come back after a while and find two different "organisms," one that had features like the top half of a sea urchin, and one that had features like the bottom half. To his astonishment, he wound up with two completely normal, healthy sea urchins (this is actually the process that produces twins; it works the same way in people as it does in sea urchins). Even more surprising, if he waited until the sea urchin embryo had divided *twice* before he separated the four resulting cells from each other, each of the four cells developed into a normal, healthy urchin. So Driesch was left with a baffling question: How can two cells attached to each other grow into a single normal, healthy organism, while cells separated from each other grow into *two* normal, healthy organisms? That is, how in the world can a thing be divisible, yet each of its parts still retain the ability to develop into an undivided whole?

One thing was clear: If any "instructions" for building heads and tails were present in a fertilized egg, they couldn't possibly be dividing themselves up into the different cells that result from cell division. Instead, any such "instructions" would have to be present in their entirety in *each* newly formed cell. But if every cell has the same "instructions," how is it that our heads don't wind up looking like our feet? Driesch concluded that even if he didn't yet have the foggiest idea about how it could be possible, "the sea urchin embryo is a 'harmonious equipotential system' because all of its potentially independent parts functioned together to form a single organism."[4]

The Emergence of Epigenetics

It took decades to figure out how new embryos can work like this, but today we know that what makes Driesch's phenomenon possible is epigenetics. Ever since his trailblazing work, we have understood that the cells of very young embryos are "pluripotent," meaning that each one has the ability to develop into any of the very different kinds of cells that make up a body, including, for example, liver cells, skin cells, or brain cells. Therefore, the resources required to build heads *and* tails (and everything else in a body) must be present in *every one* of the cells of the young embryo, the so-called embryonic stem cells. The pluripotency of these cells means that biological development must be all about the epigenetic process of activating and deactivating various DNA segments in discrete cells so that those cells end up dissimilar from one another. Epigenetic effects play several different roles in our bodies, but on a fundamental level their most important job is to cause otherwise indistinguishable stem cells to start taking on the distinctive shapes and functions that characterize mature cells of varying types.

One of the most important insights to emerge from Driesch's work is that the development of a cell is tied to its context; the same exact cell put into different situations can develop in very different ways. A given stem cell on its own might go on to become an entire individual person, but if that same cell is attached to another cell, it might go on to become, for example, a collection of neurons, the cells that process information in our brains. In this way, bodily features such as brains and hearts—with their distinctive brain cells and heart cells—materialize as we develop in utero from otherwise identical stem cells.

Thus, development depends on interactions between cells and their contexts; cells do what they do partly because of what is inside of them and partly because of what is outside of them. Phenotypes—and here it turns out not to matter whether we're talking about the characteristics of cells or the characteristics of whole people—are not determined by what is inside or outside but rather by how the inside and the outside *influence one another*. As the Nobel laureate Christiane Nüsslein-Volhard summed it up in 2006, the stuff inside of our cells, which is called "cytoplasm," "receives signals and information from the environment, including the neighboring cells. This information is transmitted to the genes . . . In this manner, the fate of a cell is dependent on both the cytoplasm and external influences."[5]

Many writers[6a–6c] trace the origins of modern epigenetics to the English biologist Conrad Waddington, who, in the 1940s, "introduced the word 'epigenetics' . . . as a suitable name for the branch of biology which studies the causal interactions between genes and their products which bring the phenotype into being."[7] Waddington started his scientific career in the 1930s, just a few decades after Driesch demonstrated the pluripotency of embryonic cells. Therefore, he understood that the genes inside of those cells must be able to respond differently in different contexts. That is, he realized that part of understanding development was going to entail understanding how genes are expressed, or regulated. This is why Waddington's way of using the word "epigenetics" remains important: It links genetic regulation to the *developmental* events that bring our characteristics into being.

So, Waddington defined epigenetics as being about *cellular differentiation*, the process by which cells develop from "generic" stem cells into specific kinds of cells, such as those constituting blood, bone, or muscle. As early as 1968, he wrote, "In relation to cellular differentiation, it is in fact conventional to say that the basic elementary process is the de-repression (or possibly switching on) of a structural gene."[8] In this statement we can already see the phenomenon that the word "epigenetics" is now typically used to refer to: the switching on or off of genes. DNA is activated or deactivated by molecules that are positioned *on* genes, so these molecules are quite literally *epi*genetic (given that the prefix "epi" means "on," "above," or "over"). In this sense, then, epigenetics is focused on the interface between genes and their contexts.

Dueling Definitions

Although modern biologists use "epigenetics" to refer to how genes are regulated by their contexts, the word has actually meant different things to theorists writing in other eras; this word has had a long and complex history. As a result, a more detailed understanding of epigenetics can emerge by considering the alternative ideas this word can convey. One relatively early use of this word was designed to draw attention to the inherently interactive nature of development.

Faced with the fact that we all begin life as a fertilized egg—which is not much more than a collection of DNA strands surrounded by cytoplasm and some proteins—it is easy to imagine that DNA is the boss in the executive suite. From this perspective, DNA builds cells and organs, and the resulting organs allow us to move around in the world, eating, drinking, and doing things like having families and building houses. In fact, in *The Extended Phenotype: The Long Reach of the Gene*, the evolutionary ethologist Richard Dawkins argued that our *environments* are, effectively, mere manifestations of our genes.[9] But Driesch's discoveries about development encourage a different perspective, one that doesn't see our bodies, behaviors, and environments as being caused by dictatorial genes in a one-way process.

The American psychobiologist Gilbert Gottlieb saw things from this different perspective.[10a-10d] For Gottlieb, an important aspect of development is the bidirectional nature of the interactions that produce our characteristics. Of course, Gottlieb understood that Dawkins was right to some extent; genetic activity influences neurons, neurons influence behavior, and behavior influences people and things in the environment. But to Gottlieb this was only part of the story. As he recognized, it is also true that people and things in the environment influence behavior, behavior influences neurons, and neurons influence genetic activity. Therefore, our traits emerge because of how various factors *interact* with one another, such as when genes interact with chemicals like hormones, hormones interact with organ systems like the brain, and the brain interacts with factors in the external world, like parents, teachers, political leaders, and economic systems.

Even back in 1998, long before "epigenetics" was the buzzword it is today, Gottlieb referred to development as "epigenetic" in order to convey the idea that genetic activity is affected by the environment and behavior. In fact, Gottlieb and other theorists in the 1990s defined "epigenetics" much more broadly than most contemporary scientists do: as a word that refers to any developmental process in which something genuinely new emerges from a previous state. For example, this broad definition would mean that we could use the word "epigenetic" to describe the developments that produce a baby's first words, because this is a situation in which something new has emerged that was not previously present. Theorists in fields as diverse as philosophy of science,[11] genetics,[12a-12c] neuroscience,[13] and developmental psychobiology[14a-14b] continue to use the word "epigenetic" in this broad way sometimes, and for a good reason: Using the word like this reminds us that development entails *bidirectional* interactions and that nonmolecular factors are just as important as molecular factors in driving development.

Other researchers have defined epigenetics in yet another way. For example, the authors of an article in the journal *Science* defined "epigenetics" as "The study of changes in gene function that are . . . heritable and that do not entail a change in DNA sequence."[15] This definition is unfortunate, because it equates epigenetics with "epigenetic inheritance," a narrow aspect of epigenetics that is controversial when talking about certain kinds of inheritance. I will discuss inheritance in Part III of this book, but by then, it will be clear that epigenetics encompasses a lot more than just "heritable" effects on our bodies. As David Sweatt wrote in a recent paper, a definition this narrow would prevent us from considering anything occurring in neurons to be epigenetic, because "neurons cannot divide . . . [so] nothing that occurs in neurons in the adult [brain] would qualify as being epigenetic by this definition."[16] Thus, defining "epigenetics" in terms of heritability is excessively restrictive.

Such narrow definitions of "epigenetics" also take the word away from its earlier meanings, as biologists Eva Jablonka and Marion Lamb explained in 2002:

> [Epigenetics] has always been associated with the interactions of genes, their products, and the internal and external environment. . . . Because of this, there is a continuity between epigenetics in Waddington's sense and epigenetics today: both focus on . . . the influence of environmental conditions on what happens in cells and organisms. It is only when epigenetics is equated solely with the inheritance of non-DNA variations that its original meaning is obscured.[17]

For these reasons, I will not restrict my discussion of epigenetics to effects that are heritable. Instead, I will almost always use the word "epigenetics" the way most contemporary scientists do: as a word that refers to interactions between DNA and other molecules in its local environment, interactions that influence gene expression.[18]

The Persistence of Biological Determinism

Driesch's work proved that biological outcomes are context dependent, and, as Gottlieb realized a century later, biological factors and environmental factors influence each other bidirectionally. But because people develop some of their traits in predictable ways—for example, most of us end up with two arms and ten toes—it is easy to forget that biology isn't calling all the shots. Even in the face of modern epigenetics, biological determinism—the old idea that biology controls the development of characteristics like intelligence, height, or personality—has proven remarkably tenacious.

For example, consider the following quotation from a recent book on epigenetics by Nessa Carey:

> There was a period when the prevailing orthodoxy seemed to be that the only thing that mattered was our DNA script . . . [but] this can't be the case, as the same script is used differently depending on its cellular context. The field is now possibly at risk of swinging a bit too far in the opposite direction, with hard-line epigeneticists almost minimizing

the significance of the DNA code. The truth is, of course, somewhere in between.[19]

This excerpt admirably captures the kind of interactionist view that modern epigenetics inspires, but notice that it still portrays the battle for control over development as being between DNA and other cellular factors; this text permits us to imagine that we can understand development strictly in terms of biology. The quotation fails to explicitly mention any influences originating in the external environment.

The persistence of "biological determinism" is worrisome, because scientists who are willing to believe that some of our characteristics are simply "innate" will not be particularly motivated to study the *origins* of those characteristics in development; if you are convinced that a child's unwillingness to share his toys simply reflects "human nature," you will have little reason to study the specific factors that contribute to the development of selfishness. As Daniel Lehrman put it in 1953,[20] concluding that a trait is innate, genetic, or instinctive "inevitably tend[s] to short-circuit the scientist's investigation" of development, because such a conclusion leads scientists to think they understand the origin of the trait, when in fact they know nothing about how the trait actually arose in development. Explanations that invoke only evolutionary or genetic factors are never sufficient explanations of trait origins,[21] and remaining mindful of this fact can help keep scientists focused on the practical goal of figuring out how to help people by discovering *how* their characteristics develop. Making these kinds of discoveries requires, first, remembering that development is open to experience and, second, concentrating on how experiential manipulations influence development. One reason epigenetics is important is because it can help us stay focused on the interactive and open-to-experience nature of development.

4

DNA

Trying to discuss epigenetics without talking about genes is like trying to discuss painting without talking about paint. So, before we can dig any deeper into epigenetics, we need to talk briefly about genes or, at the very least, define what that word means. Alas, this is easier said than done. As surprising as it might be given that we hear references to genes seemingly every day, theorists in the life sciences have yet to agree on what a "gene" is, and it appears that none of the various gene concepts they have developed are better or worse than the others. As a result, contemporary biologists switch freely between several different gene concepts, ideas that do not, unfortunately, map very well onto one another.[1a–1d] But because I will need to refer to "genes" repeatedly throughout this book, it is important to establish what exactly it is that we're talking about. The gene concept I will employ in this book holds that genes are part of the DNA that makes up chromosomes.

All of us began life as a fertilized egg. A fertilized human egg is a cell, and like all cells it has several components, but the only part that is going to concern us is the part known as the nucleus, which floats in a gel-like substance that fills up the inside of cells. The nucleus of a fertilized human egg contains very large molecules called chromosomes that a mother and father contributed to the egg. And as the egg ultimately develops into an adult made of trillions of cells, nearly all of those cells will have a nucleus containing exact copies of these very same chromosomes.

In the first half of the 20th century, scientists developed what came to be known as the classical molecular gene concept,[2] which holds that genes are located inside cell nuclei and, more specifically, that they make up portions of our chromosomes. By the 1950s, scientists knew that chromosomes were made mostly of DNA, and in 1953 Watson and Crick identified the structure of DNA as a double-stranded, twisted helix.[3] What made Watson and Crick's discovery especially noteworthy was that it explained how DNA's structure allows *information* to be passed from parents to offspring. The next chapter contains details about the structure of DNA and how it does its job, but for now it is enough to note that segments of DNA can be thought of as holding information that is used to construct proteins. For the purposes of this book, I will define "genes" as DNA segments that contain information used to construct proteins.[4]

Proteins are made of long sequences of elements that are strung together like beads on a string, and the components of DNA are likewise arranged in bead-like sequences that *correspond* to the sequences of elements that make up proteins. Thus, the sequence of DNA components represents stored "sequence information" that can be used to construct proteins with elements that are arranged in the right order.

Proteins are important because even though they are made of linearly arranged elements and might therefore seem elongated like a string, these "strings" normally bunch up in a particular way for each particular kind of protein, and the way the protein bunches up is normally related to the sequence of its elements. In this way, each kind of protein winds up with a distinctive three-dimensional shape. And, it is the specific shapes of proteins that matter, because these shapes are what allow the proteins to perform specific functions in our bodies.

For example, there are proteins embedded in the membranes that make up the outer surface of each of our cells, and these proteins allow those cells to recognize each other. So, among other things, this arrangement renders our immune system able to recognize foreign cells like bacteria that should be attacked. Other proteins give muscle cells the ability to contract, allowing us to move around (and to continue living, because our hearts are muscles and they only continue to beat because of how the proteins within them operate). Still other proteins are neurotransmitters, such as serotonin, a rock star of the protein world because of the media attention it has received for its role in mood regulation and, therefore, depression. But serotonin can't do anything unless it is able to interact with particular kinds of serotonin *receptors* in our brains, which are also proteins that are able to *recognize* serotonin in a shape-based manner (analogous to the way a keyhole's distinctive shape allows it to "recognize" a properly shaped key that can open the lock). One of the other proteins we will encounter in later chapters—because it has an important role in psychological functioning—is the "glucocorticoid receptor" protein, which is involved in modulating fearful responses in stressful situations.

The "genes" I will be referring to in this book are classical molecular genes,[5] and these have only one job: to provide information for use in the construction of proteins. Because proteins influence our characteristics, our molecular genes will always account for some of who and how we are. But because our phenotypes are built by processes that are open to the influences of nongenetic factors—diet, hormones, stress, or sensations, for example—these genes are never solely responsible for our full-blown phenotypes.

The Gene: A Concept in Trouble

Classical molecular genes are DNA segments that provide stored sequence information to "cellular machinery"[6] that is located in the cytoplasm and that physically constructs proteins. Nonetheless, this kind of "gene" is still merely a theoretical entity. In fact, the latest research suggests that although the classical molecular gene concept can be useful, it actually does not capture reality very well.[7]

Specifically, it now appears that in most cases, there are no discrete entities in our DNA that we can point to and say, "Here is the molecular gene that codes for protein X." This was the conclusion of scientists working with the National Human Genome Research Institute on the ENCODE project,[8] an undertaking designed to determine what various portions of our DNA actually do. In the end, this research challenged existing ideas about genes, in a way that led to the development of a new hypothetical gene concept,[9] one that has been added to the list of gene concepts that have been adopted (and found wanting) at various points through the years.[10] The scientists involved in the ENCODE project concluded that based on the results of their work, the "view of a gene as a discrete element in the genome has been shaken."[11]

Given how common the word "gene" is, it seems as though it should mean something specific, particularly because it is a technical word with scientific origins. But the gene concept continues to evolve. In 2000, Evelyn Fox Keller wrote, "the sheer weight of the findings . . .[has] brought the concept of the gene to the verge of collapse. What is a gene today? As we listen to the ways in which the term is now used by working biologists, we find that the gene has become many things—no longer a single entity."[12] More recently, the medical geneticist Alexandre Reymond concluded, "We have still not truly answered the question, 'What is a gene?' "[13]

So, although I will talk about genes repeatedly in this book, it is only because there is no other convenient way to communicate about contemporary ideas in molecular biology. And when I refer to a gene, I will be talking about a segment or segments of DNA containing sequence information that is used to help construct a protein (or some other product that performs a biological function). But it is worth remembering that contemporary biologists do not mean any one thing when they talk about "genes"; the gene remains a fundamentally hypothetical concept to this day. The common belief that there are things inside of us that constitute a set of instructions for building bodies and minds—things that are analogous to "blueprints" or "recipes"—is undoubtedly false.[14a-14d] Instead, DNA segments often contain information that is ambiguous, and that must be edited and rearranged in context-dependent ways before it can be used.[15] The next chapter describes some of the strange and fascinating ways in which DNA actually works. I find this material to be extremely interesting and important; nonetheless, understanding it at the level of detail provided in the next chapter will be necessary only in order to understand the other "Zooming in" chapters in the book. Readers less interested in molecular detail might choose to skip to chapter 6, "Regulation."

‖ 5 ‖

Zooming in on DNA

In the 1860s in what is now the Czech Republic, a monk named Gregor Mendel was engaged in a series of experiments on pea plants that ultimately opened the door on the modern era of genetics. To make sense of what he saw in his garden, Mendel proposed the existence of "heritable factors" responsible for determining plants' characteristics, such as how wrinkly their seeds were or whether they were green or yellow. Shortly after 1900 Mendel's theory rose to prominence and the search was on to locate his "heritable factors" within living cells.

To qualify as Mendel's factors, any candidate molecules would have required some particular properties. First, they would have needed to be transmittable from parents to offspring. Second, they would have needed to be transmittable from a fertilized egg to each of the two "daughter" cells created during cell division. And third, they would have needed to be able to influence the structure and functioning of the daughter cells, so that an organism could be built with species-appropriate features; human embryos need to develop human hearts, human bones, and human brains if they are going to grow into human babies.

In 1953 Watson and Crick discovered how DNA is structured, thereby showing it to be a molecule with the properties required to be Mendel's genetic material. The structure of DNA gives it the ability to replicate itself, thereby solving the problem of getting a complete set of chromosomes into every new daughter cell produced by cell division. In fact, after noting that the structure they were proposing for DNA "has novel features which are of considerable biological interest," Watson and Crick wrote, "It has not escaped our notice that the [structure] we have postulated immediately suggests a possible copying mechanism for the genetic material."[1] Moreover, copies of these molecules are present in each sperm and egg, making the molecules a potential vehicle for the transmission of genes across generations. And although it took some time to ascertain how DNA is able to effectively store information that contributes to the building of an organism's distinctive characteristics, it was clear within a decade that the structure of DNA gives it this ability as well. A remarkable molecule indeed.

The information in the next part of this chapter will not be new to those who have had a good introduction to biology. But in the interest of helping readers without this background to understand DNA and its operation, I offer here a primer on the basics. After that, I will discuss things like alternative splicing, non-coding DNA, and micro- and sn-RNAs, for example; anyone interested in reading subsequent "Zooming in" chapters might find this information helpful.

The Twisted Ladder: A Primer on DNA

Each chromosome is made primarily of a very long strand of DNA, intertwined with itself in a heap, like a large skein of yarn unwound and packed up into a cohesive mass. A single DNA molecule is made of two very long chemical strands twisted around each other, like a thread that, when looked at closely, is seen to be made of two distinct strands of fiber wrapped around each other to form a single strand. Some stretches along the exceedingly long strand of DNA that makes up a chromosome do not have functions that we currently understand, but other segments are structured in such a way as to be helpful for cells when they produce molecules such as proteins; as I noted at the end of the last chapter, when I use the word "genes" in this book, I will be referring to these lengths along the DNA strand.

Each of the two strands of a DNA molecule is constructed of a series of elements called nucleotide bases, which are strung like beads along the strand. These nucleotide bases—I'll usually call them "bases" to simplify things—come in four main types, and they are generally known by the first letters of their chemical names, A (for adenine), C (for cytosine), G (for guanine), and T (for thymine). Analogous to the way a sentence is an ordered sequence of meaningful elements (i.e., words), a potentially influential segment of DNA is an ordered sequence of bases strung one after another along the length of DNA. Words in English can be made of varying numbers of letters—some English words are very short, and others are very long—but the meaningful elements in a DNA sequence are always just three letters long (for example, C-A-G or T-A-T). Of course, just as a sentence can be made of a very large number of words, a gene can consist of a very large number of triplets, so that someone "reading" along the length of a DNA segment might encounter a long, ordered list of letter-bases, like so: GATGGCACCTAA ACCACCAGTGCCCAAAGTCTGTGTGATGAACTT.

Each triplet is meaningful because its presence along a strand of DNA can lead to the addition of a particular molecule onto a protein being constructed using that strand's information. Like DNA, proteins are molecules made of long chains of elements strung one after another in sequence, but whereas the elements that make up DNA are the bases A, C, G, and T, the elements that make up proteins are called amino acids (another difference is that whereas DNA is a double-stranded molecule, proteins are just a single chain of amino acids). Any particular triplet of DNA bases corresponds to a particular amino acid. To use the triplets chosen in the last paragraph as examples, the bases C-A-G, in that order, correspond to an amino acid called "glutamine," and the bases T-A-T correspond to an amino acid called "tyrosine." Remember that a protein's shape is what gives it its distinctive characteristics, and because the shape of a protein is influenced by the order of the amino acids that constitute it, this shape is affected by the order of bases in a gene (because the order of bases in the gene corresponds to the order of amino acids in the associated protein). Because protein shapes are what make them distinctive, it is the order of amino acids in a protein—and, hence, the order of bases in its corresponding gene—that make a protein like serotonin function as a neurotransmitter in a brain and a protein like hemoglobin function as an oxygen transporter in the blood.

Proteins are not actually built in cell nuclei, where chromosomes are located. Instead, any sequence information in a chromosome must be transported out of the nucleus and into the cytoplasm, where protein production takes place. Another kind of molecule—called RNA—is actually responsible for carrying sequence information from the chromosomes to the protein-producing machinery in the cytoplasm. RNA is similar to DNA in that it is made of nucleotide bases strung together to form a chain (but, like proteins, RNA is single-stranded). *Transcription* is the name of the process by which a succession of DNA bases is used to create a complementary succession of RNA bases; this process produces a strand of RNA called a *transcript*. It is RNA transcripts that actually transport sequence information from the DNA in the nucleus out to where proteins are actually constructed. Once the RNA transcript reaches the protein construction machinery in the cytoplasm, it undergoes a process called *translation* in which its sequence information is used to build a particular protein. That is, translation is a process wherein cellular machinery effectively "reads" the information extracted from a DNA strand and uses that information to build a protein.

... But Most DNA Is Not Used to Build Proteins!

If my explanations and similes here have been good, it might seem that this system is relatively straightforward, as if an incredibly intelligent engineer had designed it. But whenever a system has been designed by natural selection, we should expect it to have some odd, less-than-efficient quirks (for reasons presented in chapter 13, "Memory"). And in the current case we have a whopper of an inefficiency in the system: Only about 1.2% of the nucleotide bases found in the human genome are used in the production of proteins (or other products) that have some sort of a distinct biological function.[2] That is, the story I have just finished telling about the functioning of our genome does not apply to about 98.8%

of our DNA. This raises the obvious question: What in the world is the rest of that genetic material *for*?

Biologists refer to DNA that does not code for proteins as noncoding DNA.[3] Forty years ago, when biologists first started noticing noncoding DNA, it seemed as if all of this material had no function at all, and it was referred to as "junk DNA."[4] Although some DNA really *might* carry no meaningful information at all, there is strong evidence that most noncoding DNA actually does have a function; in fact, the scientists who ran the ENCODE project recently reported that they were able to assign "some sort of function to roughly 80% of the [human] genome."[5] In some cases, the exact same noncoding sequences are present in distantly related species; this suggests that natural selection has found a reason to retain these sequences across long spans of evolutionary time, indicating that they serve *some* function, even if we have not yet figured out what that function is. It's as if you've traveled to a foreign country, and you see the following collection of letters on a variety of different signs: "dagatengolefskinongu." That might seem like gibberish, but if you see the *exact same sequence* of letters embossed on a bicycle, a swing-set, and a pair of ice skates, you would not be considered crazy if you concluded that the sequence probably means *something*. Moreover, we know that although more than 98% of our DNA does not code for proteins, most of this noncoding DNA is nonetheless transcribed into RNA at various points in development, so it almost assuredly has some function.

As it happens, there are certain segments of noncoding DNA that molecular biologists have now been able to interpret. Over 50 years ago, the French biologists Jacob and Monod[6a–6b] reported that specific lengths of DNA in the *Escherichia coli* bacterium were used not to provide sequence information for protein production but to *regulate* protein production. These researchers reported that a particular section of DNA containing protein-related sequence information is associated with three other *non*coding sections of DNA that they called promoter, operator, and terminator regions. Their discovery—for which they won the Nobel Prize in 1965—indicated that when a sugar called lactose was present in the bacterium's environment, the protein production process would begin, yielding a protein able to digest the lactose. Because this protein is not produced when there is no lactose in the bacterium's environment, it was clear that environmental factors are able to regulate gene expression, turning protein-coding genes on when those proteins are needed, and turning them off when the proteins are not needed.

Thus, although promoters, operators, and terminators do not actually code for proteins, they are nonetheless segments of DNA with important functions. In the case of *E. coli*, when lactose is not present in the environment, a molecule called a repressor attaches to the operator region of the DNA. When the repressor is present, it renders the coding regions of the DNA unreadable, thereby saving the energy that would otherwise be spent producing an unneeded lactose-digesting protein. But when lactose *is* present, the shape of the repressor is altered in a way that ultimately leads to initiation of transcription and to the production of the lactose-digesting protein. It is now clear that the environments surrounding *our* cells are also able to control the genetic activity inside those cells, even though the mechanisms are not identical to those discovered in bacteria (the genes in human cells do not have operators, for example). But as with simpler organisms, this control is enabled by the presence of *non*coding regions of DNA that, depending on their context, can promote or terminate transcription of the *coding* regions of DNA, and thereby promote or terminate protein production. In this way, some of our noncoding DNA can be construed as regulatory regions that are never actually transcribed into RNA; instead, these regions are sites where repressor molecules or activator molecules can attach to the DNA and thereby decrease or increase protein production.

A second way noncoding DNA can contribute to gene regulation is by containing sequence information that can be transcribed to form RNA molecules that do specific things themselves, without ever needing to be translated into a protein. The DNA that "codes" for these kinds of functional RNA molecules is still called "noncoding DNA" because it does not code for a protein.[7] One such type of noncoding RNA is called microRNA; these molecules are able to attach to segments of DNA and thereby influence what happens at *other* places in the genome. Likewise, so-called small nuclear RNAs (snRNAs) help cells produce proteins accurately; together with other molecules, these RNAs form the cellular protein-building machinery. Both of these kinds of RNA molecules probably make up an extremely important "layer" of gene regulation in all but the simplest organisms,[8] even if much about their function is still unknown.[9] Nonetheless, interest in these molecules has increased, as various disorders have been found to be associated with abnormal noncoding RNAs, including some cancers,[10] Alzheimer's disease,[11] Prader-Willi syndrome,[12] and other neurological diseases;[13] I will describe some of these findings in chapter 7, "Zooming in on Regulation." In the end, the human genome probably does contain some DNA that serves no particular purpose; such DNA—which really would best be considered "junk"—could have accumulated in us during our evolution if it did not adversely affect survival or reproduction. But it is now clear that other portions of our noncoding DNA play very important roles in the regulation of gene expression.

Alternative RNA Splicing and the Demise of the Classical Gene Concept

There is at least one other place in the genomes of complex animals where noncoding DNA appears, and as strange as it sounds, this DNA is scattered liberally *within* coding DNA. This is a peculiar state of affairs, because we ordinarily do not think it makes sense to sprinkle meaning*less* information into meaning*ful* information. It is as if a perfectly good sentence like "Dawn needs serotonin receptors here" was adulterated with meaningless "information," like so: "Dawnkor ampneeds 2 dopamineserotonin recepbi er jawlfioghjtormolecules t here." I am aware that this sounds like a ridiculous, impossibly nonsensical situation, but this is, in fact, how "meaningful" information is stored in most of our coding DNA. And besides being a really fascinating story with which to end this chapter, it helps explain why the scientists leading the ENCODE project wound up needing to think up yet another new definition of the word "gene."

RNA splicing, discovered in 1977, is the name of the intriguing and surprising aspect of gene expression that takes a seemingly nonsensical segment of DNA and extracts the useful sequence information embedded within it.[14a-14b] To make sense of this process, molecular biologists have defined two different types of DNA segments that make up the majority of coding DNA. The first of these types is called an exon, because it contains sequence information that will be *ex*pressed. The other type is called an intron, because it lies *in* between exons, and will not be expressed because it does not contain information relevant to the protein (or microRNA) being produced.[15] Clearly, in order to wind up with a useful product, the introns must somehow get cut out of the sequence, so that only the information in the exons is used to produce the protein, the microRNA, or any other kind of molecule being produced.

RNA splicing occurs after transcription. That is, the original sequence in the DNA—to use our metaphorical example, "Dawnkor ampneeds 2 dopamineserotonin recepbi er jawlfioghjtormolecules t here"—is first transcribed so that a strand of RNA is produced that contains both the "information" and the "non-information" in the DNA segment. Then, cellular machinery made of proteins and snRNAs literally cuts the meaningless introns out of this RNA transcript and splices—that is, joins—the exons together to produce a mature RNA strand that can be used to build a functional product. Thus, it is as if the "kor" following "Dawn" and the "amp" preceding "needs" are removed, and the segments "Dawn" and "needs" are joined together to make one continuous meaningful sequence (in this metaphor, the words "Dawn," "needs," "serotonin," etc., are analogous to exons, and the other, nonsensical letter-strings—for example, "kor amp" and "2 dopamine"—are analogous to introns). The fact that genetic information is stored like this, with a bunch of gibberish tossed in at random, continues to strike me as bizarre. But it just gets weirder. It turns out that RNA transcripts can be spliced in several different ways that can yield strikingly different products. That is, the same segment of DNA can yield RNA that can be alternatively spliced in ways that lead to very different outcomes.

In this way, a given DNA sequence has the potential to do multiple things. To return to our analogy, "Dawnkor ampneeds 2 dopamineserotonin recepbi er jawlfioghjtormolecules t here" can be spliced to yield the meaningful sequence "Dawn needs serotonin receptors here," but if you look closely, you might be able to see how the same sequence could be alternatively spliced to yield the very different segment "Dawn needs dopamine receptors here." In fact, the same "gene" could also yield the instructions "Dawn needs 2 serotonin receptors here," or even "Dawn needs dopamine molecules there." Remarkably, a DNA segment containing exons I'll arbitrarily label "1," "2," "3," and "4" could be spliced to produce a wide variety of mature RNA strands, such as "1234," "134," "234," "14," "13," or even—reversing the order in which the exons lie on the DNA segment—"4321," "2431," "41," and so forth.[16] But would these different mature RNA molecules produce proteins that do similar things? Not at all. As scientists reported in 2008, products coded for by "individual mammalian genes . . . may have related, distinct, or even opposing functions."[17]

What, then, determines whether we get "receptors here" or "molecules there"? Context. In an early demonstration of alternative splicing, researchers[18] discovered that the same exact segment of DNA can be used in one kind of cell to produce an amino acid chain that regulates calcium and in another kind of cell to produce a neurohormone, products that do very different things. But while most alternative splicing seems to work like this—producing different products in different cells—it now appears that something even more unexpected might be at work. Somewhat mind-bogglingly, although most varying splice products are found in a person's different cell types, some of the variation appears to occur *across individuals.*[19] As hard as this is to believe, a finding like this implies that a gene in Humphrey Bogart might have done something different than that *exact same gene* would have done in Frank Sinatra.

Recent data even suggest that alternative splicing can be driven by experience. For example, when rats learn about a novel environment, cells in their brains use a particular DNA segment to produce a specific protein as they form memories of the experience. But if the rats are exposed to an electrical shock in that environment and they therefore form a memory *associating* the new environment with this punishing experience, that same DNA segment is used to produce a different form of the protein.[20] Thus, a single DNA segment—a gene—can be used to produce one product in response to one kind of experience and a different product in response to a slightly different kind of experience. Even without knowing anything about epigenetics, the existence of this kind of phenomenon should make us skeptical that there are genes that *invariably* cause particular phenotypes, independently of context.

In 1999, biologists thought alternative splicing occurs during the reading of as much as one-third of our DNA, a percentage that seemed rather high at the time. But, as it turns out, that was a wild underestimation. In 2003, one team of scientists concluded "that at least 74% of human multi-exon genes are alternatively spliced,"[21] and studies five years later indicated that alternative RNA splicing is "actually a universal feature of human genes,"[22] with different laboratories reporting that between 92%[23] and 95%[24] of human genes undergo alternative splicing.

And that's not all. Some mature RNA is constructed by joining together two or more RNA transcripts that were produced from DNA segments located rather far from one another on a single strand of DNA. Even more surprising, molecular biologists have now discovered that RNA transcripts derived from *two entirely different chromosomes* can be spliced together to form a single protein-coding sequence. In part because of the discovery of these sorts of phenomena, the leaders of the ENCODE project wrote "Clearly, the classical concept of the gene as 'a locus' [that is, a particular chromosomal location] no longer applies for these gene products whose DNA sequences are widely separated across the genome."[25]

This story should make it clear why the definition of the word "gene" has recently needed yet another revision. DNA does not in fact contain a code that specifies particular outcomes.[26] Instead, genes are used in context-dependent ways. If a DNA segment is used to produce a neurohormone in one context and a calcium-regulating amino acid chain in a different context, should we consider this sequence of DNA to be the "gene" for the neurohormone? For the amino acid chain? For both? For neither (since there are contexts in which neither product is generated)? The available data indicate that a *single* length of RNA can sometimes be edited to produce *hundreds* of different products,[27] because sequences specifying these different products are embedded in the same length of DNA. In some cases, the exons used to produce a protein even *overlap* one another, so that the bases that constitute the end of one exon are the same exact bases that constitute the beginning of the next exon! In such circumstances, it is clear that we must revise our traditional understanding of the gene as a persisting, continuous sequence of nucleotide bases that specifies a single product. I noted at the end of the preceding chapter that the information in DNA is ambiguous; this is true in the sense that, to be of any use, pieces cut from an unedited stretch of DNA must be spliced back together in the right order, in ways that depend on context. And because all of this must occur before the information in a "gene" can be used to create biologically functional molecules, genes like this are not able to determine phenotypes independently of their environments.

Recent attempts to define the word "gene" have gone so far as to imagine that the genome is like "an operating system for a living being,"[28] a simile that would permit defining the gene as a kind of "subroutine" like those used by computer scientists. But even this attempt to define what genes are had to be rejected in the wake of the ENCODE project. Of course, the ENCODE team generated their own new—although not particularly intuitive—definition of the word gene: "The gene is a union of genomic sequences encoding a coherent set of potentially overlapping functional products."[29] Perhaps this rather opaque definition will finally be . . . definitive. But for the moment, it remains the case that it has not yet proven possible to define the word "gene" in a way that satisfies all parties in the community of informed biologists.

|| 6 ||

Regulation

Like most people, I have many books on my shelves that I have never read. I am quite sure they are full of good, useful information, but I have not had the time to read them all, so the information in the unread volumes has had no effect on me. The information is there, but it might as well not be (for all the good it has done me so far!). Genetic information, too, is of little consequence when it is unused.

In the early 20th century, scientists knew from Driesch's work with sea urchins that the stem cells that make up an embryo are "pluripotent"—that is, each of these identical cells can develop into any of the more than 200 different types of mature cells in our bodies.[1] Therefore, each embryonic stem cell must contain all of the genetic information required to produce any mature cell. In addition, scientists of the early 20th century knew that as embryos develop, their cells differentiate, meaning they develop the distinctive features that are typical of the different kinds of mature cells. Finally, after differentiating, normal cells lose their pluripotency; a cell that has become a neuron stays that way, never spontaneously turning into a liver cell or any other kind of cell.

This last point was somewhat of a mystery. If mature neurons and liver cells, for example, both develop from identical stem cells, why can't mature neurons turn into mature liver cells, or vice versa? One explanation for this loss of potential could be that as cells mature and differentiate, they actually *lose* the information required to become other kinds of cells. But in 1958, Frederick Steward demonstrated that an entirely new plant can be generated from a single root cell taken from a mature plant,[2] so in these plants—and, as it turns out, in living things in general—differentiated cells have *not* lost any of their original information. This is how biologists realized that, like the information in the unread books in our libraries, the information required to become any kind of cell remains present in differentiated cells, even if that information has somehow been locked away and thereby rendered powerless.

Mid-20th-century scientists understood that for embryonic stem cells to be pluripotent, they would need to have some sort of mechanism whereby a single collection of genes could do one set of things in one cell, but a different set of things in a different cell. That is, for two identical stem cells to develop into cells as different as those in our brains and our lungs, one cell would have to use a particular portion of its information while the other cell would have to use a different (if potentially overlapping) portion. But no one had any idea of what kind of mechanism might allow cells to selectively use information in this way, so the pluripotency-differentiation problem remained a puzzle.

X-Inactivation: One X + One X Equals ... One X?

Meanwhile, researchers were struggling with another perplexing question that might at first glance seem irrelevant to the pluripotency-differentiation problem. By 1905, biologists knew that normal women have two X chromosomes in almost all of the cells of their bodies and that normal men have only one X chromosome in the corresponding cells of *their* bodies. But because the presence of specific genes was thought to correspond to the presence of specific proteins, that would mean that compared to men, women should have twice as much of the proteins specified on the X chromosome.[3] However, even though there are over a thousand genes on X chromosomes that are used to produce proteins, men's bodies and women's bodies contain about the same amounts of most of these proteins. The obvious question is, how in the world can women *not* produce twice as many of these proteins if they have twice the amount of genetic material associated with these proteins?

In a remarkable feat of insight stimulated primarily by suggestive data from mouse studies, the English geneticist Mary F. Lyon hypothesized in 1961 that one of the two X chromosomes in the cells of normal female embryos is effectively shut down early in development, and maintained in an inactive state thereafter.[4] We now know she was right: An epigenetic process leads to X-inactivation in each normal female embryo even before it implants in the uterus.[5] So, the cells in every normal woman *have* two X chromosomes—one from the woman's mother and one from the woman's father—but since one of the chromosomes was inactivated when the woman was an embryo, only the other one is functional. (More information about X-inactivation is available in the next chapter.)

The discovery that chromosomes can be inactivated suggests a possible solution to the mystery of pluripotency and differentiation, particularly if mere *segments* of chromosomes can be inactivated (rather than the entire molecule). In fact, this is how nature solved one of the most important problems that arose with the evolution of complex animals: How can a multicellular adult pass on to her offspring all of the different cell types that she herself developed over the course of her lifetime? In theory, evolution *could* have left us with a system whereby a mother passes on to her offspring a complete set of all of the different cell types in her mature body. But that would have been a much more cumbersome system than the one nature discovered for us, namely a system that effectively passes on a single pluripotent cell that can then *develop* all of the different cell types using different fragments of information, all of which are contained in a central "database" in cell nuclei. Once a system is in place to activate some genes and deactivate others, getting some stem cells to develop in one way and other stem cells to develop in a different way is not a problem. Through the study of X-inactivation, scientists came to understand that the regulation of gene expression is critically important in the process of development.

By the late 1960s, Waddington was referring to the "switching on" of particular genes to explain the process of cellular differentiation, because it had become clear that this process relies on the differential *use* of identical genetic "databases" in different cells.[6] As we develop, different genes are turned on and off in different cells in a way that leaves us with the many different kinds of cells in our bodies; that is, what makes our cell types different from each other is the fact that each type has its own distinctive pattern of gene expression.[7] Because biological development is all about cellular differentiation, focusing on development is an excellent way to learn about processes that control genetic expression. And because these processes are epigenetic, studying development is a great way to learn about epigenetics. So let us begin with the question of how chromosomes (or segments of chromosomes) can be turned on or off. Answering this question requires some familiarity with chromosomes themselves.

DNA's Entourage

Most of us have seen our genetic material pictured as chromosomes, with four limb-like blobs emerging from a narrow "waist," a sort of strange looking "X." Most of us have also seen our genetic material pictured as DNA, with its ladder-like rungs twisted into a double helix. One of the things that often confuses people is the relationship between these two depictions. In fact, they are two views of the same thing; a chromosome is made up of one very long, continuous double-strand of DNA, all bunched up into a mass with the familiar "X" shape. Another bit of news to those without much training in biology is that there is a middle level of structure between the chromosome level and the double helix level, one that turns out to be very important in how DNA *functions*.

The mechanism that permits different cells to use different DNA segments involves molecules that turn genes on and off, but that do not alter the information in DNA itself. This system allows the sequence information in DNA to remain present but unused, like the words in a book that has been locked shut. The fascinating question is how organisms solved the problem of how to make sequence information in cells *in*accessible to those cells except under specific circumstances. How do cells manage to keep secrets from themselves? The answer to this question requires learning a bit more about that middle level of structure between the double helix and the chromosome.

If you were to grasp the very end of the DNA strand that makes up a chromosome and pull it up from the bundle below, it would not come out like a straight piece of 2-ply yarn being pulled from a jumbled mass of wool. Instead, you would see that at numerous places along the pulled-out strand, it is wound several times tightly around a spool-like conglomeration of other large molecules before it continues on to the next tightly wound region (see Figure 6.1). DNA is packaged like this in the cells of all complex animals.

The large molecules making up the "spools" that DNA winds around are called histones, and they are proteins; a single "spool" is made of eight histones. One reason histones are important is because they play a crucial role in bundling DNA into chromosomes in an efficient and organized way. This is no small feat, because if we stretched out all of the DNA in a single human cell, it would be more than two *meters* long.[8] Somehow, these very large molecules must be packed into really tiny spaces, and histones enable this process.

Chromosomes are not made simply of DNA. Histones—and some other molecules that we will discuss—are all found in the chromosomes together with the DNA. In fact, the "stuff" of our chromosomes, which is called *chromatin*, contains twice as much protein as it does DNA, primarily in the form of histones.[9] And it is the non-DNA molecules that are part of our chromatin that are the focus of behavioral epigenetics research. Because these non-DNA components of our chromosomes are in actual physical contact with our DNA (and therefore our genes), they are *epi*genetic in the literal sense of the word—they are *on* our genes.

So, just as we each have a genome, we also each have an *epigenome*, an entire complement of *epi*genetic features that characterize our cells. And just as the unique characteristics of a person's genome influence that person's traits, so do the unique characteristics of the person's epigenome. In fact, a person's epigenome is every bit as influential as his or her genome.

The epigenome has the powerful effects it does because DNA that is tightly wrapped around histones is effectively silenced. Thus, in addition to their packaging responsibilities, histones are important because they influence what genes do. The information in a DNA segment can only be *used* if that information can be *read*—transcribed, to use the technical word—by biochemical "machinery" able to decipher DNA. And although histones themselves don't read the information in DNA, they are influential because transcription cannot take place when a DNA segment is wound so tightly around a "spool" that the information in the segment cannot be accessed. And when the information in a gene cannot be accessed, the proteins associated with that gene cannot be produced. This is how the epigenome can influence what chromatin does without actually changing the sequence information in the affected DNA.[10]

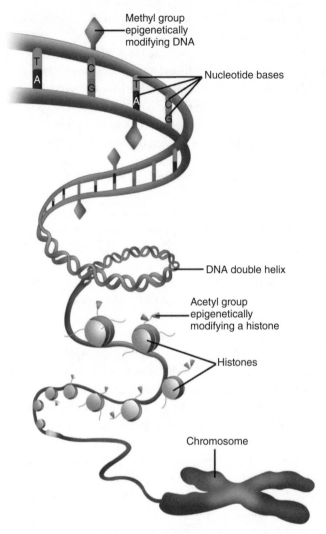

Figure 6.1 A schematic diagram of DNA pulled from a chromosome, showing nucleotide bases, the double helix wrapped around histones, and some epigenetic modifications to both the DNA and the histones.

DNA Methylation and Histone Modifications

There are several different epigenetic mechanisms that can silence or activate DNA, and most of these affect the histones; at least one interacts with DNA directly.[11] The best-understood mechanism that interacts with DNA directly is known as "DNA methylation." DNA methylation is a process by which a molecule called a "methyl group" gets attached to a DNA strand (as illustrated in Figure 6.1), much as pepper particles sprinkled on a bowl of spaghetti might stick to the strands of pasta (but do note that methyl groups form much stronger attachments to DNA than pepper does to spaghetti!). Once these methyl groups are attached to the DNA strand, the methylated section of the strand effectively closes up, becoming physically inaccessible to the "machinery" that would otherwise interact with that section;[12] in this state, the DNA strand cannot be transcribed. Therefore, processes that lead to *hyper*methylation—in which a DNA strand takes on additional methyl groups—reduce expression of genes on that strand. Conversely, processes that lead to *hypo*methylation—in which a DNA strand is stripped of some of its methyl groups—increase the likelihood that genes on that strand will be expressed. The simplified takeaway message here is: DNA methylation silences genes. Although the truth is that DNA methylation doesn't *always* silence genes,[13] it very often does, so for the purposes of this book, we will treat it as if this is a consistent effect (there will be more information on *how* methyl groups actually affect DNA in the next two "Zooming in" chapters).

Other epigenetic mechanisms affect histones, thereby influencing DNA indirectly. For example, histones, like DNA, can be methylated. But there is an important distinction between these two different kinds of epigenetic marks; in contrast to *DNA* methylation, *histone* methylation is not clearly associated with gene silencing. Instead, methylation of histones can silence *or activate* nearby genes, depending on a variety of other factors.[14a-14b] Because the effects of histone methylation are not particularly straightforward, I will refer to it infrequently; I mention it here only because we will encounter it briefly in later chapters, as it plays roles both in memory formation and in our reactions to drugs such as cocaine and some antidepressant medications.

Histones can also be affected by several other kinds of molecules.[15] The most well studied histone modification involves a collection of atoms known as an acetyl group[16] (see Figure 6.1). Histone acetylation is a process in which an acetyl group physically attaches to a histone (similar to how histone methylation involves a methyl group attaching to a histone). Histone acetylation and DNA methylation essentially have opposite effects; histone acetylation causes a section of DNA near the acetylated histone to open up, rendering that section accessible. Thus, whereas DNA methylation is generally thought to render DNA inaccessible, histone acetylation is associated with gene *activation*. This acetylation process has its direct effects on histones—not DNA—but histone acetylation is nonetheless associated with increased gene expression. And because histone acetylation is almost always associated with gene activation, we will encounter this process frequently in the coming pages.

Whether we are talking about DNA methylation or histone modifications, these processes can influence specific DNA segments while leaving other segments unaffected. Thus, different portions of chromatin can "open" and "close" independently, so that some sections can be made available for reading while other sections remain essentially hidden from the transcription machinery.[17] In this way, epigenetic modification systems are able to control gene expression in a precise way, increasing the production of proteins from specific genes alone.

Perhaps the most important difference between DNA methylation and histone modifications is that DNA methylation is much more stable. Unlike histone modifications, DNA methylation allows marking of the genome so that the phenotype of a cell can be maintained across an organism's entire life;[18] this ability to persist across long periods of time is one reason DNA methylation has been called "the prima donna of epigenetics."[19] Of course, histone modifications play critical roles in gene regulation too, but compared with DNA methylation, they are more dynamic. In both cases, the effect of the processes is to alter the configuration of the chromatin, thereby influencing genetic activity.

There are several other kinds of molecules that can mediate gene regulation as well, such as microRNAs (e.g., molecules like miR-124 and miR-222)[20a-20b] or specific proteins (e.g., molecules like CDH1),[21] but they are beyond the scope of this book, so I will not consider them further. There are also molecules other than acetyl and methyl groups that can modify histones and thereby mediate gene regulation, but I will not consider these in any detail either. I will mention histone *methyl*ation in some of the subsequent "Zooming in" chapters, but outside of these chapters, I will refer in this book exclusively to the two kinds of epigenetic processes that scientists best understand: DNA methylation and histone acetylation.

Tweaking Gene Activity

Scholars from a variety of disciplines are now closely following research on epigenetics; the field is hot. Recent studies have revealed that epigenomes "are highly organized and strikingly nonrandom with respect to histone and DNA modifications,"[22] so the patterns of epigenetic marks that constitute our epigenomes are most assuredly not some sort of cosmic accident. In addition, an important conclusion emerging from this research is that specific genes in a body are not permanently activated or deactivated. Instead, our chromatin undergoes regular changes, called "remodeling," that activates some genes and silences others.[23]

Grasping the significance of epigenetics requires understanding that genes can be switched on or off. But although we can simplify things and talk about DNA methylation "silencing" genes and histone acetylation "activating" genes, the fact is that epigenetic regulation need not work in a binary, on-or-off manner. There has actually been debate about whether genes are always either "on" or "off" like a light-switch, or if gene activity can be regulated the way a dimmer switch regulates the brightness of a light bulb.[24] Some evidence suggests that genes do operate in a binary fashion,[25a-25b] but it is not yet clear that the debate has been settled. Regardless, when we think about epigenetic effects in the context of most human phenotypes, this debate turns out not to matter much, for the following reason.

Imagine you have a group of 1,000 cells, and all of them have a given gene accessible and are therefore pumping out the protein associated with that gene; in this case, the cells will be producing a lot of that protein. Likewise, if all of the cells have repressed that gene, they will be producing very little of the protein. But if 500 of the cells have the gene accessible and 500 of them do not, the *population* of cells will be producing a quantity of protein that is midway between that produced by the fully active population and that produced by the fully silenced population. In this way, even if genes really *do* work in an all-or-none manner, we should continue to think of genetic activation as being graded;[26] theoretically, a population of genes would be able to operate at precisely 10% capacity, 37% capacity, 72% capacity, or any capacity in between. Thus, the genetic activity in populations of cells can be tweaked—up-regulated or down-regulated incrementally—thereby giving bodies much finer control over the amounts of various proteins they are generating. And this control over protein production gives bodies much finer control over their own functioning more generally.[27]

The processes that contribute to chromatin remodeling regulate what our genes are doing at any given moment, turning some of them off and turning others on, and thereby increasing or decreasing in graded ways the genetic activity in groups of cells.[28] For this reason, if we want to know why a person is currently as she is, it would be just as important to understand her epigenetic state as it would be to know about her genetic constitution. Whether or not you have a particular gene will not matter much if that gene is packaged in a way that makes it unreadable and, therefore, not functional.

Behavioral epigenetics is particularly exciting because the epigenetic states of some of our cells change in response to our experiences. Because experiences influence epigenetic states, the American developmental scientist Robert Lickliter has described epigenetics as "the study of . . . how gene expression changes during [cell differentiation], *and how environmental factors can modify how genes are expressed.*"[29] The story told by 20th-century biologists held that a person's DNA sequence could never be affected by mere life experiences, a position that relegated experiences to a secondary role in producing people's traits. But although it remains true that we are born and die with the exact same sequence information in our genetic material (for the most part), the discovery of an *epi*genetic code that *can* be influenced by environmental factors—and that can subsequently influence genetic activity—should alter our understanding of why each of us develops the characteristics we do.

|| 7 ||

Zooming in on Regulation

The first evidence that mature, differentiated cells retain the potential to grow into other cell types emerged in the 1950s from the labs of biologists, like Fredrick Steward, who were working with plants. Although these findings also implied that mature cells taken from *animals* could perhaps be used to clone those animals, it was not until John Gurdon and colleagues successfully cloned frogs in the 1960s that scientists knew for sure that "cell specialization does not involve any loss, irreversible inactivation or permanent change in the . . . genes required for development."[1] Nonetheless, another three decades passed before anyone was able to take a mature, donated cell from a *mammal* and make it behave like a pluripotent embryonic stem cell, that is, able to develop into a clone of the donor animal. In 1996, scientists in Scotland witnessed the birth of Dolly, a cloned ewe (i.e., a female sheep) whose entire genome came from a mature, differentiated cell taken from a donor ewe's mammary gland.[2] Because decades of failures preceded this success, many biologists had presumed that differentiated cells from complex animals would never be able to be returned to a pluripotent state; some explicitly thought cloning mammals would be impossible.

There are several things to learn from scientists' adventures in cloning. First, developing into an adult mammal does not entail irreversible changes in the animal's genetic information;[3] the genetic information required to grow a whole animal remains present even in mature, differentiated mammalian cells, just as it does in the cells of plants or frogs. Perhaps as important is the realization that the Scottish team succeeded because they implanted Dolly's genome into an unfertilized egg (one that had been emptied of its own genome); that is, they put Dolly's DNA into a very specific environment that contributed to her development. As the scientists noted in their breakthrough paper, their results were "consistent with the generally accepted view that mammalian differentiation is almost all achieved by systematic, sequential changes in gene expression brought about by interactions between the nucleus and the changing cytoplasmic environment."[4] A gene's context always matters.

Second, cloning research has taught us that although the word "clone" evokes mental images of identical copies of animals, clones are not indistinguishable from each other; they merely have the same DNA as their parent and as any other clones of that parent. But because phenotypes are not determined by the genome but rather develop via gene-environment interactions, clones differ from one another in noticeable ways. Clones can look and act very differently than their genetically identical relatives, as revealed in anecdotal reports about the strikingly different appearances and personalities of calf clones[5] or about the very different coat-color patterns of the first cloned house cat and the "parent" that donated her genome.[6] In the case of the cat, the conspicuous differences between her and her genome-donating mother are due to well-documented epigenetic effects, described below.

Third, the cloning research in Scotland revealed a way to turn back the hands of the biological clock, returning mature cells to an earlier state like the one typical of embryos. More recent research has revealed an even simpler way to reset the clock of differentiated cells. This technique, developed in Shinya Yamanaka's lab in Kyoto, Japan,[7] entails taking DNA that codes for specific gene products and inserting that DNA into a differentiated cell;[8] once these products are built by the cell, they have the effect of "de-differentiating" the cell, that is, of returning it to a pluripotent state. In this way, a mature cell can effectively be made young again.

Yamanaka's breakthrough was so important that he and John Gurdon were awarded a Nobel Prize in Physiology or Medicine in October 2012. Because the kinds of stem cells his team created are capable of becoming neurons, beta cells of the pancreas, or whatever other kinds of cells we might want them to become, they have enormous potential to help people lacking particular cell types. Such people might be lacking these cell types because they have a degenerative disorder (e.g., Parkinson's disease, in which particular types of neurons have died), an autoimmune disorder (e.g., type 1 diabetes, in which beta cells have died), or some other condition associated with cell death (e.g., a severe heart attack, after which cardiac muscle cells have died).

These kinds of stem cells were first cleared for use in human beings in July 2013; in a subsequent trial planned in Japan, researchers aimed to treat six patients with age-related vision loss using transplanted stem cells derived from the patients' own skin.[9] This technology is too new to have yet yielded demonstrable benefits, but its promise is immense, in terms of both lives and money saved. For example, type 1 diabetes alone generates a burden on the US economy of nearly one billion dollars every 4 years,[10] so a technology that would allow type 1 diabetes sufferers to produce their own insulin—from new beta cells inside of their own bodies— could do even more than radically improve lives; it could also save an enormous amount of money. When we consider the many other disorders that could potentially be treated with these kinds of stem cells, the significance of Yamanaka's work is obvious.

This kind of innovation grew from research on epigenetic influences on development, because cellular differentiation is a developmental process entailing epigenetic change. And as documented in the forthcoming chapter "Hope," research on epigenetics has also transformed how some researchers think about the development of schizophrenia, addiction, mood disorders, obesity, cancer, and other conditions. Of course, it should not surprise us that studying development is yielding valuable insights into human disorders. Our phenotypes arise in development, and most of the diseases that plague us have their roots in development, too. If we discover those roots, we might learn how to influence development in a way that prevents the diseases in the first place.

Epigenetic Imprints: A Difference Between Maternal and Paternal DNA

The first disease to be recognized as involving epigenetics is a disorder known as Prader-Willi syndrome.[11] Although we have learned a lot about this condition since it was first identified in 1956, we have not yet learned how to prevent it. A relatively rare disorder, Prader-Willi syndrome is characterized by mental retardation and the tendency to overeat; some patients also exhibit obsessive behavior, poor gross motor skills, or aggression.[12a–12b] For over 20 years, scientists have known that this condition is associated, in about two-thirds of cases,[13a–13b] with the deletion of genetic material on the 15th chromosome inherited from a patient's father.[14] The fact that Prader-Willi syndrome might be a fundamentally epigenetic disease dawned on researchers as they thought about something very strange in the foregoing statement: Why should it matter if the genetic abnormality was on the chromosome that came from the father rather than the mother? The corresponding chromosomes in men's and women's bodies (other than the sex chromosomes, of course) are not fundamentally different from one another, so the finding that a factor such as parent-of-origin actually *matters* was very surprising.

As it happens, mammals have evolved an epigenetic way to track the parental origin of some of their chromosomes. In some cases, chromosomes that come from mothers and fathers really are interchangeable. But in other cases, epigenetic marks distinguish chromosomes that originated in a male from those that originated in a female; such chromosomes are said to have "imprinted" regions. Imprinting can block or enhance the expression of gene products in some species,[15] but in the examples I will be considering in this book, imprinted regions are always epigenetically silenced, and therefore unexpressed. Regardless, imprinting in a particular region of DNA is always related to the parent who provided the chromosome.

Taken as a whole, maternal and paternal contributions to a new organism's genome do not function equivalently.[16a–16b] The fact that ordinary (i.e., non-sex) chromosomes from fathers and mothers do not function in the same way became apparent after some pioneering experiments on mice in the 1980s. This work demonstrated that both maternal and paternal chromosomes are required for survival. Even if an embryo has a full complement of chromosomes, if all of the chromosomes were provided by male donors *or* if all of the chromosomes were provided by female donors, the embryo will not survive to birth;[17] receiving one set of maternal chromosomes and one set of paternal chromosomes is critical. This sort of effect suggests that a disorder like Prader-Willi syndrome—which is associated specifically with a paternal chromosome—might be related to imprinting. Accordingly, the existence of a parent-of-origin effect in Prader-Willi patients drew attention to imprinting, and ultimately alerted scientists that specific imprints can be associated with specific human disorders.[18]

The DNA segment missing in most Prader-Willi patients is normally found on the 15th paternal chromosome, where it is used to produce important snRNAs; when this segment is deleted, these snRNAs cannot be produced. What complicates this situation is that in normal people, the equivalent segment of the 15th *maternal* chromosome is imprinted and unexpressed.[19] Because this segment has been epigenetically silenced, it is unable to compensate for the abnormality on the corresponding paternal chromosome.

This story could give the impression that Prader-Willi syndrome is essentially a genetic abnormality, because after all, the patients I have described are all missing some of the DNA sequence information found in normal people. But the fundamentally *epi*genetic nature of this disorder was revealed when researchers discovered that some Prader-Willi sufferers actually have two 15th chromosomes that contain *all* of the normal sequence information. Thus, despite how it first appeared, Prader-Willi syndrome does not depend on the deletion of genetic information; it sometimes occurs in people who are deletion-free. But this leaves us with a perplexing question: How can people with two normal 15th chromosomes develop this syndrome?

It turns out that these individuals are abnormal in a different way. Although normal people receive one 15th chromosome from their father and one from their mother, Prader-Willi patients *without* genetic deletions somehow wind up with two normal 15th chromosomes *both of which came from their mother*[20] (this is, of course, an abnormal occurrence). Because both of these chromosomes are imprinted (i.e., epigenetically silenced) in the region where maternal 15th chromosomes are *normally* imprinted, the required snRNAs are not expressed and the patients develop symptoms that are indistinguishable from those of patients with a genetic *deletion* on their 15th paternal chromosome. Therefore, the presence of even *two* normal maternal 15th chromosomes cannot compensate for an abnormal or absent paternal 15th chromosome. Like Benjamin Franklin's silver in the mine, having the required genetic sequence in your genome is of little value if epigenetic modifications like imprinting leave that information inaccessible.

Until relatively recently, diagnosing Prader-Willi syndrome was challenging because there is an entirely different disorder called Angelman syndrome[21] that is associated with abnormalities in the very same chromosomal region implicated in Prader-Willi syndrome. In contrast to Prader-Willi, Angelman syndrome is characterized by developmental delays that are even more severe, and by movement or balance disorders, frequent laughter, and jerky "hand-flapping" movements.[22] This raises the excellent question: How can two entirely different disorders arise from abnormalities in the very same chromosomal region?

We now know that Angelman syndrome develops when sequence information on the *maternal* 15th chromosome has been deleted, because the corresponding region of the normal paternal 15th chromosome is imprinted and unexpressed. Thus, Prader-Willi and Angelman syndromes are like mirror-image disorders; they typically involve *deletions* of DNA segments on the *p*aternal and *m*aternal 15th chromosomes, respectively, and *epigenetic silencing* of those same DNA segments on the *m*aternal and *p*aternal 15th chromosomes, respectively. Recent studies suggest that the critical sequence information is actually located in adjacent, rather than identical, places on the corresponding chromosomes,[23] but in both cases, the disorders develop whenever the required segment cannot be used, *either* because it has been deleted *or* because it is present on the 15th chromosome provided by the "wrong" parent, and is therefore imprinted and unavailable for use. In this way, normal human development appears to require accessible DNA segments on both a maternal *and* a paternal 15th chromosome.

The Case of the Calico Cat: Epigenetic X-Inactivation in Normal Females

Epigenetic silencing does not just contribute to disorders like Prader-Willi or Angelman syndrome; instead, most epigenetic modifications of chromatin are actually normal occurrences that contribute to healthy development. The role of epigenetic silencing in normal development is most conspicuous in the process of X-inactivation. The mechanism by which one of a woman's two X chromosomes is silenced is now relatively well understood, and its interesting effects are readily observable in specific circumstances.

Imprinting and X-inactivation both involve epigenetic modifications of chromatin, but they are different in several ways. First, men and women both have some chromosomal regions that are normally imprinted, but only women experience X-inactivation. Second, X-inactivation occurs early in the development of an embryo;[24] in contrast, imprinting occurs in sperm and eggs, that is, before a new embryo is even conceived.[25] Third, as important as imprinting might be, it seems to affect fewer genes than X-inactivation does;[26] X-inactivation silences more than 1,000 genes—not *all* of the genes on the X chromosome, but still a very large number.[27, 28] Finally, by definition, imprinting involves the epigenetic alteration of DNA in a parent-specific manner; whether a particular chromosome was provided by a father or a mother matters very much in imprinting. In contrast, X-inactivation proceeds without regard to the X chromosome's maternal versus paternal origin;[29] as long as one of the X chromosomes is inactivated, development can proceed normally.

For this reason, determining which X chromosome will be inactivated is always a random process;[30] in any given cell of a female mammal, the inactivated X chromosome could be the one that came from the mother or the one that came from the father. Therefore, all normal female mammals are so-called epigenetic mosaics with respect to their X chromosomes. That is, the X chromosomes in some of their cells are in one epigenetic state while the X chromosomes in other cells are in a different epigenetic state. Calico cats illustrate this phenomenon very well, because in these house pets, you can actually *see* the effects of epigenetic mosaicism.

Calico cats are easy to identify, because they always have more than one color of fur arranged in patches across their bodies. These cats are virtually always female, and their unusual coloration is a visible indication of the random X-inactivation that has occurred in their cells.[31] One gene on the feline X chromosome is used to produce pigment in specialized skin cells called melanocytes; these cells collaborate with other cells to give rise to colored hair. Depending on the sequence information present in this gene, it can contribute to the development of black, white, or orange-ish hair. Because male cats have only one X chromosome, they normally have a solid coat color; all of their melanocytes do the same thing, so all of these cats' hairs are the same color. A female cat can have a solid coat color as well, as happens when both parents pass on a gene associated with the same hair color. But whenever the DNA that a female cat has inherited from her mother and the DNA she has inherited from her father contains differing sequence information at the relevant location on the X chromosome, a calico will result.

Imagine a newly conceived female cat embryo that has inherited one X chromosome containing sequence information associated with orange fur and another X chromosome containing sequence information associated with black fur. Early in this embryo's development, one of the X chromosomes in each of her cells will be epigenetically inactivated at random; in some cases it will be the X chromosome with the "black gene," and in others it will be the X chromosome with the "orange gene." The end result will be that some of her melanocyte stem cells will have an active "black gene" and others will have an active "orange gene." When these stem cells divide, they will pass on their epigenetic state; thus, the daughter cells that descend from a melanocyte stem cell with an active "orange gene" will likewise have an active "orange gene" (and an inactivated "black gene" on the other X-chromosome). In this way, calico cats wind up with groups of related cells in a given region, all of which produce fur of the same color. Thus, all of the hairs in one area will have the same color, but nearby could be an area populated by cells descended from a different melanocyte stem cell, and these cells would all produce fur of the other color. In fact, when you look at a calico cat, you are, in effect, actually *seeing* the results of the random epigenetic inactivation of one type of "pigment gene" in some of her cells and the random epigenetic inactivation of a different type of "pigment gene" in her other cells.

It is telling that a particular calico cat's coat-color pattern does not change as she ages; it means that X-inactivation is extremely stable. Once the choice has been made in a given cell to inactivate one of the X chromosomes and not the other, the inactivated chromosome will remain the inactive one permanently.[32] This same sort of random-and-permanent X-inactivation process occurs in human females just as it does in cats, but we ordinarily can't *see* the resulting mosaicism, because genes associated with pigmentation in women are located on chromosomes other than the X chromosomes.[33]

This account of calico patterning explains why the first-ever house pet produced by cloning—who was named CC, for "Carbon Copy"—did not look like the beloved pet her human owner was seeking to reproduce.[34] The cell nucleus that gave rise to CC came originally from a cat named Rainbow, who, as her name suggests, was calico. Because the coat-color patterns of calico cats develop because of an *epigenetic* effect (i.e., random X-inactivation), it should not surprise us that CC, who has the exact same genome as Rainbow, nonetheless did not wind up with Rainbow's coat-color pattern (or general appearance). Even if two individuals have identical genomes, if they have dissimilar *epi*genomes they can wind up with very different phenotypes. Despite her evocative name, CC was definitely not a "Carbon Copy" of Rainbow, probably to the dismay of her owner. (If you're interested in seeing how CC and Rainbow looked, there are some great comparison photographs available on the Internet; you can find them easily by searching Google for "CC and Rainbow.")

The Mechanics of X-Inactivation: Some General Features of Epigenetic Silencing

The mechanism by which an X chromosome is inactivated is very interesting, and it illuminates some general features of epigenetic silencing that are worth noting. In the early 1960s, researchers[35a–35b] realized that in the cells of some mice, a portion of an X chromosome can sometimes break off and become attached to another chromosome. Sometimes when this happens, the other chromosome shuts down, as if it was inactivated (something that would normally never happen to that chromosome). This discovery suggested that some portion of the X chromosome might have a role in the inactivation process. After a particularly good candidate region was located on the X chromosome—later called the X-inactivation center[36]—it became the focus of intense study.

This work revealed that a portion of the X-inactivation center can be used to produce an RNA transcript that is expressed by some X chromosomes, *but only those that are about to be inactivated.* That is, although an X-inactivation center is present on all X chromosomes, X chromosomes that remain active do not *express* this RNA transcript; only to-be-inactivated X chromosomes have the relevant segment transcribed.[37] This finding strongly suggested that the transcript generated by the X-inactivation center was responsible for inactivating the very chromosome that generated it! And sure enough, an X chromosome that has somehow lost the critical segments of the X-inactivation center cannot be inactivated.[38a–38b] Moreover, the abnormal *presence* of these segments on some *other* chromosomes can lead to the inactivation of portions of those chromosomes.[39] Together, these findings made it quite clear that the transcript generated by the X-inactivation center can somehow inactivate chromosomes.

The transcript generated by the X-inactivation center struck the scientists who discovered it as truly weird. First, it contained signals throughout its length that instructed any protein-constructing machinery that might be attempting to translate it to stop the translation process right away. Second, the transcript was found to never leave the cell nucleus. Keep in mind that in the early 1990s when this transcript was discovered, biologists believed that RNA's sole function was related to protein construction, and because proteins are not constructed in cell nuclei, an RNA transcript that stays in the nucleus can't be used to build proteins. So, as you can imagine, this newly discovered transcript was a real head-scratcher; what possible use could it be if it has nothing to do with protein construction? But because it was obviously playing some sort of important role in X-inactivation, it was subjected to a lot of additional research and given the name X-inactive specific transcript (XIST, which, once it was discovered, could obviously be said to "exist," making its abbreviated name quite appropriate). Since then, many other noncoding RNAs have been discovered, but XIST was among the first to hint that untranslated RNA could have very important roles in the epigenetic control of DNA.

After XIST is expressed from an X chromosome, it immediately attaches itself to that chromosome and covers it, rendering the sequence information in the X chromosome less accessible to transcription machinery. But XIST does not silence the X chromosome all by itself. Instead, the presence of XIST seems to attract other molecules to the histones in the region, which produce other epigenetic modifications that make transcription increasingly difficult. Ultimately, promoters for the genes on the X chromosome become methylated, which attracts repressive proteins that reduce the likelihood of transcription even further, maintaining the X chromosome in an inactive state. One group of scientists active in this research area put it like this: "Spreading of Xist RNA leads to conversion of the chromosome to a silent . . . configuration. This X inactivation involves multiple epigenetic changes."[40]

This sort of process, in which particular kinds of epigenetic events cause other epigenetic events, which cause yet *other* epigenetic events, and so on, is characteristic of epigenetic regulation. For example, it is possible that DNA methylation silences genes simply by interfering with the ability of transcription machinery to access the DNA. But it appears that a second mechanism of silencing-by-methylation is also available, one that entails a multistep process commonly used in organs like the brain, where gene expression is relatively dynamic.[41] In this second mode, methyl groups serve to attract specific proteins that then recruit several *other* proteins including so-called corepressor complexes and enzymes;[42] these enzymes modify histones, removing acetyl groups and adding methyl groups in a way that ultimately closes up the chromatin and leads to gene deactivation.[43] In the case of X-inactivation, it is a combination of DNA methylation and histone modifications that silence most (but not all) of the genes on the X chromosome.[44] In the end, an X chromosome that has expressed XIST winds up slinking off to the side of the nucleus while becoming compacted into a small, ineffectual, nearly silent blob of chromatin.

For anyone armed with a basic understanding of DNA, histones, methyl groups, and the like, the new science of behavioral epigenetics is surprisingly accessible.

PART II

WHAT DO WE KNOW?

8

Epigenetics

When I was a senior in high school, one of the colleges I was interested in attending was Northwestern University, in Evanston, Illinois. Wanting to get a better feel for the place, I talked my parents into letting me make the six-hour drive to Evanston, but because I had never taken such a long road trip on my own before, my parents asked me to find a friend to join me for the drive. Fortunately, a couple of the guys in my classes were interested in Northwestern, too, so we made a plan to hit the road together.

One of my travel buddies that spring was Spencer Fine. Spencer was well known at our high school, in part because he was an identical twin, and, as is typically the case with identical twins, Spencer and his brother Scott were an unending source of fascination for lots of our classmates. Many people are taken aback when they encounter twins, probably because we are all so used to encountering unique individuals. But for me, what was striking about Scott and Spencer was how *non-identical* they were. Sure, they looked so similar that no one would have mistaken them for anything other than identical twins; on first meeting them, it could be difficult not to stare, doing a feature-by-feature comparison of their appearances. But after knowing them for a few years in high school, none of our classmates was ever confused about which twin we were talking to. And in my experience, this is almost always the case. "Identical" twins look more similar than most nontwin siblings do, but for those who know them well, a case of mistaken identity would be highly unlikely. The physical similarities can be so striking that we focus on them, but there can be no denying that "identical" twins are *not* identical, regardless of the name we have given this type of twin-pair.

Technically, these types of twins are known as *monozygotic* (or MZ) twins, because they develop from a single fertilized egg (a zygote) that is formed when a single sperm fertilizes a single egg. Because of this shared history, MZ twins share 100% of their DNA, and this explains (at least in part) why they are so similar to each other. Although we currently do not understand what causes twinning in most cases, the existence of twins gives us a sort of "natural experiment" that generations of psychologists have sought to exploit in their efforts to assess whether "nature" or "nurture" is the more important contributor to our traits. A cottage industry still exists that is devoted to answering this question with twin studies, but recent scholarly work in epigenetics and other disciplines has made it clear that traditional twin studies will never provide a good answer to this question, because it is an ill-formed question; nature and nurture both contribute in essential ways to the building of our traits. Nonetheless, a newer type of twin study is beginning to give us clues about how we become who we are.

In 2005, a team of researchers at the Spanish National Cancer Centre in Madrid (along with an international collection of collaborators) published a report on an important study of the epigenetic statuses of 40 pairs of MZ twins.[1] Looking at both DNA methylation and histone acetylation across the twins' genomes, the researchers discovered that the *young* identical twins had patterns of epigenetic markings that were extremely similar one another. But as the twins got older and accumulated the distinctive experiences that characterize individual lives, their epigenetic states diverged; the twins who "were older, had different lifestyles, and had spent less of their lives together"[2] showed evidence of noteworthy differences in DNA methylation and histone acetylation throughout their genomes. The implication of this study is that our lived experiences leave "marks" on our DNA, and these marks affect how our genes are expressed.[3a-3c]

Other studies of identical twins have been conducted since 2005, but they have not all generated the same conclusions. For instance, two studies reported that MZ twins are *born* with differing epigenetic profiles, differences that in some cases reflect differences in the twins' prenatal environments.[4a-4b] In addition, one of these studies reported that—unlike in the Madrid study—the epigenetic differences present at birth did *not* increase as individuals aged. But at least five other studies[5a-5e] have found that DNA methylation patterns *do* change with age. So even if the epigenetic profiles of MZ twins really do differ at birth, the implications of the Spanish National Cancer Centre study remain valid: Our experiences affect what our genes do.

Because epigenetic alterations change how our genes are expressed, it should not surprise us that individuals are unique, identical twins included. We each have a distinctive set of experiences, and since those experiences influence the activity of genes that alter the structure and chemistry of our bodies' cells—thereby altering the structure and functioning of our bodies themselves—we each look and act like unique individuals, even in the rare situation where two individuals share the same DNA. This is why "identical" twins are not, in fact, identical.

Such epigenetic differences have also been noted in MZ twins who are discordant for certain disorders, including schizophrenia;[6] in cases of discordance, one member of an MZ twin-pair is normal, but the other twin has the disease. Discordance like this is a relatively common occurrence that was difficult to explain before we understood the importance of epigenetics. It now appears that epigenetic differences can help explain at least some instances of discordance.[7]

Some Striking Effects of Epigenetics

As interesting as the MZ twin data are, it is still true that MZ twins are often different from each other in *relatively* subtle ways. In contrast to these studies of human beings, experiments on other organisms have demonstrated that epigenetic effects can be every bit as bold as genetic effects. As we saw in the preceding chapter, the coat-color patterns of calico cats reveal how noticeable epigenetic effects can be.

Studies of very obvious epigenetic effects are enlightening because even though most of us are comfortable with the idea that our experiences influence how we think, feel, and act, we usually assume that *conspicuous* differences in the shapes of our bodies, the structures of our faces, and other aspects of our physical appearances are influenced primarily by genetic factors. After all, one of the reasons cats and dogs look so different from one another is undeniably because they have different genomes! But studies of epigenetic effects in plants and animals—effects that, by definition, leave genetic sequence information unchanged—have shown that epigenetic marks can profoundly influence even gross physical structures.

In a notable demonstration in 1999, a trio of scientists in the UK published photographs of toadflax flowers, which ordinarily appear in nature like yellowish snapdragons.[8] Alongside a photograph of an ordinary toadflax flower, these researchers displayed a photograph of a so-called "peloric mutant" toadflax flower, which looks like it could be a completely different species (see Figure 8.1). In fact, Linnaeus—the father of modern biological classification—characterized this naturally occurring mutant back in 1749, so the fact that the mutant was a toadflax-gone-wrong was no news to anyone. The surprise that led to this paper

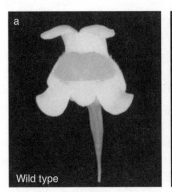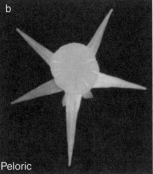

Figure 8.1 A photograph showing the face view of a wild toadflax flower and the face view of a peloric mutant toadflax flower. Reprinted by permission from Dr. Enrico Coen, Dr. Pilar Cubas, and Macmillan Publishers Ltd.; original image printed in Cubas, P., Vincent, C., & Coen, E. (1999). An epigenetic mutation responsible for natural variation in floral symmetry. *Nature, 401,* 157–161.

being published in *Nature*, the preeminent science journal in Europe, was that the difference between the ordinary and mutant versions of these flowers was strictly *epi*genetic, not genetic. The unusual shape of the mutant flower reflects the presence of a methylated (and, therefore, silenced) gene, a gene that normally contributes to the development of the ordinary flower. Clearly, an epigenetic alteration can so radically affect the gross shape of an organism that the effect can be as extreme as the effects of genetic mutations.

We can see similarly radical effects of epigenetics on gross body shape in some animal species. For example, although it is too early to say for *sure* if epigenetic differences might account for the different appearances of modern humans and Neanderthals, a fascinating recent study has suggested that this might be the case. By comparing methylation maps generated from Neanderthal DNA and modern human DNA, a group of scientists at the Hebrew University of Jerusalem (along with an international collection of collaborators) discovered thousands of DNA regions that were differentially methylated, some of which could potentially account for the different anatomies of these two species of humans.[9]

Honeybees are another animal species in which we can see significant effects of epigenetics on anatomy and behavior, and they are a particularly interesting example, because large numbers of female larvae in a colony are genetically identical. Remarkably, although the sisters in a given colony are all clones of one another, they do not all share the same fate. Most of them develop into worker bees, but a small number become queens, who look and behave very differently than their identical twin siblings. Relative to workers, nonvirgin queens are twice as large with much longer abdomens, they have life spans that are 20 times longer, and their behavioral repertoires are distinctly different. Even their bodily organs differ;[10] whereas workers have sting barbs in their rears and pollen baskets on their hind legs, queens have neither. In contrast, queens have mature ovaries, so they can reproduce; workers do not, so they are infertile. Because queens and their sisters share identical genes, an environmental factor must account for these disparities, and in fact, queens consume a distinctive diet, one that makes all the difference.

Before discussing the regal diet and its epigenetic effects, this is a great spot to notice the difference between "causing an outcome" and "accounting for a different outcome." Faced with this situation—eat diet A and you're a worker, eat diet B and you're a queen—it is tempting to think that it must be their diets alone that cause workers to develop pollen baskets and sting barbs; after all, all of the bees are genetically identical and the *only* difference in their environments is dietary. But it can't possibly be the case that diet A single-handedly causes pollen baskets to develop, because if I suddenly started feeding *you* the diet that turns female honeybee larvae into workers, you would not develop pollen baskets on your legs! Pollen baskets develop because of the *interaction* of this diet with a bee's genome. Thus, the *difference* between queens and workers is *accounted for* by the difference in their diets, but the diets themselves do not single-handedly cause the bees' behavioral or other phenotypes.

The reason this is worth noting here is because it seems to be easier for us to keep in mind the distinction between *causing a trait* and *accounting for differences in traits* when the difference-maker is environmental, as diet is in this example. If the situation is reversed and it's a gene that makes the difference, we seem inclined to forget about this distinction and assume the gene alone has causal power. Imagine, for instance, that a geneticist discovers a gene that is present in everyone with disease X but absent in everyone without disease X. In this case, many people would conclude that the geneticist has discovered a gene that single-handedly causes the disease. But just because the presence of this newly discovered gene can *account* for the disease phenotype doesn't mean the gene *causes* this phenotype independently of environmental factors. In fact, genes cannot single-handedly cause the development of a phenotype any more than diets can. The truly complex reality is that neither genetic nor environmental factors *independently* cause phenotypes. A general lesson we can draw from studying how diets influence bees' bodies is that traits are as they are for both environmental *and* genetic reasons.

Diets are clearly important for bees. Early in the larval stage in the lives of female bees, worker bees nurse the larvae with a substance called royal jelly, secreted by a gland at the top of each worker's head. After three days on this diet, the nurses switch most of the developing bees to a different "worker diet,"[11] but they continue providing incipient queens with copious quantities of royal jelly. Female larvae that keep eating royal jelly differentiate into queens, and they continue to eat royal jelly for the rest of their long lives, long after their twin sisters (and even most of their own offspring!) have died.

There is still a lot we don't understand about these processes,[12] but ongoing research has begun to clarify the story. It appears that a protein in royal jelly increases concentrations of a hormone in female larvae, which contributes to their differentiation into queens.[13] But how can a single protein that an animal eats cause its body to develop so differently than it would otherwise? Ten years ago, researchers looking at gene expression patterns in developing queens and workers discovered that although these bees share identical genomes, queen-destined larvae *use* their genomes very differently than do worker-destined larvae.[14] These findings suggested that dietary factors might have effects that alter genetic expression in the larvae, thereby driving development down different pathways.

In fact, it is now evident that epigenetics *is* the missing link. When scientists manipulate epigenetic states directly using injections of specially designed molecules, larvae that are injected develop into queens just as surely as if they were fed a diet rich in royal jelly.[15] Ultimately, this research proved that becoming a queen requires demethylation of DNA that is normally methylated in worker bees. Currently, there are still several pieces of the bee puzzle that are missing;[16] for instance, it remains unclear whether the protein present in royal jelly produces epigenetic effects in a direct or indirect way. But one thing is certain: Diet radically changes bees' bodies and behaviors by influencing genetic expression through epigenetic mechanisms.

Getting Our Environments Under Our Skin

Can dietary experiences change the way *our* genes are expressed, as they change the way bees' genes are expressed? Some of the strongest evidence that diet can alter mammalian bodies through epigenetics as conspicuously as it can alter honeybees' bodies comes from studies of a particular breed of mice[17a–17b] that we will consider in chapters 15 and 16, both of which will address the topic of nutrition. Other important lines of evidence suggest that a relatively *wide* variety of experiences can influence gene expression in mammals. Besides diet, other factors on this list (each of which will be considered at least briefly in later chapters) include environmental chemicals,[18a–18b] commonly abused drugs,[19] exercise,[20a–20d] and specific parenting behaviors.[21] Ten years ago, before scientists had much data indicating that mammals' experiences influence their epigenetic states, Rudolf Jaenisch and Adrian Bird—two leaders in what was then an emerging field—put a hunch into words, speculating that "epigenetic mechanisms seem to allow an organism to respond to the environment through changes in gene expression."[22] They went on to predict that future research would enable us "to understand, and perhaps manipulate, the ways in which the genome learns from its experiences."[23] In 2014, we are still far from manipulating genomes like this, but scientists now acknowledge the pervasive influence of the environment on genetic functioning in mammals.

The discovery that the environment affects the epigenome raises an important question: How can environmental factors get "inside of us" to affect our genetic activity? The honeybee example alerts us to one way this could work; in that case, the protein in royal jelly led to an increase in hormone concentrations in the bees' bodies. Similarly, mammals' experiences—our experiences—can cause hormones to be released in our bodies, and these molecules can then move into the vicinity of DNA, where they can produce epigenetic effects.

Our environments also influence our internal states by stimulating our sensory organs; seeing and hearing, for example, both produce changes in our bodies that can have epigenetic consequences (as will become apparent shortly). Because stimulation arising in the environment can affect biological activity at several levels—at the level of the neurons in our sensory organs, at the level of the hormones in our bloodstreams, at the level of the genes in our cell nuclei—an essential part of how we come to be as we are will always be what we experience, that is, the contexts that our minds, bodies, cells, organs, and genes find themselves in. This perspective encourages us to think about how factors *interact* to produce our characteristics, and more specifically, how nongenetic factors influence genetic expression. These interactions regularly occur very early in life, as when the development of a bee larva is affected by the presence of royal jelly in her diet or when the development of a newborn mouse is affected by how the mouse is mothered. But the accumulating evidence suggests that our experiences in adulthood affect how our genes function as well.

Most days, I wake up in California, go about my business, and ultimately wind down at home before going to sleep for the night. When I wake up the next day, things proceed pretty much as they did the day before. This cycle reflects a circadian rhythm, a temporal pattern that repeats once each day. In addition to creating our sleep-wake cycle, this rhythm produces cyclical changes in characteristics like our core body temperatures and the concentrations of hormones in our bodies. Remarkably, this rhythm persists even when a person is isolated from cues about what time of day it is; this is why it seems as though we have an internal biological clock that runs independently of whatever is going on around us. It is clear that maintaining the rhythm is important; disrupting it can seriously damage a person's health, contributing to a variety of conditions, including depression, insomnia, coronary heart disease, and cancer.[24] And we now know that the reason this rhythm is so influential is because upward of 10% of our genes are expressed cyclically, being transcribed only in specific periods during our 24-hour days.[25]

Might a person's biological clock be dependent on her DNA? Interestingly, scientists have known for over 40 years that fruit flies have a DNA segment that helps maintain circadian rhythms,[26] and we now know mammals have similar segments. These genes are components of machinery distributed throughout our bodies, machinery that makes up a body's circadian clock.[27] Individual cells have their own clocklike rhythms,[28] but the rhythms of these cells are regularly synchronized by specific neurons in a brain area known as the hypothalamus. These neurons function as pacemakers; they do this by producing specific proteins in a time-locked manner, such that the number of proteins in these cells peaks regularly, once every 24 hours.[29]

Experiments on mice have shown that mammalian circadian rhythms are maintained by the turning on and turning off of various genes in a temporal pattern that measures out our 24-hour days—genes are turned on, proteins are constructed, protein concentrations increase, genes are turned off, protein levels fall off, and so on, repeating anew each day.

If every day was a normal day for me, this system might work very well for keeping track of time. But on an especially good day, I might wake up in California, pack, and head to the airport to catch a 1 p.m. flight to Paris. When my flight lands, it will be 9 a.m. in France, but it will feel like 12:00 a.m. to me, because it actually *will* be midnight at that moment in Los Angeles. So, I'll be ready to go to sleep, but everyone else in Paris will be just starting to enjoy their morning croissant. This is what jetlag is all about (and not, as some people think, a general sense of tiredness you get from traveling on a jet—a 3-hour flight from north to south will not produce jetlag, but a 3-hour flight from east to west will). If my circadian rhythms really were internally set by the activities of some unresponsive DNA in my hypothalamic neurons, I would be out of luck: No matter how long I stayed in Paris, I would always be wide awake at 11:00 at night and ready to crash after sunrise. Fortunately for all of us, we do adjust to local time after a while, but that raises a question: How are we able to adjust in this way? What can *reset* a biological clock that, left to its own devices, will just keep running on a 24-hour cycle for a lifetime?

The answer appears to be "light."[30] Researchers have explored this question using hamsters, because their circadian clocks are much like people's. Exposing hamsters to light when they *expect* it to be nighttime produces genetic activity in their hypothalamic pacemaker neurons; therefore, we can conclude that these neurons are receiving signals from the eyes about light exposure.[31] Likewise, when a person experiences light at an abnormal time of day—as when a tourist sees the sun even though her brain expects it to be dark because the sun has already set back at home—the light enters her eyes and strikes cells in her retinas, which send neural signals to her hypothalamic pacemaker neurons; upon receiving these signals, genes in those neurons begin churning out proteins in a cascade of events that leads to the resetting of her circadian clock. But what does this have to do with epigenetics?

For a body to match its rhythm to a local time zone, a feedback mechanism must exist that detects light, responds to it, and then detects the effect of the response; such a mechanism would allow an organism to flexibly fit its behavior to its solar context. And because epigenetic changes could be a part of such a mechanism, neuroscientists have explored whether epigenetics might have a role in matching biological and astronomical rhythms. In fact, there are DNA segments that regulate the activity of genes associated with our circadian clocks, and acetylation of histones associated with those segments influences the activity of these clock-related genes. Moreover, when mammals are exposed to discrete light pulses, histones associated with expression of these clock-related genes become acetylated, making it clear that epigenetic mechanisms help regulate our circadian clocks.

To demonstrate the role of histone acetylation in circadian clock functioning, a team of researchers in Kyoto injected an experimental drug into the brains of some mice.[32] The drug they used facilitates histone acetylation and thereby activates genes. As expected, the injections produced increased clock-related gene activity, a result that led the authors to conclude, "The rhythmic transcription and light induction of clock genes are regulated by histone acetylation and deacetylation."[33] The independent discovery of a protein that methylates histones in response to a clock-resetting stimulus[34] further underscores the role of epigenetics in maintaining circadian rhythms and, perhaps more importantly, in synchronizing those rhythms with environmental events.[35] (Details on the epigenetic modification of histones are available in the next chapter.)

By adjusting their epigenetic state daily, mammals are able to match the rhythms of gene expression to the rhythms of the natural world, ensuring that their bodily activities—in terms of behavior, physiology, and gene expression— remain in harmony. The finding that epigenetic mechanisms can be used like this suggests that our epigenetic states might be in a near-constant state of flux and that these mechanisms might efficiently bring about rapid biological change in response to stimulation. In fact, it has become clear that input to a neuron— regardless of whether that input comes from other neurons or directly from the environment—can alter the epigenetic state of that neuron's DNA, thereby ultimately altering how the neuron functions.

This is extremely important, as it provides a way in which our experiences can alter how our brains operate. Of course, we have all always known that our experiences affect our minds, and therefore, our brains; but work on epigenetics has revealed a *mechanistic* way in which the things we learn, and information about our environment, can be physically incorporated into our brains. Thus, we now know that epigenetic mechanisms play crucial roles in learning and memory,[36] psychological processes that entail changing the brain in response to environmental events (as detailed in chapters 13 and 14, on memory). So, epigenetic changes can influence the brains—and therefore, the minds—of children and adults, and they can occur specifically in response to environmental events.[37a–37b] This is why behavioral epigenetics is so exciting: It is the link between our genes and our environments, the link that allows our experiences to shape our brains and make us who we are.

A note of caution is in order here. Several popular news magazines have published articles on epigenetics in the last few years, including *Time*[38] and *Newsweek*.[39] These pieces have alarmed some writers who have expressed skepticism about behavioral epigenetics, claiming that the field is "hotly contested,"[40] the subject of "hype,"[41] and possessed of a "seductive allure" responsible for the discipline possibly "getting ahead of itself."[42] In some cases, uncertainty is warranted. For example, it will be a while before we fully understand the physical ways in which our experiences dynamically alter our epigenetic states; in particular, researchers still haven't agreed on the mechanism that allows DNA to be *de*methylated as a result of an experience[43] (although I will describe an excellent candidate mechanism in the next chapter). And there is still an enormous amount of work to do before scientists understand how—and under what conditions—epigenetic alterations can be transmitted to descendant generations. In the chapter titled "Caution," I will further consider where skepticism about behavioral epigenetics is warranted. But no one needs to be skeptical of one of the major take-home messages emerging from behavioral epigenetics research, namely, a message about genetic determinism: The information in our genes *cannot* single-handedly determine the nature of our characteristics, because genes work in *collaboration* with environmental, epigenetic, and other nongenetic factors to build our phenotypes. Caution is warranted whenever we are getting a glimpse of a previously unseen reality, as we are when we study behavioral epigenetics. But there is no need to be overly cautious when it comes to rejecting genetic determinism, because it has been obvious for many decades that genetic determinism should be rejected.

9

Zooming in on Epigenetics

I am a nerd. It pains me to admit it, because I grew up in a time before the nerds got their revenge, and I would much rather have had my peers in high school think I was friend-worthy. But although I was interested in all sorts of nonnerdy things, I thought science was cool, too. And I still do, which is why I use the present tense when proclaiming my nerdiness. So even though I think epigenetics is important because of what it says about who we are and how we should live our lives—respectable, big-picture, philosophical questions—I'm also interested in the details about how it all works. When I began to read about these details, I was stunned; I could never have imagined anything this complicated. In fact, the very intricacy of the system boggles the mind and inspires awe for the designer of the system. Being the biologically informed nerd that I am, I am confident we have natural selection to thank for these astonishing systems, but I can forgive anyone who has not studied evolution for looking at this collection of workings and concluding that there simply has to have been an intelligent designer responsible for something this beautiful.

The chapter "Regulation" introduced DNA methylation as a gene-silencing mechanism and histone acetylation as a gene-activating mechanism. There, I used a peppered-spaghetti metaphor that might have been useful on one level, but that left a lot to be desired on other levels. For one thing, that metaphor doesn't give any indication about how these epigenetic processes actually work. Of course, most people do not need to know how they work, but if you want to understand how scientists develop medicines or other manipulations that might actually improve people's lives, you need to know some specifics. There are two things to be aware of before we start, though. The first is that researchers have only just begun to solve this puzzle, so there are several areas where we still have remarkably little understanding. The second is that although we *do* now have inklings about a small fragment of the whole, this small fragment has revealed a system *so* detailed that I will only be able to scratch its surface here. By the end of this chapter, you will have read about arcane things like histone deacetylases, ubiquitylation, and hydroxymethylcytosine, and you might feel like your head is spinning from the details. Even so, this really is just the surface. The good news is that the information in this chapter is as complex as any in this entire book, so it will be enough to carry you through to the book's conclusion.

To appreciate the importance of epigenetic modifications, it will be helpful to first know a bit about how genetic transcription normally occurs. Transcription begins when molecules called "transcription factors" become attached to locations on DNA called "regulatory sites." Because regulatory sites are just DNA segments themselves, they are made of distinctive sequences of nucleotide bases that are able to "bind" transcription factors; that is, transcription factors can become attached to DNA at these spots. When a transcription factor binds to a regulatory site, that begins transcription of the gene associated with that site. So, regulatory sites are appropriately named: Each one regulates the expression of a particular gene. Of course, it would simplify matters considerably if regulatory sites were always nearby the genes they regulate, but this isn't how it works. Instead, some regulatory sites are near the genes they regulate, but some are located at quite a distance down the DNA strand. Amazingly, genes on some chromosomes are regulated through interactions with regulatory sites on *other* chromosomes. That is, sometimes a site on one chromosome regulates the activity of a gene located on an entirely different chromosome.[1a–1b]

As if this is not sufficiently complex, natural selection has *not* made transcription factors and regulatory sites analogous to simple keys and locks, in which a single key can open one and only one lock, and a single lock can be opened by one and only one key. Instead, the situation is more like one in which some keys can open several kinds of locks, and some locks can be opened by multiple kinds of keys. As described in a current molecular biology textbook,

> A single gene may be controlled by many different DNA regulatory sites that bind a variety of different transcriptional factors. Conversely, a single transcription factor may become attached to numerous sites around the genome, thereby controlling the expression of a host of different genes.[2]

To complicate matters further, some transcription factors interact with one another when they are in close proximity on a DNA strand, and these interactions can further influence how a gene is transcribed. Again, the textbook provides a helpful way to think about it:

> The regulatory region of a gene can be thought of as a type of integration center for that gene's expression. Cells exposed to different stimuli respond by synthesizing different transcription factors . . . the extent to which a given gene is transcribed presumably depends upon the particular *combination* of transcription factors [that are present at the regulatory site—or sites—for that gene].[3]

Thus, we can think of some DNA segments as information processors, because they effectively take different signals as input and generate a response in terms of increased or decreased gene expression.[4]

Because transcription in a particular chromosomal location is controlled by what is going on at a different location, control of gene expression depends on *where* on a DNA strand an epigenetic modification occurs. This is true regardless of whether we're talking about modifications of histones or of DNA itself. Generally, the epigenetic modifications discussed in this book occur in regulatory sites, not in DNA regions that actually contain sequence information. Epigenetic factors affect the expression of a gene by altering the ability of transcription factors to bind to the regulatory sites that regulate that gene's activity.

Some Nuts and Bolts of Chromatin Remodeling

As I noted in the chapter "Regulation," methylation is the primary process known to epigenetically alter DNA itself, but modifying histones with various kinds of chemicals can also influence gene expression. Histones can be methylated and acetylated, but they can also be phosphorylated or ubiquitinated by attaching phosphate groups or ubiquitin proteins to them, respectively. All of these processes affect gene expression. But because phosphorylation, ubiquitination, and other kinds of histone modifications have not been as well studied as histone acetylation or methylation,[5] I will focus in this book almost exclusively on DNA methylation, histone methylation, and histone acetylation.

And now, how histone acetylation works, in a four-paragraph nutshell. DNA has a negative electrical charge, whereas histones are positively charged; because opposites attract, this means DNA is usually drawn tightly against the "histone spool" it is wrapped around. You can think of DNA and histones as curvy, flexible magnets that are very strongly attracted to one another. As a result of the cramped configuration that results from this arrangement, transcription factors are less able to access the information in the DNA.[6] Each of the "spools" around which DNA is wrapped is actually made of four *pairs* of different histones that are closely associated with one another (see Figure 9.1). It's reasonable to think of this octet of histones as a single solid spool—which is why I will keep using the word "spool" to refer to this structure—but this image is off base in two important ways.

First, the histones that make up a spool are not all the same. If you took eight blobs of Play Doh—two red, two green, two yellow, and two blue—and rolled them all together into a spool shape, you'd wind up with a spool, but it would be made of eight noticeably different parts. This is why biologists typically refer to specific histones with a number, such as H3 or H4; the numbers tell you which histones in an octet are being referred to.

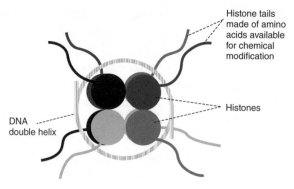

Figure 9.1 A schematic diagram of the arrangement of histones around which DNA is wrapped. Histones have amino acid tails that extend out beyond the DNA.

Second, unlike a single blob of Play Doh, a single histone isn't a homogeneous substance. Because they are proteins, each histone is made of a long string of amino acids crumpled into a characteristic shape. And although most of the amino acids constituting the histones are crammed together into a globelike shape that forms a part of a spool, each of the eight histones in a spool has a tail end that sticks out—in fact, way out—beyond even the DNA strand that is wrapped around the spool. These eight tails are significant, because each one is made of a large number of amino acids strung together, and these amino acids can form strong bonds with other chemicals, such as acetyl, methyl, or phosphate groups.

Histone acetylation, as I have noted, generally activates gene expression,[7a–7b] but there is ongoing debate about how it does this. One hypothesis is that adding acetyl groups to specific amino acids in the tails of specific histones reduces the positive charge of those histones. As a result, the nearby DNA becomes less "magnetically" attracted to the histone, and voilà: The new freedom from the histone allows transcription factors to access regulatory sites on the DNA and start up the RNA/protein production process.[8] A second hypothesis is that the acetyl groups serve as docking stations of sorts, which recruit yet other proteins to the region, proteins that then contribute to chromatin remodeling.[9]

Adding an acetyl group onto the correct amino acid in the tail of the correct histone is not necessarily as easy as I've made it sound. For one thing, there are four different kinds of histones, and for another, a histone tail is made of more than one kind of amino acid, including amino acids such as lysine, arginine, or serine. And it is not just that a histone tail contains a variety of different amino acids; a single tail might contain *several* of a given type of amino acid, and acetylating one of those amino acids might not produce the same effect as acetylating another one. For instance, the H3 histone has at least seven lysines in its tail that can be acetylated,[10a–10b] and although each lysine is identical to the others, the fact that they are in different *positions* in the tail matters a lot. And just as important as *which* lysine might be modified is the question of *how many* of the lysines might be modified; for instance, we know that methylating one, two, or three lysines can produce different biological outcomes.[11]

So, the specific effects of epigenetic marks depend on things like which histone is modified (H3 or H2A?), which chemical group is doing the modifying (an acetyl group or a methyl group?), which amino acid is being bound (the lysine in position 9 on the tail of H3, or the lysine in position 27 on that same tail?), and how many amino acids are modified (are we seeing monomethylation or trimethylation?). Clearly, there is a lot going on here. And the fact that different combinations of modifications can have different effects means that processes like acetylation cannot be allowed to occur haphazardly.

Scientists have discovered that there is a family of proteins that can acetylate histones in an orderly fashion. Because these proteins transfer acetyl groups onto histones, they are called—reasonably enough—"histone acetyl-transferases"; mercifully, they are often just called HATs. Proteins that function as HATs can perform very specific functions, thereby overcoming some of the problems inherent in an incredibly complex system in which slightly different modifications produce different effects. For example, one HAT preferentially modifies the lysine at position 9 on H3, whereas a different HAT preferentially modifies the lysine at position 14 on that same histone.[12] Researchers are still exploring how all of this works, but the existence of HATs that can do very specific jobs clarifies the situation a bit.

The fact that we can reset our biological clocks after we fly across time zones— and that our diets and other experiences can influence gene expression—means that our cells must be able to both start and end genetic activity when and where it is required. So as hard as HATs must work when they acetylate histones, their work must be reversible. And sure enough, just as there are HATs to acetylate histones, there is another group of proteins able to *un*do all of that work. These proteins are called histone *de*acetylases, and, like HATs, they are generally known by an abbreviation: HDACs (pronounced "H-dax").

HATs and HDACs work in opposition; HATs are associated with gene activation and HDACs are associated with gene repression. But unlike HATs, which acetylate histones in very specific ways, most HDACs are relatively nonspecific; they remove acetyl groups from pretty much anywhere on any histone. In some cases, they can be picky, taking acetyl groups off of only particular lysines in particular histone tails,[13] but mostly, HDACs do not have specific targets, a reality that has implications for drug companies trying to design medications with precise effects on our epigenetic states (as we will see in the chapter "Hope"). But regardless of the ability of HATs and HDACs to act in specific ways, histone acetylation and deacetylation are both processes of interest to psychologists because they are dynamic and regulated by factors in the environment.[14]

Burgeoning Complexity: The Histone Code Hypothesis

Generally speaking, histone *methyl*ation is a lot like histone *acetyl*ation. But partly because methyl groups do not neutralize histones' positive electrical charge, histone methylation is less clearly associated with particular effects on gene expression.[15] In fact, histone methylation can be associated with gene activation *or* repression.[16, 17] But because mono-, di-, or trimethylation of lysines can produce different outcomes—and because certain proteins can distinguish very effectively between the presence of one, two, or three methyl groups in a particular spot on a histone[18]—histone methylation is common and thought to be important.

The fact that methyl groups have different effects than acetyl groups, that one methyl group has a different effect than three methyl groups, that modifying the fourth lysine of histone 3 does something different than modifying the ninth lysine of histone 3,[19] and that modifying histone 3 is different than modifying histone 4, means that there is an enormous number of different combinations of histone modifications that could be used to fine-tune genetic activity; this suggests that there is an extremely complex *system* involved in gene regulation.[20] In a recent study of 39 different kinds of histone modifications—and this is just a fraction of the number of histone modifications that are available, because at least 50 different kinds have already been discovered[21]—4,339 different combinations were detected,[22] *but this was in just one type of cell.* And because different genes are expressed in different cell types, the number of combinations of histone modifications used in human bodies is probably quite a bit larger than this.

To help get a feel for this situation, consider Nessa Carey's very nice metaphor about how histone modifications affect gene expression:

> Imagine a chromosome as the trunk of a very big Christmas tree. The branches sticking out all over the tree are the histone tails and these can be decorated with epigenetic modifications. We pick up the purple baubles and we put one, two or three purple baubles on some of the branches. We also have green icicle decorations and we can put either one or two of these on some branches, some of which already have purple baubles on them. Then we pick up the red stars but are told we can't put these on a branch if the adjacent branch has any purple baubles. The gold snowflakes and green icicles can't be present on the same branch. And so it goes on, with increasingly complex rules and patterns. Eventually . . . we wind the lights around the tree. The bulbs represent individual genes. . . . [Now imagine that somehow,] the brightness of each bulb is determined by the precise conformation of the decorations surrounding it. The likelihood is that we would really struggle to predict the brightness of most of the bulbs because the pattern of Christmas decorations is so complicated.[23]

And in fact we currently understand very little about how specific combinations of histone modifications influence gene expression.

Nonetheless, the sheer number of *possible* combinations of histone modifications has led some biologists[24a–24b] to propose the existence of a "histone code" that would rival the DNA code for importance in influencing our characteristics. The existence of a histone code remains a hypothesis at this point, and as the molecular biologist Catherine Dulac pointed out when discussing this "highly debated" hypothesis, "a single histone mark, or [even] a defined combination of marks, is not simply predictive of a given transcriptional outcome."[25] Still, the possibility that there is a previously undiscovered code buried in our chromosomes is tantalizing indeed.

More on DNA Methylation, The Prima Donna of Epigenetics

The only other class of epigenetic modifications I will refer to regularly in this book is DNA methylation. As noted earlier, DNA methylation is normally associated with gene silencing; this effect occurs when methyl groups are attached to the DNA in the regulatory region of a gene. More specifically, when a methyl group is attached to the nucleotide base designated by the letter "C," a new kind of base is created; thus, some segments of DNA are now understood to actually be made of *five* bases, A, C, G, T, and the methylated C, designated "mC."[26] When we say that a particular region of DNA is highly methylated, what we mean is that several of the C bases in that region have been converted to these mC bases. And very often, when there are a lot of mC bases in a regulatory region of a gene, that gene is relatively unexpressed.

Most of the methylated regions in the human genome are methylated similarly in everyone, but a proportion of these regions are variable,[27] meaning that some people have methylated DNA in these regions and some people do not. These are regions of particular interest to behavioral scientists, because it is possible that these differences could explain differences in people's behavioral phenotypes. As we will see in the chapters "Primates" and "Zooming in on Nutrition," respectively, in some cases the extent of methylation in a particular region is influenced by specific experiences an individual has had,[28a–28b] but in other cases it appears to be random.[29] In still other cases, DNA methylation is influenced by genetic mutations[30] or other natural variations in individuals' DNA sequences;[31a–31b] that is, a DNA segment can carry sequence information that influences its own methylation status.[32a–32b] As a result, a person's epigenetic state is likely to reflect gene-environment interactions, so scientists in the future might discover that individual animals' epigenomes don't all respond in the same way to those animals' experiences.

DNA methylation is much more stable than any histone modification. The existence of molecules like HATs and HDACs testifies to the fact that histone modifications are dynamic; they can be implemented and are reversible. In contrast, because DNA methylation is so stable, many researchers believe its function is less about "turning off" a gene than about maintaining an already-inactivated gene in a silent state.[33]

We encountered an example of how this can work in "Zooming in on Regulation." When one of the two X chromosomes in a female mammalian embryo is going to be inactivated, it first produces the noncoding RNA called *XIST*, which covers the chromosome and renders most of its genes relatively inaccessible to transcription machinery. Next, a variety of repressive histone modifications are implemented.[34] But such modifications could potentially be undone, so the system next calls in a protein able to methylate DNA itself. This methylation quiets the genes on the chromosome even more, and in a more permanent way.[35] The methyl groups on the DNA then attract HDACs and other proteins that effectively shut down most of the chromosome even further.[36, 37]

Although DNA methylation is very stable, it is not irreversible.[38] When you think about it, it would have to be this way given the sex-specific nature of imprinting, which entails marking the DNA with methyl groups. Otherwise, how could a genomic region in my mother's DNA be marked as having come from her father (i.e., a male parent), yet be passed on to me having been marked properly as originating in my mother (i.e., a female parent)? There will be more about this in the chapter "Multiplicity," but for now, it is enough to understand that methyl marks have to be removable, somehow.

In fact, DNA is demethylated a couple of times in the life cycle, including once right after conception; the extensive erasure of epigenetic marks after conception is one reason it was assumed for decades that epigenetic marks could not possibly be inherited. But even if DNA *can* be demethylated, DNA methylation is often very stable, being transmitted faithfully from dividing cells to all of their "daughters," across organisms' entire lives. As Carey put it, "the chemical bond between a methyl group and the . . . DNA is so strong that for many years it was considered completely irreversible."[39]

I will close here with an acknowledgment of a controversy surrounding behavioral epigenetics. We know that histone acetylation and deacetylation are both dynamically regulated by environmental factors,[40] and one reason this is widely accepted is because of the existence of proteins that acetylate and deacetylate histones, namely HATs and HDACs. In contrast, although we know of the existence of proteins that transfer methyl groups on to DNA, no one has yet discovered an enzyme that everyone agrees is able to *de*methylate DNA in mammals.[41] Thus, the idea that our experiences might lead to DNA demethylation is viewed with suspicion in some quarters.[42]

As I just indicated, demethylation does occur, via an active process that takes place shortly after conception.[43] In addition, demethylation can occur via a second, passive process; when DNA is replicated during cell division, the newly created DNA is normally methylated in a way that mirrors the "parent" strand, and *failure* to methylate the new strand like this effectively amounts to a kind of passive demethylation.[44] Nonetheless, demethylation later in life remains controversial,[45] because biologists consider *passive* demethylation to be impossible in nondividing cells like mature neurons, which are the very cells of primary interest to behavioral epigeneticists. *Abnormal* demethylation can occur after exposure to certain drugs[46] or environmental toxins,[47] but to date, we remain ignorant of a mechanism by which DNA is known to be actively demethylated in response to normal experiences.[48, 49]

In a rather exciting development for epigeneticists, reports have appeared in the last 5 years of a new "sixth" base in DNA that could very well play an important role in active DNA demethylation.[50a–50c] This base is generated when another chemical group is attached to a methylated C base, yielding a new base called hydroxymethylcytosine, or hmC for short. Although the function of this base is still unknown,[51] hmC is present in relatively high concentrations in neurons[52a–52b] and embryonic stem cells,[53] and appears to reflect another epigenetic mechanism that involves the direct modification of DNA.[54] Perhaps more importantly, several researchers have speculated that hmC bases might serve to *tag* DNA segments in a way that prompts cellular machinery to subsequently demethylate the segment in an active way.[55a–55e] Among the evidence supporting this speculation is the finding that when experimentally produced DNA that contains hmC bases is introduced into mammalian cells, it undergoes active demethylation; in time, the hmC bases are replaced with unmethylated C bases.[56] In addition, it has been shown that hmC is present in the brains of human fetuses at places in the genome that are ultimately demethylated (and therefore, active) in adult brains.[57] Finally, recent studies have revealed that depriving monkeys of their mothers early in life is associated with altered hmC concentrations in regulatory sites in DNA taken from the monkeys' brains in adulthood; importantly, these regulatory sites are known to be related to psychological abnormalities.[58] Thus, many scientists are increasingly comfortable with the suggestion that there may be a two-step active DNA demethylation process that involves first converting mC bases into hmC bases, and then replacing the hmC bases with ordinary, unmethylated C bases, leaving a segment of DNA less methylated than it was.

As we will see, some of the most exciting findings in behavioral epigenetics involve experience-based demethylation of DNA, so ignorance of exactly *how* normal experiences might produce active DNA demethylation has exposed behavioral epigenetics to some controversy. Nonetheless, we should acknowledge that even though biologists have not yet discovered a mechanism that everyone agrees can demethylate DNA in response to experiences, that doesn't mean such a mechanism doesn't exist. Frances Champagne at Columbia University in New York is currently one of the leading researchers in behavioral epigenetics, and as she sees it, the very fact that experimentally controlled experiences can produce hypomethylation in certain regions of DNA means that there is not anything fundamentally askew in her field. Instead, she argues, our ignorance about *how* experiences lead to methyl groups being removed from DNA just means there are still pieces of the puzzle we have not yet discovered. I find Champagne's argument compelling: "There's a chemical reaction. DNA methyl groups are coming off. So there has to be [some mechanism] . . . to do it."[59] Accordingly, it is just a matter of time before someone solves this part of the problem.

10

Experience

The students who attend the college where I am a professor have a lot of heart. Almost to a person, they volunteer in our community, aiding people in need. Because many of the classes I teach are on child development, a lot of my students are interested in helping children, so they often take on internships that involve tutoring kids, working with adolescents in juvenile detention, or otherwise helping out individuals at risk for unhappy outcomes. The stories my students tell me are sometimes horrific; the neglect and abuse suffered by some of the children my students work with is almost inconceivable to me, because my parents treated me well and because it would feel very unnatural to me to not attend to a child's needs. But it is clear from my students' encounters that some children have very difficult lives.

For most of us, it is only common sense that these kinds of awful developmental experiences have consequences. That is not to say that neglect and abuse necessarily and always produce permanent psychological scars. I have known individuals who had really nasty parents who nonetheless emerged as healthy adults. And there is plenty of empirical evidence of this phenomenon as well; psychologists have conducted extensive studies of unexpected resilience, and this work confirms that in some circumstances, some people are able to achieve healthy outcomes despite the presence of risk factors early in their development.[1] But risk factors are aptly named, because children exposed to them often grow up to be less well off than children unexposed to such factors. To give just one example, children who experience abuse or neglect early in life have an increased likelihood of ultimately developing psychiatric disorders like anxiety and depression.[2a–2b]

Because it has always seemed like common sense to me that how we are treated as children influences how we act and feel when we are older, I have always been somewhat unimpressed by the effects Harry Harlow observed in his famous research in the late 1950s and early 1960s. In this classic work of psychological experimentation, Harlow separated rhesus monkeys from their mothers and reared them in bare wire cages, thereby discovering that such monkeys developed "detachment from the environment, hostility directed outwardly toward others and inwardly toward the animal's own body, and inability to form adequate social or heterosexual attachments to others when such opportunities are provided in preadolescence, adolescence, or adulthood."[3] Because of the close evolutionary relationship between people and other primates, everyone understood that Harlow had proven that some aspect of a human mother's interactions with her children plays an important role in allowing those children to develop normally. But seriously, how could anyone have expected anything else?

Of course, I'm not being fair to Harlow here. His work did not simply demonstrate the obvious, but instead helped to prove that what matters is not the fact that mothers are sources of nourishment for their babies, but that they are also sources of what Harlow called "contact comfort."[4] The importance of touch for normal development has since been demonstrated unequivocally in human newborns by researchers like Tiffany Field, who has repeatedly shown that exposing premature babies to massage therapy leads to more weight gain,[5] reduced stress behaviors,[6] and reduced pain responses,[7] among other effects. Clearly, regardless of whether or not I think this kind of human contact is self-evidently important for babies, scientific research on the effects of human contact is valuable, having already improved the lives of countless preemies.

Although there is value in proving that an early experience is associated with a particular developmental outcome, figuring out *how* that experience produces its effects is even more important. Because I am a social scientist, I find it interesting and significant that early exposure to poverty is associated later in life with poor health[8] and impaired psychological well-being,[9] but I do not find such revelations to be especially surprising. Findings like this leave unanswered the really crucial questions. *How* do the situations or events we experience early in life have their effects on us years later? Is there some mechanism we can discern that will allow us to see how these things work? That is, is there a way in which our experiences in childhood cause physical changes inside of us, so that these experiences effectively get under our skin?

There is a reason I think these are the truly crucial questions. If you know neglect in childhood is associated with anxiety in adulthood, for instance, all you can do is try to convince parents they should not neglect their children. But if you know *how* neglect leads to anxiety, you'll probably have many other avenues of recourse. The importance of pursuing the *mechanistic* causes of developmental outcomes is apparent when you think about it abstractly. If you know that condition N (neglect) is associated with an undesirable outcome A (anxiety), all you can do is try to influence N. But if you discover that N causes D, which causes W, which causes P, . . . which causes outcome A, you have the potential to avoid that undesirable outcome by intervening at any of the preceding four steps.

This kind of causal series—in which one event causes the next in a very long chain—is so common in living things that biologists have a specific word for it: a cascade. Because our biological and psychological traits are caused by cascades of events, the American developmental scientist Linda B. Smith has written that development can be "determined, not by some prescribed outcome . . . but as the product of a history of cascading causes in which each subsequent change depends on prior changes."[10] Discovering *how* experiences contribute to a developmental outcome can be exceptionally valuable, because this kind of discovery typically highlights multiple possible ways to influence the outcome.

The Long-Term Effects of Early Experiences

In a truly extraordinary line of research conducted at McGill University in Montreal, a team of researchers has discovered one way in which our early experiences can influence gene expression and thereby influence later behavior.[11a-11b] This team—led by developmental psychobiologist Michael Meaney and biochemist Moshe Szyf—has discovered a system that can seem almost unfathomably complex.[12] But although the system *is* astonishingly complex, I will be able to convey the basic ideas behind the work here.

All of this groundbreaking work has been conducted with rats. Although most of us would prefer to believe people have very little in common with rats, the fact is that as mammals, we're actually rather closely related. Of most importance are the facts that (1) newborn rats are altricial, like we are—that is, they are born unable to fend for themselves—so mother rats take care of their babies, and (2) their nervous systems are very much like ours. As a result, they are an excellent species to study if you are interested in learning how various mothering behaviors might influence behavioral outcomes in offspring.

Thanks in part to work done by researchers like Harlow and Meaney, the psychobiology of stress had been studied extensively by the end of the 20th century. By then, we knew that exposing infant monkeys and other primates to stressors, such as maternal neglect or harsh, unpredictable discipline, could lead to abnormal behaviors in adulthood.[13a-13c] In addition, we understood quite a bit about the neural systems and neurochemistry underlying these effects. We also had reason to believe that similar mechanisms in rats and primates are responsible for how early stressful experiences contribute to abnormal, dysfunctional states—that is, pathology—later in life.[14] This meant that researchers could begin trying to figure out how genes were involved in these processes by doing studies on rodents.

In 1997, researchers in the Meaney lab reported that close observations had revealed naturally occurring variations in how mother rats interact with their new offspring. All mother rats intermittently lick and groom their pups in association with nursing, but they do not all do this to the same extent; even if the amount of time they spend in contact with their offspring is equivalent,[15] some of the mothers spend more time licking and grooming their pups (Meaney and his colleagues refer to licking and grooming as LG). The news that led to this research being published in *Science*—the preeminent science journal in the United States—was that pups exposed in the first 10 days of life to low levels of LG grew up to be adult rats with increased levels of stress reactivity. That is, pups reared by low LG mothers grew up to be adults that did not tolerate mild stressors as easily as did pups reared by high LG mothers. Specifically, the rats reared by low LG mothers behaved fearfully when placed in open spaces, were more likely to startle in response to surprising stimuli, and took longer to start eating when they were fed in a novel environment.[16a-16b] Thus, early experiences affected the rats' later behaviors. In addition, they also affected the rats' neural and hormonal responses to stress, a story I will tell in detail in the next chapter.

Whenever differences in mothers' behaviors are related to phenotypic differences in their offspring, we must immediately acknowledge that the mothers' behaviors need not have contributed to the offspring's phenotypes at all. If there is a genetic factor in the mothers that can affect their behavior *and also* be inherited by their offspring, the offspring's phenotype might reflect the presence of the genetic factor, not the mother's behavior per se. So, the only way to be certain that it was LG per se that was influencing the rat pups' subsequent development was to do a cross-fostering study. These kinds of studies entail taking newborn rats and effectively adopting them out to a foster mother.

In just such a study,[17] researchers in Meaney's lab took female pups born to high LG mothers and placed them, within 12 hours of their birth, in the nest of an adult female rat known to be a poor groomer. Likewise, high LG mothers were given "custody" of female pups that had been born to low LG mothers. In the end, it was the experience of LG that mattered; even if a pup was born to a high LG mother, if the pup was not licked and groomed much as a newborn, she grew up to be a more fearful adult. Conversely, the pups born to low LG mothers were licked and groomed a lot by their foster mothers, and as a result, they grew up to be less fearful adults.

Interestingly, the pups' early experiences influenced more than just their fearfulness. Female rats raised by high LG mothers also became high LG mothers themselves once they grew up and gave birth to their own litters, *even though their biological mothers had been low LG mothers.* The complex system that allows these kinds of early experiences to affect later mothering behaviors is only now beginning to be understood,[18] but Meaney has noted that this research demonstrates the possible existence of "nongenomic transmission of individual differences in maternal behavior from the mother to her female offspring."[19] That is, this research suggests that we might "inherit" some of our parents' characteristics in a nongenetic way. Given biologists' traditional position that only genetic information can be transmitted from ancestral to descendant generations,[20a-20b] the discovery of a nongenomic mode of intergenerational transmission is a very important one.[21]

These experimental results are very interesting, of course, but if you recognize our evolutionary brotherhood with the rodents, you might be as unimpressed as

I was when I first learned about the effects of Harlow's isolation of baby monkeys; *of course* parents' behaviors have long-term effects on their offspring! The reason Meaney's work is important is because his team took the next step and asked the *how* question: Is there some sort of *physical* effect of early experience in infancy that we can detect in the offspring's brain and that can cause behavioral differences in adulthood, even after so much time has passed? As you will have likely guessed, the answer to this question is a resounding "yes," and the mechanism responsible for the effect is epigenetic. Meaney and his team have done a brilliant job of following the clues, and have pieced together an extremely thorough account of how the experience of LG in infancy is registered in a brain in a way that leads to gene silencing and altered behavior among adult rats.

Mothering, Methylation, Memory, and More

The Meaney team's data indicate that experiences early in life, during a specific developmental period, are capable of influencing DNA methylation. To telegraph their findings, the group titled their seminal paper on this research "Epigenetic Programming by Maternal Behavior."[22] Personally, I don't like their use of the word "programming" here, because it implies a sort of automation that unfolds in a context-independent and inevitable way. In fact, there are compelling reasons to believe early experiences do *not* cement destiny like this; experiences later in life also shape the brain.[23] But this quibble aside, there can be no doubt that the epigenetic effects Meaney and his team discovered have managed to answer the long-standing, interesting, and very important question about a *mechanism* by which early experiences can influence developmental outcomes.

Specifically, newborn rats that experience low levels of LG have more methylation in particular genomic regions in cells from a particular area of the brain. Consequently, these rats produce less of a particular kind of protein in their brains, a protein that helps normal rats respond to stressful situations. This protein is known as the GR protein, and the cells affected by the experience are in an area of the brain known as the hippocampus (not to be confused with the hypothalamus, the brain area containing the pacemaker neurons described in the chapter "Epigenetics"). Details about how LG produces long-term effects on GR protein production in the hippocampus are available in the next chapter. For now, it is enough to reiterate that for Meaney's rats, something about experiencing low levels of licking and grooming in the first 10 days of life led to increased methylation of—and therefore, reduced expression of—a DNA segment involved in producing the stress-moderating GR protein. Thus, by the time they reached adulthood, the offspring of low LG mothers produced fewer of the normally present GR proteins, because the GR gene had been epigenetically silenced in the cells of the hippocampus. And importantly, these effects were apparent even in rats that were reared by adoptive mothers who treated them differently than their biological mothers would have. So, it was the mothers' licking and grooming per se that caused these effects on methylation,[24] and these effects produced altered behavior into adulthood.

Subsequent research has shown that licking and grooming affects more than just how rats respond to stress when they are adults; these kinds of maternal behaviors also positively influence how offspring perform on cognitive tests, including tests of attention[25] and spatial learning.[26] Licking and grooming also appears to promote the formation of synapses (i.e., neural connections) in the hippocampus.[27] So far, no one has demonstrated that these effects on cognition are mediated by epigenetics, but it would be a good bet that additional research will provide this proof. After all, as we will see in the chapter "Memory," a different line of inquiry has already provided evidence that epigenetic systems are involved in learning and memory.[28] But before considering these cognitive processes, the chapter "Primates" will explore recent findings that have supported what the Meaney team expected from the outset: The kinds of epigenetic events responsible for the LG effect in rats seem to characterize the development of human brains and behaviors, too.[29]

11

Zooming in on Experience

Every 4 years, Americans elect their president, and prior to these elections, we see images of the candidates a lot. Often, one of the candidates is an incumbent who won the election as a younger person 4 years earlier. I have always found it striking how a term in the Oval Office seems to age the occupants; Bill Clinton in particular appeared to change from a relatively young, energetic man into a significantly more tired version of himself in the late 1990s. Although others have taken note of this phenomenon and suggested that perhaps it might reflect the stressfulness of the presidency, available data suggest that presidents do not wind up with shorter lives than the rest of us,[1] and there is no good scientific evidence that Barack Obama's head would be any less gray if he had settled for an easier job.[2a–2b] But presidents' appearances and life spans notwithstanding, it is quite clear that in the long run, chronic stress can kill.[3]

Stress reactions are very odd things, because at the right time and in the right magnitude, they are lifesavers, but at the wrong times and in the wrong magnitudes, they are dangerous. In the course of our normal lives, we all encounter sudden, unexpected, and potentially threatening events that cause us to become alert and vigilant; these effects are caused by the same processes in the stress system that provide the physiological resources to help us fight or flee from a threat.[4] If we didn't have access to the resources required to run away from a threatening grizzly bear when we need those resources, that would be a bad situation indeed. Unfortunately, the elevated heart rate, blood pressure, and respiration rate that accompanies stressors can be problematic if they persist in *non*threatening situations. This kind of chronic stress can wreak havoc on our cardiovascular systems.[5] When it comes to dealing with everyday hassles, the name of the game is homeostasis: finding a way to efficiently return to a calm, baseline state once the threat has been addressed.[6]

Like many other organisms, we have evolved an extremely complex system that allows us to respond to perceived internal and external threats to our well-being, whether those threats are real or not.[7] This system includes behavioral and physiological components that are interconnected.[8] Many organs play roles in stress responses, and the brain is central in these processes.[9] In addition, a number of hormones and neurotransmitters perform essential functions, communicating information about the states of various organs and systems throughout the body.

A Stress Response Loop

Responding to a perceived stressor begins with the release of neurotransmitters from a particular branch of the nervous system and from the adrenal glands, located just above the kidneys.[10] These neurotransmitters include one called epinephrine, but it's more widely known as adrenaline because of the adrenal glands that secrete it—no big surprise that adrenaline is released when a person encounters a grizzly bear.

In response to the release of adrenaline, a part of the hypothalamus releases a hormone called CRH (see Figure 11.1), short for corticotropin-releasing hormone (you might recall that the hypothalamus is the brain area involved in the functioning of our biological clocks; the reappearance of the hypothalamus at this point in our story is no accident, because levels of our primary stress hormone vary with our circadian rhythm). Corticotropin-releasing hormone is a small protein,[11] which, when injected into the brain, directly causes the stress response that animals exhibit when they encounter threats in the natural world.

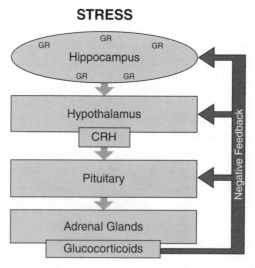

Figure 11.1 A schematic diagram of the hypothalamic-pituitary-adrenal (HPA) axis. The HPA axis controls stress reactions (as well as regulating several other bodily processes) and makes use of negative feedback. The letters "GR" in the oval representing the hippocampus denote glucocorticoid receptors, which can be activated by glucocorticoids in a way that diminishes the body's stress response.

Thus, CRH is one of the principal tools our brains use to create stress responses.[12] So when Michael Meaney wanted to study how early experiences influence stress responses in adulthood, it made sense to start with the established finding that when infant rodents are deprived of exposure to their mothers, they grow up to be adults characterized by increased CRH gene expression and increased stress reactivity.[13]

In the late 1990s, researchers in the Meaney lab reported that adult rats that were reared by low LG mothers produce more CRH than adult rats that were reared by high LG mothers.[14] Thus, being licked and groomed infrequently early in their lives influenced the neuroendocrine (i.e., neural and hormonal) stress responses of these rats when they were tested as adults. In addition, the more fearful *behaviors* of rats raised by low LG mothers are mediated by increased release of CRH.[15a–15c] For a rat raised by a low LG mother, increased release of CRH means more activation of the *a*drenal glands (which, together with the *h*ypothalamus and the *p*ituitary gland make up the so-called HPA axis); as Meaney and his colleagues put it, "the greater the frequency of maternal licking and grooming during infancy, the lower the HPA response to stress in adulthood."[16]

Release of CRH from the hypothalamus signals your adrenal glands to release the steroid hormone *cortisol* into your bloodstream; the more stress you experience, the more CRH is produced in your brain, and the more cortisol is produced by your adrenal glands. Cortisol has several functions, including increasing the amount of energy available to our bodies in the form of blood sugar (i.e., glucose). Perhaps obviously, a system that can increase a body's access to its energy resources can be very useful in threatening situations, when survival might very well depend on access to that energy. But because another of cortisol's functions is to suppress the immune system, chronic stress also increases susceptibility to viral or bacterial illness, among other unpleasant outcomes.

This is why it is bad for animals to stay in a stressed state; to remain healthy, we need to *no longer* experience stress responses once a threat is no longer present. So, an efficient HPA axis is one that can react rapidly to stressors *and*, after any threats have dissipated, revert quickly to a healthy baseline.[17] The mechanism we have evolved to accomplish this is known as a negative feedback loop. On a conceptual level, this works like the thermostat in your house: When the temperature goes up, the system works to bring it back down (and vice versa). In the case of the HPA axis, cortisol is the link in the negative feedback chain that helps bodies return to normal after a threat has been neutralized. When the hypothalamus detects a lot of cortisol, it slows down its production of CRH and thereby "instructs" the adrenal glands to stop making cortisol. This is how our brains are able to detect our stress levels and settle us down once the situation permits. *How* cortisol is able to do this is a complex story, but it is a story worth understanding, because "good mothering" has its long-term effects on baby rats—and in all likelihood, on people, too—by influencing how this complex system operates.

Glucocorticoid Receptors: The Indispensable Interactants

Cortisol is just one member of a class of steroid hormones known as glucocorticoids. As a biologically astute detective might guess from their name, glucocorticoids are involved in regulating the levels of *gluco*se present in our bloodstreams, they are produced in the *cortic*al regions of our adrenal glands, and they are steroid hormones—gluco-cortic-oids. Cortisol is the most important of our glucocorticoids, but knowing the name of this class of hormones is helpful, because it turns out that the way cortisol provides negative feedback to the hypothalamus is through the presence of a protein called the glucocorticoid receptor—the GR protein referenced in the preceding chapter.

Glucocorticoid receptors are proteins that have just the right shape to enable them to bind to glucocorticoids, including cortisol. These receptors are present inside most of our cells—including in the neurons of the hypothalamus and the hippocampus—and their presence enables those cells to respond to cortisol (and other glucocorticoids). The hippocampus is consequential in our story because activity here can influence how the hypothalamus responds to stress. Ordinarily, GRs just float around "unactivated" in the gel-like interior of whatever cell they're located in, but when they encounter a glucocorticoid, they latch onto it and form a composite unit made of both molecules. This "activated" glucocorticoid-GR complex has a couple of remarkable properties. First, after the complex forms, the cell actively transports it into the cell's nucleus. Second, once inside the nucleus, the complex is able to bind to DNA, so it can function as a transcription factor. This is why steroid hormones in general are so powerful: In collaboration with their receptors, they directly alter genetic expression.

Glucocorticoid-GR complexes can do different things in different cells, and in some cases, we still do not understand how they work.[18] They appear to play roles in the transcription of a wide variety of genes,[19] including some that have no known function;[20] one recent study found these complexes binding at over 4,300 different locations in the human genome,[21] and although glucocorticoid-GR complexes *activate* transcription at some of these sites, they *repress* transcription at other sites. Even more confusing, different people don't always respond in the same ways to the *same* glucocorticoid,[22] so the actions of these molecules in our bodies really are unbelievably complicated. As the British pharmacologist Julia Buckingham wrote in a recent review article on glucocorticoids, "the picture is far from clear. . . . While difficult to interpret, the data . . . illustrate admirably the amazing complexity of glucocorticoid action and the resultant capacity of steroids to exert very fine control over a broad range of physiological and pathophysiological functions."[23]

As a result of this state of affairs, I cannot tell you exactly *how* glucocorticoid-GR complexes in the hippocampus cause the hypothalamus to produce less CRH, but we know for sure that they do. When these complexes are formed in hippocampal cells, we find reduced expression of CRH genes in those cells and decreased release of CRH from the hypothalamus.[24a–24b] And the behavioral consequence of this reduced release of hypothalamic CRH is a reduced stress response (see Figure 11.1).

Armed with this background, you are now in a position to understand how cortisol's interaction with GR proteins allows for the negative feedback required to keep our stress response systems in check. After the scary creak in your house late at night causes adrenalin and cortisol to shoot through your body—bringing you to a high state of alertness and preparing the energy needed for your muscles to deal with whatever it is that stepped on the floorboard—you sit bolt upright in bed, listening carefully for another sound. When you don't hear one (houses do "settle," after all), your system returns to normal because the cortisol travels in your blood up to your hypothalamus, binds to GRs in hypothalamic cells, and travels with the GRs into those cells' nuclei; there, the GR-cortisol complexes down-regulate the production of CRH and thereby tell your adrenal glands to stop producing so much cortisol . . . because in the end, no one was actually in your house and it's safe to go back to sleep.

The Mechanisms of Mothering

The Meaney team's important finding was that early exposure to licking and grooming produces diminished stress reactivity later in life, and the mechanism responsible for this effect involves GRs. It turns out that the adult offspring of high LG mothers produce *more GRs* in their hippocampal cells, leading to greater glucocorticoid feedback sensitivity.[25] In this way, these rats' early experiences lead them to be more sensitive to the presence of cortisol in their systems, and to dampen down their stress responses more efficiently once they are no longer in a threatening situation. We can be confident that licking and grooming produce their effects by altering GR production in the hippocampus, because experimentally eliminating the difference in GR levels in high versus low LG rats eliminates the differences in their stress reactivity when they are adults.[26]

This is a beautifully elaborated, mechanistic explanation of how early experiences influence a psychological characteristic later in life, and many scientists would be satisfied just to know they discovered a brain difference in adults that can be traced to differing experiences early in life. But Meaney and his team took this research a step further, by asking the next question: *How* does being licked and groomed early in life lead rats to have more hippocampal GRs in adulthood? Because increased numbers of GRs must reflect increased *expression* of genes that code for GRs, the obvious place to look would be epigenetics.

So, Meaney's team extracted DNA from their rats' hippocampal cells, and they looked specifically at the DNA region that serves as the promoter for the GR gene. And in the crowning achievement of this line of research to date, they found that rats exposed to low LG mothers had significantly more DNA methylation here than did rats exposed to high LG mothers.[27] As a result, rats that did not receive much licking and grooming when they were pups grew up to be adults with fewer hippocampal GRs, because the promoter region for the gene involved in producing these GRs had been epigenetically rendered inaccessible. With fewer GRs in the hippocampus, a rat experiencing stress would be less able to respond to the presence of cortisol in its bloodstream; its hypothalamus would continue pumping out CRH and it would have a significantly more difficult time recovering from the stressful experience.

As I noted in the last chapter, the team also conducted a cross-fostering study to see if the increased stress reactivity associated with low LG mothering was due to the low LG experience per se. This study found that rats exposed to low LG mothering exhibited not only increased behavioral stress, but also increased GR promoter methylation *even though their biological mothers were high LG mothers*. In fact, the methylation levels found in the hippocampal cells of these "adopted" rats were indistinguishable from those found in rats raised by their own LG mothers. So it really was the licking and grooming that produced the observed differences in DNA methylation.

An analysis of the *timing* of methylation corroborated this conclusion. Before the rats were born, they were all in similar epigenetic states. The epigenetic differences present in adulthood first appeared between the day after the pups were born and their 6th day after birth, so their experiences in that first week of life were the critical factor. Specifically, the experience of being licked and groomed arouses newborn pups and causes the release of adrenaline in their bodies; this adrenaline leads to the release of thyroid hormones that get into the newborns' brains, where the hormones trigger serotonin activity in hippocampal cells,[28a–28b] activity known to influence genetic functioning in those cells.[29a–29b] Once exposure to low levels of licking and grooming left week-old rats with highly methylated GR gene promoters, those promoters stayed methylated into adulthood, because DNA methylation is relatively stable. Thus, the research team concluded that maternal care in the first week of life can "directly alter the methylation status of the ... promoter of the GR gene."[30]

DNA methylation is typically associated with reduced histone acetylation, and the Meaney team observed this epigenetic effect of experience as well. Taken together, the epigenetic effects they detected support the conclusion that a rat's experience with licking and grooming in infancy affects DNA methylation, which alters chromatin structure in a longer-term way, influencing the ability of the rat's DNA to produce GRs, thereby shaping its stress reactivity much later in life. If such a finding can be generalized, it would mean that *our* early experiences can influence gene expression into adulthood, a conclusion that would provide a long-sought mechanism for the way in which our early experiences help mold us into the people we become.

The Epigenetic Effects of Stress in Rodents: Other Molecules, Other Brain Regions

Recent studies have provided supporting evidence that these kinds of effects can be detected in other species, in other hormone systems, and in response to experiences even earlier in life. Working with mice rather than rats, a German team led by Dietmar Spengler studied another hormone—called AVP (for arginine vasopressin)—that the hypothalamus releases along with CRH when an animal experiences stress.[31] When AVP is released, it starts a cascade of events that leads to the release of cortisol from the adrenal glands. Rather than studying individual differences in mothering behaviors as the Meaney team did, Spengler's group stressed some of their mice by separating them from their mothers for 3 hours per day early in their lives. This kind of experience is worth studying, because as Harlow discovered,[32] maternal deprivation over a period of months has significant effects on monkeys; in human beings, too, "emotional neglect" in childhood is correlated with stress hormone concentrations in adulthood.[33] Testing the deprived mice later in life revealed a variety of behavioral effects indicative of stress, including memory deficits. In terms of physiology, the stress of separation also led to an overactive HPA axis and an increased responsiveness to potent stressors,[34] effects that resulted from increased expression of the AVP gene in hypothalamic cells.

A close look at the DNA from these cells revealed that compared with control mice, mice separated from their mothers periodically after birth had less methylation of DNA regions associated with AVP. As would be expected, such hypomethylation would mean that *more* AVP was produced, which is consistent with the finding that adult mice deprived of their mothers in infancy were hyperresponsive when placed in stressful circumstances. Additional work revealed that the hypomethylation observed was related to how neurons in the hypothalamus acted at the time the young mice were separated from their mothers. So here, too, we have a detailed and mechanistic explanation for a long-term effect of early experience. The researchers in Germany concluded that early-life stress "can dynamically control DNA methylation in . . . neurons to generate stable changes in *Avp* expression that trigger neuroendocrine [e.g., cortisol] and behavioral alterations that are frequent features in depression."[35]

Yet another study revealed that when pregnant mice were subjected to stress early in gestation, the male offspring they ultimately bore went on to be adults that behaved in maladaptive ways when stressed.[36] In addition to coping poorly with stress, these offspring were found to have fewer GRs in their hippocampus, a finding consistent with their increased stress-sensitivity. Moreover, epigenetic analysis of their hippocampal tissue revealed that, as expected, the DNA segments associated with the GR gene were more methylated than those segments were in mice not exposed to prenatal stress. Thus, experiences *prior* to birth also appear able to influence epigenetic states and adult behaviors in rodents.

An important point to note here is that in Meaney's studies of rats and in the study of pregnant mice, *increased* methylation was associated with increased stress, but in the study from Germany, *decreased* methylation was associated with increased stress. This is not as strange as it seems when you think about it, because the methylated DNA in the former studies was associated with the GR gene whereas the methylated DNA in the latter study was associated with the AVP gene. Remember, adding AVP into the system causes the production and release of *more* cortisol from the adrenal glands, whereas the presence of more GRs in the system causes the production and release of *less* cortisol from the adrenal glands. So there is a consistent story being told here, but one of its morals is that there is no straightforward evaluation we can make about methylation. Methylation— and any accompanying change in gene expression—is neither inherently good nor inherently bad; it all depends on which DNA segments are being affected.[37] This lesson applies fairly widely of course; cortisol, too, is neither good nor bad, because it helps us a lot when we are faced with a threat but it can hurt us a lot if it stays in the system in high concentrations when it is no longer needed.

Finally, the epigenetic effects of early experience are not limited to the hypo- thalamus or hippocampus, and they influence more than just the GR and AVP proteins. This conclusion is supported by a study of rat pups whose mothers were so stressed out that they treated their newborns abusively, by frequently stepping on them, dropping them, dragging them, or handling them roughly. As a result of this maltreatment, the offspring grew up to have altered patterns of methylation in their brains.[38] Specifically, compared with nonabused rats, rats exposed to abu- sive mothering for just a half-hour per day for the first week of their lives wound up with more methylation in DNA segments associated with a protein called brain- derived neurotrophic factor, mercifully known to scientists as BDNF. This pro- tein supports the growth of new neurons and contributes to the ongoing survival of existing neurons; since DNA methylation down-regulates genes, there was less of this important protein produced in the abused rats' brains.

We can draw three important conclusions from this study. First, the effects of abusive mothering were seen in rat pups the day after the abusive treatment ended, but, as in the Meaney studies, they were also seen when those rats had matured to adolescence and adulthood. So, the effects of the early experience were detect- able in methylation patterns throughout the life span of these animals. Second, early experience can influence the methylation of DNA associated with proteins like BDNF that are *not* specifically associated with stress responses. Third, early experience can influence the methylation of DNA in cells beyond the hypothalamus or hippocampus; the epigenetic effects of *maltreatment* in rats was found *in the prefrontal cortex,* a brain area implicated in several higher cognitive and social behaviors, such as the planning of complex, goal-directed activity.[39]

There is now a consensus building among behavioral epigeneticists that early experiences are able to influence the expression of a wide variety of genes in a wide variety of brain areas and that such effects can be detectable many years after the influential experiences. There is every reason to think that the Meaney group's findings regarding rats' stress responses are just the tip of the iceberg. The system we (and our mammalian relatives) have evolved for responding to stressors is very complex, so there is still a lot to learn about how it all works. But it is now clear that studies of epigenetics will change how we think about the effects of our experiences on our bodies, brains, and minds.

It has been obvious for decades that our stress system is responsive to our experiences; that is one of the points of having this system! What is important about the rodent work discussed in this chapter is that it provides novel evidence that these effects do not have to happen in real time. Instead, an experience at one point in life can influence gene expression at a later point in life, meaning that some epigenetic alterations effectively serve as retained *records* of previous experiences.[40] So not only can our experiences get under our skin—they can get lodged there, too, for better or for worse.

12

Primates

One evening many years ago, I was preparing my home for the arrival of some guests when I was faced with the task of opening a large bag of M&Ms. I know: This is not a real puzzle for most people, but I had grown bored of opening bags in the normal way, and I thought it would be more fun to just squeeze the bag until the air inside popped open its top and released the intoxicating smell of the candy within. (Yes, this is embarrassing to admit.) Of course, it was the bottom of the bag that popped open, and in an instant, my kitchen floor was covered with M&Ms. What made this a memorable experience for me, though, was how my big, furry dog, James Taylor, reacted to this display of stupidity. He didn't jump up from where he was sitting across the room. Instead, he just looked me in the eye and started thumping his tail on the floor, like that was the most hilarious thing he had ever seen.

Obviously, I am inclined to anthropomorphize at times—to attribute human characteristics to nonhuman animals. Several philosophers have argued that this is an occupational hazard for behavioral scientists; these philosophers have warned us that because we cannot possibly know anything for certain about animals' internal, subjective states, it is bad practice to assume we share qualities of mind such as a sense of humor. At least one philosopher of science, Brian Keeley, disagrees, having argued persuasively that "the alleged sin of anthropomorphism is largely a myth; that there is nothing in principle wrong with attributing human properties to nonhuman animals."[1] Even so, comparative psychologists generally try to avoid *assuming* that nonhuman animals have mental lives like our own. In a 2004 paper on what studies of animal development can tell us about human development, Gottlieb and Lickliter wrote, "We should be certain about one aspect of animal models: the question of the utility of animal models for understanding human psychological and behavioral development *is not tenable*, if by animal model we mean we are modeling *identical* ... human psychological, social, and behavioral phenomena."[2] That is, as similar as we might be to our mammalian relatives, we cannot assume we share identical psychologies. People are not monkeys, and rats are not human.

But just because we cannot assume animals have mental or behavioral states identical to ours does not mean we lack identical physiological or molecular states. In fact, because all mammals—including rodents, like mice and rats, and primates, like monkeys, apes, and humans—evolved from a common ancestor, some of the features that characterize both primates and rodents have been "conserved," a word biologists use to refer to features that have remained unchanged across evolutionary time. For example, the hormone released by our brains when we are stressed—CRH, for those who read the preceding chapter—is *identical* to the hormone released by rats' brains when they are stressed;[3] this means that the genetic sequence used to produce this protein has been conserved from 75 million years ago, when it was present in the last common ancestor of rats and people.[4] In the sentence after the one quoted above, Gottlieb and Lickliter acknowledged this difference between the psychological and the molecular levels of analysis and went on to note that in contrast to animals' behavioral characteristics, their "genetic, physiological, and anatomical" characteristics might be much more comparable to ours. Nevertheless, they ended this passage with an appropriate warning:

> Even at the nonbehavioral level caution needs to be exercised. For example, the same genes express themselves differently in different species, so just because one is dealing with identical genes does not guarantee the fidelity of the underlying match between species when similar phenotypes or outcomes of development are under consideration.[5]

Clearly, discoveries about the epigenetic effects of experiences in rats cannot be taken as evidence that things work the same way in us. To determine whether the Meaney team's discoveries apply to people, we're going to need some investigations of people.

Studying Suicides: An Entry into Human Behavioral Epigenetics

Unfortunately, studying the epigenetic effects of experiences in people is not so easy. The first thing to remember is that epigenetic control of gene expression was initially recognized in connection with the problem of differentiation, that is, how the cells of a new embryo change into the differing kinds of cells we're made of. One thing we know for sure about epigenetics is that the epigenetic states of different cell types are different from one another, because epigenetic mechanisms were nature's solution to the differentiation problem. For years, scientists have assessed people's genomes by examining DNA in so-called buccal cells (pronounced like "buckle") that have been swabbed from the insides of the people's cheeks; all of our cells contain the same genetic information, so if you want to get access to that information, looking in *any* cell will do. But if you are interested in *epigenetic* information, a cell from the inside of a cheek is going to provide a different picture than a cell from the inside of a brain.

So the question is: Which kinds of cells are likely to show the epigenetic effects of experience? The answer might be obvious: Cells that are able to "*learn*" from their prior experiences by altering their own structures and functions in response to those experiences.

As soon as we ask ourselves which cell types would be most likely to have this sort of ability, one good answer pops to mind: neurons. After all, if you are interested in learning, the brain is an outstanding place to start. And in fact, if we look at the Meaney team's groundbreaking research, the cells they chose to study were from the brain. But if you want to confirm that the Meaney team's research is applicable to people, you're immediately faced with a difficult problem: How can you get brain cells from people? Of course, you can't—healthy people generally won't let you sample their brains—and studying cells from people's cheeks would probably not help your cause, because there is no reason to think these cells would alter their functioning as a result of experience.

Fortunately, scientists are a resolute lot. In fact, it *is* possible to get brain samples from people—even people free of any neurological disease—but only if you are creative enough to figure out where to look. Two groups of scientists came up with the same resourceful solution to this problem in the late 2000s: Examine the brains of people who have committed suicide.[6a–6b] In both cases, the researchers assessed DNA extracted from cells in the cerebral cortex, the most recently evolved outer layer of the brain, which is involved in many higher cognitive functions.

Both studies revealed different methylation profiles for the suicidal people compared with people who died suddenly of other (non-disease-related) causes. Specifically, suicide victims in both studies had more methylation in particular DNA regions that have been theoretically linked to suicidal behavior. Interestingly, although these research teams—one primarily in Canada, one in Europe—studied different DNA regions in cells taken from different parts of the cortex, they reported similar epigenetic effects, suggesting that there are multiple genes and brain areas involved in suicide (which should not surprise us, because suicide is a rather complex behavior). Although both teams acknowledged that their findings were merely correlational, the Canadian researchers concluded, "DNA methylation aberrations may be an underlying cause of major depressive disorder and suicide,"[7] and the European researchers concluded that their "study reinforces the mounting hypothesis that DNA methylation is involved in psychiatric conditions . . . and represents one of the first demonstrations that alteration of gene-specific DNA methylation in the human brain is associated with suicidal behavior."[8]

As interesting as the results of these studies were, however, they revealed something about the relationship between epigenetic states and suicide, not about how *experiences* influence epigenetic states. To see if the kinds of findings the Meaney team reported in rats might also apply to human beings, a different sort of approach was required, an approach ultimately hit on by . . . the Meaney team. In 2009, Patrick McGowan and his colleagues in Meaney's lab reported on a study of DNA extracted from the brains of people in three different categories: suicide victims who experienced abuse when they were children (i.e., "sexual contact, severe physical abuse and/or severe neglect"[9]), suicide victims who did not experience child abuse, and a control group of never-abused people who died suddenly as a result of accidents, not suicide.[10] Importantly, McGowan and his colleagues examined cells from the hippocampus, the same brain area that was affected in rats when they were licked and groomed as pups. In addition, these researchers studied methylation of the human DNA segment that corresponds to the DNA segment Meaney and Szyf originally studied in rats: the segment involved in initiating transcription of the GR gene, a segment known as the GR promoter.

The study provided evidence that early experiences are related to epigenetic states in people. Specifically, suicide victims who experienced abuse as children had GR promoters that were highly methylated relative to the GR promoters of nonabused people, regardless of how the nonabused people died. So, these data were similar to those obtained in rats;[11] that is, there was reduced expression of stress-moderating proteins in the brains of people who had experienced bad parenting years earlier. Do not be confused by the fact that the people in this study were suicide victims, because unlike in the Canadian and European studies, in McGowan's study, suicide per se could not account for the observed effect; child abuse did. The team concluded that their results successfully "translate previous results from rat to humans and suggest a common effect of parental care on the epigenetic regulation of" genes involved in human stress responses.[12] Thus, they wrote, "epigenetic processes might mediate the effects" of children's experiences on gene expression, and "stable epigenetic marks such as DNA methylation might then persist into adulthood and influence the vulnerability for psychopathology"[13] (i.e., mental disorders). So, this finding made it look like *our* early experiences, too, might influence the epigenetic states of the DNA in our brain cells, thereby affecting our behaviors many years later.

There Will Be Blood

Although these results are striking, they are still unsatisfying in some ways. Because these effects were detected in the brains of suicide victims, we have to wonder if the abuse these people experienced as children was so extreme that it produced effects that would not be seen in the brains of people exposed to less severe bad parenting. More generally, correlational studies like this, in which people's experiences are not expressly manipulated by an experimenter, do not permit us to conclude that specific experiences *cause* specific epigenetic outcomes. In addition, studies like this require scientists to wait until research participants are dead before they collect their data; if we want to know about how early experiences affect *living* people, we have to proceed in some other way. Luckily enough, there are body parts besides brains that are worth studying in connection with behavioral epigenetics, and one of them is reasonably accessible: Blood.

Back in the late 1980s, researchers at Ohio State University began to explore how the stress of preparing for academic examinations affects students. At the time, it was already known that stress can impair a body's ability to fight infection.[14] Because blood contains specialized white cells that are part of the body's immune system, the researchers compared white blood cells taken from relaxed students to white blood cells taken from those same students a month later, when they were involved in stressful 3-day examinations.[15] The comparison revealed that when students were taking exams, their white blood cells expressed fewer of the proteins that help those cells recognize and attack bacteria and viruses. Thus, these cells were rendered less able to perform their immune functions when the students were stressed.

This finding suggested that stress probably influences genetic activity; the scientists at Ohio State concluded that interactions between stress and immune responses "may be observed at the level of gene expression."[16] Although the epigenetic mechanism responsible for such effects was not yet the subject of study in the late 1980s or early 1990s, the existence of this kind of phenomenon makes blood cells a good candidate to consider when seeking cells that might register experience in an *epigenetic* way. Not only is the DNA in blood cells accessible; DNA in these cells also behaves differently in different contexts. This is why contemporary researchers think at least some blood cells might be able to serve as a kind of stand-in for brain cells,[17a-17b] even if brain and blood cells might not react to experiences in identical ways.[18a-18b] Can white blood cells reveal whether specific experiences influence specific epigenetic states in living people?

People Say We Monkey Around

The best way to attack this question would be to manipulate a person's experiences and then look to see whether those experiences influence the epigenetic state of the DNA in that person's blood cells. But ethical concerns prohibit human research that involves the kinds of manipulations used by rodent researchers, so there is no way to prove conclusively that specific *detrimental* experiences—with, say, maternal deprivation—influence the epigenetic states of living people. If we want to *prove* that blood cells show epigenetic effects of these kinds of experiences, the best we can do is manipulate the experiences of some our close primate relatives, such as monkeys. This approach isn't perfect, because monkeys aren't people; but even so, the results of this kind of work can shed some light.

In an extremely important study of the effects of maternal deprivation on DNA methylation, a group of researchers led by Nadine Provençal and Moshe Szyf collaborated with Stephen Suomi, who was one of Harry Harlow's research assistants many decades ago and is now the director of the comparative ethology lab at the National Institute of Child Health and Human Development outside of Washington, DC; their goal was to conduct an *experimental* investigation of the epigenetic effects of maternal deprivation on rhesus monkeys.[19] These researchers raised a small number of monkeys in a stressful, Harlow-style maternal deprivation situation. In addition, they let an equal number of "control" monkeys grow up in normal social groups, where they were raised by their biological mothers. Because the monkeys in this study were randomly assigned at birth to either the mother-deprived group or the mother-reared group, this research provided an impressive level of experimental control.

When these monkeys were 7 years old and had just reached adulthood, the researchers examined DNA taken from both their blood and brain cells. Consistent with the results of the McGowan team's work with human suicide/abuse victims and the Meaney team's work with rats, this study revealed patterns of DNA methylation that varied depending on how the monkeys were reared. Because this research team looked for epigenetic effects across the *entire* genome, they reported hundreds of locations in blood DNA—and thousands of locations in brain DNA—where methylation levels were related to maternal deprivation. In both blood and brain cells, the experience of maternal deprivation *caused* hypermethylation in some DNA locations and hypomethylation in others, leading to an inescapable conclusion: "Differential rearing leads to differential DNA methylation in both prefrontal cortex [i.e., brain] and T cells [i.e., specific white blood cells]."[20] Notably, although there was some overlap in the affected regions of the genome in the blood cells and the brain cells, the experience of deprivation did not alter DNA methylation patterns in the blood in exactly the same way as it altered DNA methylation patterns in the brain. Thus, although this experiment demonstrated the feasibility of studying the epigenetic effects of experiences using blood samples, the results suggested that we cannot assume that effects detected in blood DNA necessarily mirror effects in brain DNA; instead, it appears that these cell types can react in different ways to the same experience.[21, 22]

Another line of research has revealed that giving monkeys a different sort of experience can also produce epigenetic effects.[23] When they are *adults*, some female rhesus monkeys experience a distinctive kind of social stress. Because rhesus monkeys normally form dominance hierarchies, there are always lower-ranked individuals in a given community that yield to higher-ranked individuals in competitive encounters, and in some circumstances, these lower-ranked individuals experience chronic stress.[24] This raises a question: If we study animals that occupy different rungs on the dominance ladder, will we be able to detect the epigenetic effects of stress in these monkeys' blood?

A group of collaborators from the University of Chicago and Emory University tried to answer this question by controlling where individual monkeys stood in a group's dominance hierarchy;[25] in this way, they hoped to learn more about the epigenetic effects of primates' experiences. By introducing individual monkeys into a social group at specific times, the researchers were able to effectively assign dominance ranks to randomly selected individuals. Then, while controlling other environmental variables, they could search for the effects of dominance rank on gene regulation. Importantly, these scientists were also able to get blood samples more than once from some of the monkeys, so they were able to examine the epigenetic effects of *changing* from one rank to another.

The results of this experiment were striking. First, the Chicago/Emory team found that by looking at the expression of about 1,000 different genes in specific kinds of white blood cells, they could do a good job of predicting the dominance rank of the monkey that provided the blood. Second, when they looked at the *function* of the various genes associated with rank, they found that many of them were involved in immune system activities. Third, they found that when monkeys moved into a new rank, their gene expression profiles changed as well, indicating that gene expression patterns can be *plastic*—they can be responsive to changes in social status. And finally, they found that DNA methylation patterns differed for the high- versus low-ranking monkeys, consistent with their different gene expression profiles. These researchers concluded, therefore, that epigenetic changes might account for some of the associations between dominance rank and gene expression.

Along with the Provençal team's study, this experiment provided some of the strongest evidence yet that experiences can influence epigenetic states—and gene expression—in animals that are closely related to us. The Chicago/Emory group concluded:

> Our results reinforce the idea that sensitivity to the social environment is reflected in changes in gene expression in the immune system, supporting an increasingly widely recognized link between neural, endocrine [i.e., hormonal], and immune function. Moreover, our results demonstrate that these associations also appear to be highly plastic. Not only were gene expression data sufficient to robustly predict relative dominance rank but gene expression profiles also tracked dominance rank shifts closely enough to allow us to predict different rank positions for the same individuals across time. These observations indicate that any

causal relationship between dominance rank and gene regulation likely begins with rank.[26]

So in these monkeys, social status caused the gene expression patterns, not the other way around.

In this study, the experiences of *adult* monkeys influenced gene expression, indicating that it is not just *early* experiences that influence DNA methylation. Instead, it now appears that a social experience can influence epigenetic status in adulthood, and that such effects "may include natural components of social structure, such as dominance rank."[27] This is very important, as it implies that the things we do to reduce social stress might have the potential to influence genetic activity. And if this is true for monkeys, it is probably true for human beings as well. In fact, there is already some evidence that the ways in which we try to enhance our sense of well-being affects the activity of our genes.[28]

Early Experiences, Epigenetic Effects: Correlational Studies of Human Blood

To recap briefly, studies of suicide victims have suggested that people's early experiences might influence the epigenetic state of the DNA in their brains, and studies of monkeys have shown that their experiences influence the epigenetic state of some of the DNA in their brains *and* blood. Because it is unethical to conduct certain kinds of experiments on human beings, we cannot *prove* that detrimental experiences early in life cause epigenetic effects in people, but armed with evidence that experiences affect epigenetic states in monkeys' blood cells, we can at least look to see whether people's epigenetic states are *correlated* with their experiences. To date, several correlational studies of DNA extracted from human blood have been conducted, and because the data from these studies converge nicely with data collected in experimental studies of monkeys, a relatively clear picture is emerging regarding the effects of experiences on epigenetic marks.

In fact, the possibility of studying blood has already been a boon to behavioral epigeneticists working with human populations. For example, the researchers who conducted the Spanish National Cancer Centre study of identical twins, which I described in the chapter "Epigenetics," examined a specific type of white blood cell, as well as muscle cells taken from participants' quadriceps and buccal cells swabbed from the inside of their cheeks.[29] In all three cases, the results were the same: As the twins aged and spent more time leading different lives, their epigenetic profiles diverged.

Recently, a spate of studies like this one has demonstrated that we can learn a lot about epigenetics by studying cells taken from twins.[30a–30c] To choose just one example, a team of Australian researchers recently looked at methylation of four DNA segments in cells taken from *newborn* twins' umbilical cords and placentas; these researchers also examined buccal cells swabbed from the inside of the newborns' cheeks.[31] Interestingly, the epigenetic states of these DNA segments were somewhat different *at birth* for the individuals in a given twin-pair, and more so for fraternal than for identical twins.[32] Thus, genetic factors and the intrauterine environment both appear to contribute to newborns' epigenetic states. In addition—and in contrast to the Spanish study—the Australian team reported that the umbilical, placental, and buccal cells they examined had different amounts of methylation, highlighting why it is important to choose the right cell types to study (and why epigeneticists continue to debate the nature of the relationship between DNA methylation in brain tissues, blood, and buccal cells[33]). But as significant as these sorts of discoveries are, they do not help us understand whether *specific* experiences influence the epigenetic states of specific DNA segments in living people.

Two other studies came closer to this goal by analyzing DNA taken from blood cells in newborn babies' umbilical cords; both found correlations between prenatal exposure to maternal depression and DNA methylation. The researchers who conducted the first of these studies reported that babies born to women who experienced depression late in their pregnancies had abnormally high levels of methylation at a specific location in the GR promoter, a location thought to be associated with babies' stress reactions.[34] And as predicted, when tested at 3 months of age, these babies had larger stress responses than did babies born to nondepressed women. The researchers who conducted the second study were particularly interested in the serotonin system, because a molecule that interacts with serotonin— a molecule called the serotonin transporter—seems to be involved when people develop anxiety and depression.[35] And, as hypothesized, these researchers found that women who were depressed in their second trimester gave birth to infants who had *less* methylation on the serotonin transporter promoter.[36] The scientists who conducted these two studies acknowledge that their work was correlational and cannot *prove* that experiences influence DNA methylation in human infants; nonetheless, they pointed out that discovering these kinds of correlations between maternal mood and newborn babies' epigenetic states "is a first step towards a more complete understanding of how early life experience, genotype, and epigenetic processes contribute to development."[37]

Studies of associations between specific experiences and epigenetic states in human blood cells have now become more commonplace, and together, these studies have contributed to the emerging scientific consensus that our experiences can influence what our genomes do. One line of research has followed up on McGowan's study of brain tissue from abuse/suicide victims by looking for epigenetic correlates of child abuse in the blood of living people. In one such study, people who experienced sexual or physical abuse before they were 16 years old had significantly more methylated serotonin transporter promoters in adulthood than did nonabused adults, suggesting that child abuse might have long-term effects on overall methylation levels.[38] Similar conclusions were drawn in the wake of another study on the relationship between childhood maltreatment and methylation of GR promoters in blood-derived DNA; this study found that the more a person was abused as a child, the more highly methylated their GR promoters were in adulthood.[39] Finally, two additional studies examined the epigenetic correlates of child abuse across the entire human genome, and both studies found *hundreds* of DNA regions that were methylated abnormally in adults who were abused as children.[40a–40b] Taken together, the available data suggest that maltreatment in childhood affects DNA methylation, effectively registering the experience of abuse in the human body.[41]

Importantly, these kinds of effects can be expected to have functional consequences. In fact, a team of researchers recently reported that the methylation of serotonin transporter promoters in blood- and saliva-derived DNA is correlated with the way in which a living person's amygdala—a brain region involved in processing emotional events—reacts when they are shown photographs of threatening faces.[42] If future studies also find associations between DNA methylation and brain functioning, methylation could be implicated as a mechanism by which harmful early-life experiences can physically cause later psychopathology.[43]

Tragically, it appears that maltreatment might be able to affect one's epigenetic state even if it occurs before birth. In a study conducted in Germany, researchers examined the relationship between a woman's experience of domestic violence during pregnancy and the epigenetic state of her child many years later.[44] In addition to obtaining blood samples from female volunteers and their 10- to 19-year-old children, the researchers asked the mothers to report memories of violent experiences at the hands of their partners around the time of their child's birth.[45] Although the mothers' experiences of domestic violence were not related to the extent of methylation of their *own* GR promoters, those experiences were positively related to methylation of their offspring's GR promoters. Thus, the researchers concluded that "methylation in the offspring is directly affected by adverse experiences of the mother during gestation,"[46] presumably via changes in the intrauterine environment that result from the mother's own stress reactions to violence. Caution is warranted when evaluating studies like this that rely on memories rather than objective measures of domestic violence. But if these results prove replicable, they would support the hypothesis that a *fetus's* experience with maternal stress can affect that child's gene expression not just at birth, but many years later.

Loneliness, Poverty, and Oppression

Clearly, several kinds of experiences may have epigenetic effects in human beings. The experience of child abuse appears to be associated with increased methylation of GR and serotonin transporter promoters. Exposure to domestic violence in utero may be associated with increased methylation of GR promoters. Other experiences in utero might also be influential, as prenatal exposure to maternal depression seems to be associated with increased methylation of GR promoters. Moreover, we now have experimental evidence that abuse in childhood—or social stress in adulthood—can *cause* differential methylation patterns in nonhuman primates. Together, the emerging evidence implies that a variety of social stressors can affect our epigenetic states,[47] and that these effects can sometimes persist for years.[48]

Twenty-five years ago, scientists already knew of the connection between social relationships and health. An influential article written in 1988 announced that people without close relationships—lonely people—are at increased risk of *death*, and concluded that a lack of social relationships constitutes "a major risk factor for health rivaling the effects of well-established health risk factors such as cigarette smoking, blood pressure, blood lipids, obesity, and physical activity."[49] Might there be reason to think that stressors like loneliness, poverty, or oppression can influence the activity of our genes?

The jury is still out on these questions, but data have started to trickle in. For instance, one study revealed that people who feel chronically lonely have different patterns of gene expression in white blood cells compared with people who feel socially well integrated.[50] Although the researchers who conducted this study did not look at differences in DNA methylation or histone modifications, they did trace the altered gene expression patterns to reduced GR activity in immune system cells. Thus, in all likelihood, loneliness produces some of its biological effects by triggering epigenetic activities.

Another group of researchers has reported a correlation between gene expression patterns in healthy adult research participants and their socioeconomic status (SES) earlier in life.[51] Specifically, these researchers discovered a relationship between being poor in the first 5 years of life and the expression, 20 to 35 years later, of over 100 genes in white blood cells, even though all participants' occupational statuses and stress levels were similar at the time of the study. Here too, the data revealed reduced GR activity in the studied cells. Thus, studies like these have illuminated how differential gene expression is related to factors such as social support or economic resources, even if they have not actually provided solid evidence that specific epigenetic alterations like DNA methylation are responsible for the effects.[52]

Pushing the envelope, a study published in 2012 found actual epigenetic effects of exposure to disadvantaged socioeconomic conditions.[53] To explore

the possibility that people respond to these conditions with epigenetic modifications, a team of scientists led by Moshe Szyf analyzed DNA from the blood of
45-year-old men. In addition to finding relationships between the men's current
methylation profiles and their current socioeconomic statuses, the researchers
found a relationship between the men's current methylation profiles and their
socioeconomic statuses when they were very young. Specifically, the researchers found methylation levels in nearly 1,200 DNA regions to be associated with
childhood SES alone, a remarkable finding so many years after childhood's end.
The team concluded, "Our finding of a methylation signature of early-life [SES]
in adult blood DNA . . . is consistent with epigenetic mechanisms contributing
to the association between early-life [SES] and adult health."[54] Of course, a single study like this must be considered preliminary, but there is increasing conviction among biologically oriented behavioral scientists that SES in childhood
can have long-lasting effects on psychological, physiological, neural, and genetic
functioning.[55]

Because SES is correlated with ethnicity, this line of research raises the question of whether health disparities that characterize different ethnic groups might
actually reflect epigenetic modifications that result from exposure to impoverished environments. In fact, the American anthropologists Christopher Kuzawa
and Elizabeth Sweet have argued that the persistent disparity in cardiovascular
disease between black and white Americans might be traceable to epigenetic
effects of childhood environments.[56] Although DNA methylation in white blood
cells appears to be correlated with ethnicity per se,[57] black and white Americans
are also known to have different incidences of low birth weight and prematurity,
factors that reflect social stress and that could conceivably be associated with
methylation levels in newborns.[58] Although Kuzawa and Sweet's argument is
based on circumstantial evidence, they make a compelling case for their hypothesis that epigenetic effects of stress reflect a mechanism that takes social influences and incorporates them into our bodies in a durable way.[59] Ultimately, they
argue that this kind of "embodiment of social and material environments through
developmental and epigenetic processes helps explain the persistence of . . . [car-
diovascular disease] disparities across racial categories."[60]

Research on the epigenetic effects of experience in human populations is just getting underway,[61] but the results so far have been encouraging. A survey of the initial
data certainly gives the impression that these effects are probably widespread, and
of considerable consequence as we try to understand why people are as they are. In
fact, many scientists now share a collective sense of the significance of epigenetics,
a dawning awareness that has inspired a large-scale international research project
dedicated to mapping the human epigenome.[62] According to its website,

> The Human Epigenome Project aims to identify, catalogue and interpret
> genome-wide DNA methylation patterns of all human genes in all major

tissues. Methylation is the only flexible genomic parameter that can change genome function under exogenous influence [e.g., the influence of the environment]. Hence it constitutes the main and so far missing link between genetics, disease and the environment that is widely thought to play a decisive role in the [origin] of virtually all human pathologies.[63]

Eventually, this project is likely to rival the Human Genome Project in terms of complexity, scope, and importance.[64]

There is a lot still to learn, of course; by one estimate in 2012, "deeper characterization of everything the genome is doing is probably only 10% finished."[65] But the data available to us today are intriguing, and they suggest that our genes and environments are engaged in a kind of conversation that is ongoing throughout our lives. The characteristics we wind up with—from our temperaments to our diseases—emerge from the collaborative actions of both genetic and environmental factors. And we can be fairly certain at this point that at least one of the languages these collaborators use when they communicate is epigenetics.

|| 13 ||

Memory

The Oscar for Best Original Screenplay in 2004 was awarded to a wonderful and very strange movie called *Eternal Sunshine of the Spotless Mind*. A science fiction-flavored dramedy, its central premise is that a corporation called Lacuna, Inc., has developed a new technology that can be used to obliterate specific memories, thereby allowing a heartbroken person to move on after a failed love affair. The movie raises the very good point that however painful some of our memories might be, destroying them is not necessarily a very bright idea. But we don't need to dwell on the issue, because after all, the notion of selective memory destruction is just science fiction.

Or is it? The surprising truth is that the science of memory has advanced so rapidly in the last couple of decades that some neuroscientists have begun to think that focused deletion of specific memories might actually be possible.[1] In fact, researchers working with Joseph LeDoux at New York University have found that by injecting specific drugs into specific areas of rats' brains at specific times and in the context of specific experimental protocols, they seem to have erased distinct memories while leaving all other memories intact.[2a–2b] Of course, this doesn't mean a real-life Lacuna, Inc., will soon be marketing brain spa-treatments, but the fact that the neuroscience has already gotten this close to the science fiction is astonishing. If you had asked me in 2004 if specific memories would ever be "deletable" like this—without damaging anything else in the mind—I would have said I was doubtful.

I would have been skeptical back then in part because memory has always seemed so *mental* to me, about as ethereal as any psychological experience could be (and therefore not particularly amenable to any sort of physical, electrical, or chemical "surgery"). Several other psychological phenomena—to choose just a few examples, visual attention, fear, and the sensation of taste—make such obvious use of the body that it seems intuitively reasonable that they reflect *physical* events in the body. But memories feel like something else entirely. Mere introspection about memory can make Descartes-style mind-body dualism seem sensible.

The level of detail neuroscientists now have about the physical bases of memory is mind-boggling; the next chapter will consider several of these details, but it will only scratch the surface. The number of researchers responsible for our current understanding is enormous, too. Nonetheless, some of the most important work on the neuroscience of memory was recognized when the Nobel Prize in Physiology or Medicine was awarded to Eric Kandel in 2000 (along with Arvid Carlsson and Paul Greengard).

In his acceptance speech to the Nobel Foundation, Kandel explained how his attention was originally drawn to "the hippocampus, the part of the mammalian brain thought to be most directly involved in aspects of complex memory."[3] However, because of how complicated the human hippocampus is, Kandel decided it was "necessary to take a very different approach—a radically reductionist approach." He concluded that he needed

> to study not the most complex but the simplest instances of memory storage, and to study them in animals that were most tractable experimentally . . . [This conviction reflected his belief that] elementary forms of learning are common to all animals with an evolved nervous system [so] there must be conserved features in the mechanisms of learning at the cell and molecular level that can be studied effectively even in simple invertebrate animals.[4]

Kandel's reductionist approach ultimately led to a series of studies on a type of sea slug called *Aplysia* . . . and ever since, the study of learning and memory has been informed by molecular understandings that have brought us to the threshold of a new era in memory research, one in which the selective deletion of memories is no longer unthinkable and in which epigenetics are understood to play a significant role. Kandel calls his decision to take a radically reductionist approach to memory "a leap of faith for which I have been rewarded beyond my fondest hopes,"[5] because in the end, he was right that some important aspects of memory are no different in slugs than they are in people.

The Intimate Relationship Between Genes and Long-Term Memories

Before we can ask about the role of epigenetics in memory formation, we have to first ask if there is a role for *genes* in memory formation, a prospect that is not intuitively obvious. But work in Kandel's lab has made it clear that genes do play critical roles when memories are formed, that is, when a nervous system produces a record of an animal's previous experiences.

Assessing memory in slugs is not as easy as asking them if they remember the last time you took them out for an ice cream cone. Instead, to study memory in these animals, Kandel took advantage of the fact that *Aplysia*—like most complex animals—can learn to respond to a neutral stimulus that wouldn't ordinarily produce a response. In this kind of learning, a neutral stimulus is presented some time after a noxious stimulus. For example, in his breakthrough work, Kandel shocked one part of the *Aplysia's* body and then later touched another part; although the touch would not have produced a startle response in a slug that had never been shocked, slugs that *have* been shocked react to the touch with a startle response. Kandel argues that this means "the animal remembers the shock."[6]

Some people might bristle at Kandel's suggestion that this sort of phenomenon is akin to a conscious memory of a parent's face, a warm summer afternoon, or the events leading up to a tragic accident. But on the grounds that even primitive learning requires slugs' nervous systems to retain a record of their prior experiences, Kandel believes that such learning has important elements in common with our conscious memories. At the very least, we should acknowledge that these commonalities mean that Kandel-style studies of simple kinds of "information retention" could have broader implications that might bear on the more complex "information retention" that constitutes our memories.

Expounding in his Nobel Prize acceptance speech on the "remembered-shock" phenomenon, Kandel turned to perhaps his most important early discovery: "The duration of this memory is a function of the number of repetitions of the noxious experience."[7] Specifically, exposing a slug to one shock produces a kind of "short-term memory" that lasts for minutes, but exposing it to four brief shocks each day for four straight *days* produces startle responses when the slug is touched over the next three *weeks*. Thus, this more extensive experience produces a kind of "long-term memory" for the shocking events.[8]

Regardless of whether Kandel's research applies very narrowly to particular kinds of learning or more broadly to memory in general, the next discoveries that came out of his lab were amazing. Using an antibiotic that inhibits protein synthesis, his team was able to show that a slug forms short-term memories of a single shocking experience *even when its neurons are unable to produce new proteins*. In contrast, this antibiotic *prevents* a slug from forming *long*-term memories in response to multiple shocks, meaning that establishing such memories *requires* the construction of new proteins.[9] Because many behavioral scientists had concluded by the mid-1960s that *people*, too, have distinct short-term and long-term memory capacities[10]—and because they knew by then that some antibiotics could obliterate memories in mice[11]—this work raised the inspiring possibility that Kandel's team had discovered distinctive mechanisms underlying short- versus long-term memory formation in mammals. And in the case of long-term memories, genetic factors appeared to be playing important roles.

Here's how it works. Shocking an *Aplysia* a single time leads to biochemical changes in the sensory neurons that detect the shock, changes that lead those neurons—and the slug itself—to behave differently for a short period of time after the shock. Specifically, the single shock causes the sensory neurons to release an increased amount of neurotransmitter the next time they are stimulated. This kind of memory does not require the construction of new proteins, because proteins already present in the sensory neurons can produce the required biochemical changes.

In contrast, shocking an *Aplysia* four or five times over a more extended period causes the sensory neurons to *grow new connections*—they form new synapses—with the other neurons in the area.[12] These changes require the construction of new proteins and can last for weeks even if they are not reinforced, so they are understood to be a physical instantiation of a long-term memory. If we accept the contention that this kind of "behavioral memory" is related to our explicit, conscious memories, then the implication is that the memory you have of going swimming in Walden Pond in the summer of 1998 is in your brain because the microstructure of your brain *changed* after the experience so as to *physically represent* the things about that day that you remember. Regardless of the nature of the relationship between explicit and behavioral memories, there is now a consensus among neuroscientists that the synaptic connections in our brains are not fixed, but rather are dynamically remodeled as we interact with our environments.[13]

The discovery that long-term memory formation requires the construction of new proteins tells us something important about the mechanism that installs such memories in our brains: Genes are centrally involved. In fact, shocking an *Aplysia* four or five times activates specific molecules in sensory neurons; these molecules then make their way into the neurons' nuclei, where they attach to DNA and fire up the transcription machinery, beginning the process of gene expression (and ultimately, protein production). The title of Kandel's lecture to the Nobel Foundation, "The Molecular Biology of Memory Storage: A Dialogue Between Genes and Synapses,"[14] is evocative precisely because installing long-term memories in a brain requires the production of new proteins, and therefore, the activation of specific genes.

Tinkering with Information Retention: Epigenetics and Memory

From Kandel's lecture, we can already see how long-term memory formation should be described as an epigenetic process, because to produce the proteins needed to install a new long-term memory in a brain, molecules must become attached to DNA. From this perspective, memory formation involves a kind of gene-environment interaction in which experiences cause physiological changes that influence gene expression. But this is "epigenetic" only according to a rather broad definition of that word; so far, I have not yet described a role in memory formation for DNA methylation, histone acetylation, or any other sort of epigenetic machinery, for that matter. Nevertheless, it is now clear that epigenetic processes in our brains—effects akin to those that regulate our biological clocks—*are* involved in learning and in the formation of at least some kinds of memories.[15]

When you start thinking about it, it makes a lot of sense that epigenetic processes are involved in memory, because a memory/epigenetics connection would have the fingerprints of natural selection all over it. François Jacob (whose Nobel Prize–winning work on gene regulation I described in "Zooming in on DNA") wrote a beautiful essay in 1977 that described how to recognize those fingerprints. He wrote:

> Natural selection has no analogy with any aspect of human behavior. However, if one wanted to play with a comparison, one would have to say that natural selection does not work as an engineer works. It works like a tinkerer—a tinkerer who does not know exactly what he is going to produce but uses whatever he finds around him whether it be pieces of string, fragments of wood, or old cardboards; in short it works like a tinkerer who uses everything at his disposal to produce some kind of workable object. . . . The tinkerer . . . always manages with odds and ends. . . . none of the materials at the tinkerer's disposal has a precise and definite function. Each can be used in a number of different ways. In contrast with the engineer's tools, those of the tinkerer cannot be defined by a project. What these objects have in common is "it might well be of some use." For what? That depends on the opportunities.[16]

Because engineers do not tinker like this, engineered items strike us as planned, logically assembled, and made of components that are perfect for the job they do. In contrast, if a biological feature seems like it was made of bits and pieces that serve other functions in other contexts, it is because it is a product of natural selection.

Epigenetic modifications are precisely the kind of mechanism nature would select when creating a memory system, because in some ways, they have always been all about memory. As we've seen, differentiated cells have their distinctive features because they have distinctive gene expression profiles, profiles that reflect their epigenetic state. And whenever such cells divide, they pass on their distinctive epigenetic states to their "daughters," thereby guaranteeing that the daughter cells will be of the same cell *type* as the parent cells.[17] For example, any time a liver cell is going to divide to produce two new liver cells, it does so in a way that *preserves information* about which genes should and should not be active in a liver cell.[18] This is what ensures that all of the newly created cells in your liver will be liver cells, and that you'll never inadvertently begin developing a bunch of acid-secreting stomach-lining cells in your liver (which would definitely be a very bad plan)! In this way, epigenetic marks in a new generation of cells preserve information that was present in an earlier generation of cells. And there is a sense in which cellular "information preservation" can be thought of as a kind of cellular "memory."

Obviously, there are important differences between the sort of cellular "memory" carried by epigenetic marks and the sort of psychological memory that our brains use to retain factual and autobiographical information. But remember, natural selection is a tinkerer: Since it already had a system at its disposal for retaining information in the context of cell division, it would be likely to take advantage of that fact and recruit that system for use in a different context.

This sort of maneuver is so typical of natural selection that evolutionary biologists have given it its own name: exaptation. In a classic paper, Stephen Jay Gould and Elisabeth Vrba defined exaptations as features that are currently adaptive "but were not built by natural selection for their current role."[19] The first example they offer is feathers, which are adaptive in modern birds because they enable flight. However, because feathers were present on some flightless dinosaurs, several theorists have argued persuasively that feathers must have originally evolved for some purpose *other* than flight, perhaps to help dinosaurs regulate their body temperatures. Having appeared for other reasons, though, feathers were then available to be co-opted for use in flight, making feathers-for-flight a prototypical example of an exaptation and demonstrating how natural selection reuses features that evolved to solve one problem when it is confronted with an entirely different problem.

Because evolution works like this, cellular "memory" and cognitive-behavioral memory might be more than merely analogous; they might actually share important features as a result of having evolved from the same molecular systems. In fact, several of the molecular mechanisms involved in the regulation of cell differentiation are also employed in the storage of memories,[20] suggesting that perhaps memory might really best be thought of as an exaptation. Thus, the neurobiologist David Sweatt—along with his colleague Jonathan Levenson—concluded a 2005 paper on epigenetic mechanisms in memory formation by explicitly stating, "We propose that the [brain] has co-opted mechanisms of epigenetic tagging of the genome for use in the formation of long-term memories."[21] Unpacking that idea a bit, they asked:

> Are the basic epigenetic mechanisms that are important for information storage during development also important for storing memories that manifest themselves behaviourally in the adult? We predict that these

mechanisms are conserved in the adult nervous system, where they have been co-opted to serve the formation of behavioural memories.[22]

In the years that have followed that prediction, data supporting the idea that epigenetic mechanisms are involved in memory have begun piling up rapidly.

Some of the initial data indicating a role for epigenetics in memory came from Kandel's lab at Columbia University. Specifically, he and his collaborators found that when *Aplysia* sensory neurons are stimulated in a way that leads to the formation of a long-term memory, the chromatin in the nuclei of those neurons is epigenetically altered via histone acetylation.[23] Subsequent work with genetically engineered mice suggested that histone acetylation plays important roles in long-term memory formation in mammals as well.[24]

Since then, several studies on epigenetics and memory in ordinary rodents have been conducted by members of Sweatt's research team at the University of Alabama at Birmingham. One of these experiments found that for ordinary rats, histone acetylation is activated early in the process of forming long-term memories,[25] confirming the importance of epigenetic processes in normal mammalian memory formation. The neuroscientists in Alabama knew just where to look in normal rat brains for epigenetic effects of long-term memory formation: the hippocampus. After all, this brain structure has been known for over 50 years to be involved in the formation of long-term memories.[26]

Hippocampus: The Memory Forge

The hippocampus came to prominence among memory researchers in the 1950s, when William Scoville and Brenda Milner reported adverse effects of a neurosurgical procedure that had been performed on a 29-year-old man named Henry Molaison. Molaison was described in the report as having worked as a "motor winder" after graduating from high school, but by the time he arrived in Dr. Scoville's office, he was suffering from severe epileptic seizures. No one was ever able to determine for sure what was causing them, but the seizures started as relatively minor attacks when he was 10 years old, a short time after he fell off of a bicycle and was knocked unconscious for five minutes. Sadly, the seizures grew worse with time, and by the age of 16 they included convulsions, tongue-biting, and loss of consciousness. Although doctors first attempted to treat Molaison's symptoms with heavy doses of anticonvulsant medications, his condition deteriorated until he was effectively incapacitated.

In 1953, Molaison chose to undergo a radical experimental operation intended to reduce the severity of his seizures; there were no other promising treatment options available to him at that time. The operation was a success, in that it did decrease the intensity of his seizures. But regrettably, the operation also produced one very serious side effect: the loss of recent memories.[27] Because of this side effect, Henry spent the remaining five decades of his life participating in an ongoing series of studies of memory. To preserve his anonymity while he was alive— he died in 2008—scientists referred to him only as H.M., a nickname that by the late 20th century was famous among students of psychology.

H.M. is important to psychologists because the surgery conducted to alleviate his seizures damaged both his brain and memory systems in remarkably specific ways. The operation entailed the removal of *both* his right and left hippocampi. Beginning 20 months after the surgery, H.M. underwent a series of psychological tests that revealed a higher than normal IQ, no abnormal personality characteristics, and no perceptual disturbances; the side effect of the operation was limited to memory loss.

However, H.M.'s amnesia was of a very particular variety. After the surgery, he still remembered his childhood and young adulthood, and he still had possession of all of his learned skills; what was lacking was his ability to form *new* memories. In 1957, Scoville and Milner described it like this:

> After operation this young man could no longer recognize the hospital staff nor find his way to the bathroom, and he seemed to recall nothing of the day-to-day events of his hospital life . . . Ten months ago the family moved from their old house to a new one a few blocks away on the same street; he still has not learned the new address, though remembering the old one perfectly, nor can he be trusted to find his way home alone. Moreover, he does not know where objects in continual use are kept; for example, his mother still has to tell him where to find the lawn mower, even though he may have been using it only the day before. She also states that he will do the same jigsaw puzzles day after day without showing any practice effect and that he will read the same magazines over and over again without finding their contents familiar. This patient has even eaten luncheon . . . without being able to name, a mere half-hour later, a single item of food he had eaten; in fact, he could not remember having eaten luncheon at all. Yet to a casual observer this man seems like a relatively normal individual, since his understanding and reasoning are undiminished.[28]

H.M. could not even remember if he was just having a conversation with you, let alone who you were. And because this deficit persisted as the years went by, H.M. wound up an old man with virtually no memories at all from the 55 years following his operation, but with "vivid and intact"[29] memories from his youth.

This sorry tale makes it obvious why the hippocampus is recognized as being centrally involved in memory formation, but it tells us more than that. The fact that H.M. did not lose his early memories means that the brain areas involved in *forming* new memories are different from the brain areas involved in *storing* memories. Thus, the hippocampus is crucial for the formation of a new memory, but it is not where that memory will actually be stored in the long run. Instead, in a separate process known as consolidation, memories that depend on the hippocampus for formation ultimately shift to a longer-term dependence on regions in the cerebral cortex, where they are stored;[30] after a matter of weeks, maintenance of a memory no longer requires the involvement of the hippocampus.

Making Mouse Memories

Because of this knowledge, when Sweatt and his colleagues wanted to know if the formation of long-term memories in rats entails histone acetylation, they knew that the right histones to examine would be the ones in the nuclei of hippocampal cells. But before they could study the memory formation process, they needed to have an effective technique for installing a new memory in a rat's brain. As with slugs, so with rats: You can't just ask them about their memories of their grandfather.

The primary method experimentalists use to assess rodents' memories is called the contextual fear conditioning paradigm. Sounds bad—and for animal lovers like me, it is—but it serves the purpose very well. The idea is relatively simple, born as it was from the Pavlovian notion of classical conditioning. In this paradigm, a rodent is put into a neutral, nonscary "training chamber" and allowed to explore for a couple of minutes before receiving a shock. To test its memory, it is simply returned to the chamber 24 hours later; if it reacts to being put in this context again by freezing—an indication of fear—it must have formed some type of memory associating the chamber with the shock. When Levenson and colleagues examined chromatin from hippocampal cells of rats who had this experience, they discovered that the process of forming this kind of associative memory involves histone acetylation and associated changes in the structure of chromatin.[31] Thus, epigenetic events have their fingers in the memory-formation process, just as they are involved in physiologically registering some early-life experiences and in regulating biological clocks.

Researchers also use two other methods to test the epigenetic effects of learning and memory in rodents. One method entails giving animals experiences running in mazes, a procedure that allows scientists to study their *spatial* memories. The other method is called latent inhibition. In many ways, this method looks a lot like contextual fear learning; animals are still put in neutral chambers, shocked, and then tested by being reexposed to the chamber. But in latent inhibition, they learn something different.

In the latent inhibition paradigm, an animal is given more than just a couple of minutes of experience with a never-before-encountered training chamber;

instead, it could be given perhaps *sixty* minutes to run around inside the chamber, shock free. If the animal then receives a shock, it will typically *not* form a memory associating the shock and the chamber, because the previous shock-free hour in the chamber inhibits the formation of such a memory. Thus, the animal acquires a memory that the chamber is basically safe. It's a lot like what would happen if you spent a single night tossing in your bed for hours; that experience probably wouldn't leave you permanently associating your bed with sleeplessness and dreading bedtime forevermore. Instead, all of your *previous* experiences with your bed would inhibit that new "lesson," so you would be able to go back to your bed the next night and sleep soundly. Latent inhibition appears to work this way in all mammals, presumably as an evolved mechanism that keeps us from forming unwarranted associations.

One of the more thought-provoking findings of research in this area has been that these various kinds of learning and memory involve different kinds of epigenetic modifications. For example, although they are both forms of long-term memory, contextual fear learning and latent inhibition are associated with the acetylation of different histones in a given eight-histone "spool."[32] This finding led Levenson and Sweatt to infer that "there might be a histone code for memory formation, whereby specific types of memory are associated with specific patterns of histone modification."[33] In addition to utilizing different histones for different types of memory, this code might also utilize different sorts of modifications, because it is now clear that memory formation involves histone *methyl*ation as well as acetylation.[34] Scientists currently understand very little about how such a code might work, but in a recent review article, Jeremy Day and David Sweatt concluded that "overwhelming evidence indicates that histone modifications in the [brain] are essential components of memory formation and consolidation. Indeed, multiple types of behavioral experiences are capable of inducing histone modifications in several brain regions."[35]

A Heresy: The Dynamic Regulation of DNA Methylation

You may recall that biologists have traditionally considered histone modifications to be considerably more dynamic than DNA methylation; even in Meaney's demonstrations that experiences can affect DNA methylation, the changes observed were relatively permanent. However, newer research in the neurosciences suggests that even if DNA methylation is *typically* permanent, there are some very important exceptions to the general rule, particularly in the nervous system.[36] In fact, it has started to look as though synaptic activity can influence DNA methylation, and, therefore, that such methylation is *dynamically* regulated in our brains.[37a-37c] It is too early to know for sure if *all* input to a neuron can alter the behavior of the DNA in that neuron and thereby lead to alterations in how the cell functions, but this is certainly a possibility.

Another exciting discovery that has emerged from this line of research is that our neurons appear to be able to use epigenetic modifications for different purposes in different brain areas. Because DNA methylation is *relatively* stable, it makes intuitive sense that it would be involved in the long-term storage of memories in the cerebral cortex. And as expected, DNA methylation in the cells of the cortex is essential for the maintenance of very long lasting memories.[38] But surprisingly, DNA methylation also appears to be involved in the initial *formation* of memories in the hippocampus, just as histone modifications are.[39] Because the hippocampus is involved in forming memories but is not where those memories will ultimately be stored, DNA methylation in the hippocampus has to be relatively transient, despite its reputation for ageless stability. Day and Sweatt summed it up like this:

> Contextual fear conditioning produces *transient* changes in DNA methylation in the hippocampus, but *prolonged* changes in DNA methylation in the cortex. Our speculation is that there are actually two different mechanisms, one that participates in consolidation (hippocampus) and one that participates in storage (cortex). Together, these mechanisms could allow for *plasticity* in hippocampal circuits to enable rapid consolidation and *stability* in cortical circuits to promote the long-term maintenance of memory. As the hippocampus is needed to form new, subsequent memories, its epigenetic mechanisms may have to be plastic to allow the system to reset after it has served its function.[40]

Then, in a frankly speculative end to this discussion, Day and Sweatt offer a guess about what might lie on the horizon for memory researchers, a conjecture that I find very exciting somewhat astonishing:

> DNA [methylation] marks generated in the hippocampus may be "heritable" . . . in the sense that the hippocampal circuit, driven by altered DNA methylation, downloads epigenetic marks from the hippocampus to the cortex. . . . in a broad sense, transient methylation marks in the hippocampus would drive the establishment of persisting methylation marks in the cortex. We could call this "systems heritability" of epigenetic marks.[41]

Regardless of whether this speculation proves prophetic, it seems that biologists need to start rethinking any dogmatic assumptions about the stability of DNA methylation.[42] According to Day and Sweatt, such methylation appears to be "a critical molecular component of both the formation and maintenance of long-term memories"[43] and it appears to have a role "in generating and maintaining experience-driven behavioral change in young and old animals."[44] In this way,

DNA methylation can reflect the experiences we have between conception and death.

Taken together, the available data on epigenetics and memory suggest that "long-term behavioural memory regulates, and is regulated by, the epigenome."[45] This conclusion would surprise an earlier generation of biologists, who failed to recognize roles for epigenetics in any processes other than development. The memory data imply that epigenetic marks are responsive to the experiences we have as mature individuals and that epigenetic mechanisms have important, dynamic roles to play in the formation of adult animals' memories.[46] Thus, like our genomes, our epigenomes contribute to who we are; but unlike our genomes, they appear to be dynamic, and influenced by the experiences we have over the course of our lifetimes.

There is a lot still to learn about memory. In addition to the kinds of distinctions I have raised in this chapter—between long-term versus short-term memory, behavioral memory versus explicit, conscious memory, memory formation versus memory storage, contextual fear memory versus spatial memory—psychologists now recognize differences between autobiographical memories, memories for facts, and unconscious memories for skills such as bicycle riding; we also know that memory *retrieval* is a process that is different from both memory formation and memory storage, and studies of some of these processes are just getting underway. Clearly, "memory" is a very broad term. But the strides made in this field in the last 30 years have been astounding, and the dawn of the age of epigenetics holds great promise for additional breakthroughs.[47] It might be a while before we can systematically delete a traumatic memory from a person's mind à la Lacuna, Inc., but in the meantime, details about the processes constituting our memory systems have started to accumulate, and scientists have begun to test epigenetic manipulations that can have incredible effects, such as enhancing memory in normal animals,[48] eliminating the kinds of memory impairments seen in neurodegenerative disorders like Alzheimer's disease,[49] and helping animals recover lost memories.[50] Of course, understanding how these things work requires a closer focus on the details of memory, the subject of the next chapter.

14

Zooming in on Memory

Psychology classes in college have a reputation for being easy, which is almost certainly undeserved; just because students *have* their own mental lives doesn't give them automatic insight into how and why people in general think, feel, and act as they do. We often don't even understand our own behaviors and emotional reactions, let alone other people's. The fact is, our minds are as they are in part because our brains are as they are, and if there is any truth to the oft-repeated factoid that the human brain is the most complex thing in the known universe, then understanding the mind should be pretty difficult. I'd give my field even odds in a toughness race with rocket science. Consider a collection of words and phrases sampled from just the first page of an article I cited at the end of the previous chapter:

> HDAC2 . . . CK-p25 mice, which inducibly and forebrain-specifically overexpress p25 . . . . [which] aberrantly activates cyclin-dependent kinase 5 (CDK5) . . . β-amyloid accumulation, reactive astrogliosis . . . the 5XFAD mouse . . . *GluR1, GluR2, NR2A and NR2B* (also known as *Gria1,Gria2, Grin2a and Grin2b*), as well as *Nfl* (neurofilament light chain, also known as *Nefl*), *Syp* (synaptophysin) and *Syt1* (synaptotagmin 1) . . . chromatin immunoprecipitation . . . β-actin, β-globin and β-tubulin.[1]

It's like a veritable tossed letter-salad (or at best, a crazy Lewis Carroll poem)! And this is just scratching the surface. The available information related to the study of memory alone seems fathomless; the study of psychology as a whole should be recognized as challenging for even the best students.

Having said that, this book is, mercifully, neither a comprehensive monograph on the science of memory nor a psychology textbook. And although the information already available regarding the epigenetics of memory is copious and intricately interrelated, the previous chapter already conveyed about as much information as anyone needs to know to understand why research in this domain is exciting. In this "Zooming in" chapter, I will focus on why and how certain novel experimental manipulations successfully influence memory in rodents, manipulations that might ultimately prove therapeutic for human beings. Among the kinds of people that could potentially benefit from such innovations are those with Alzheimer's disease, post-traumatic stress disorder, or the memory deficits that are associated with normal aging into one's 80s.

Better Memory Through Chemistry: Manipulating Histone Acetylation

In the previous chapter, I described Kandel's discovery that shocking a sea slug several times causes gene expression and the production of proteins. How this happens has been worked out in detail.[2] When neurotransmitters stimulate a sensory neuron, the neurotransmitters cause receptors to initiate a long cascade of events in which the receptor proteins affect other chemicals, which affect other proteins ... and so on. Proteins near the end of this cascade move into the nucleus of the neuron, where they interact with still other proteins that activate a transcription factor that plays an essential role in the formation of long-term memories. Once this transcription factor has attached itself to DNA, it recruits yet another protein, known as CREB binding protein (CBP), and together the CBP and the transcription factor initiate the gene transcription required for the formation of long-term memories.[3]

CBP is vital to long-term memory formation because of two of its distinctive abilities. First, it is able to attract transcription machinery to the DNA.[4] Second, it is a HAT—a histone acetyltransferase,[5a-5c] which means that it is able to acetylate histones and thereby remodel chromatin in a way that promotes gene expression. In addition to participating in long-term memory formation, CBP has other important functions in the body; in fact, people with genetic mutations that hinder normal CBP production develop a disorder known as Rubinstein-Taybi syndrome, a condition characterized by skeletal abnormalities as well as cognitive deficits.[6] Animals lacking *any* normal copies of the gene used to construct CBP are unable to survive at all,[7] so this is obviously a very important protein.

To study how CBP abnormalities contribute to the cognitive deficits that are typical of people with Rubinstein-Taybi syndrome, scientists created genetically engineered mice with only *one* normally functioning CBP gene (healthy mice have two copies of this DNA segment).[8] As would be expected, these mutant mice have some physical characteristics like those seen in people with Rubinstein-Taybi syndrome, such as skeletal abnormalities and growth retardation.[9] Crucially, although these mice are normal in terms of their activity levels, anxiety, and motivation, they exhibit long-term memory deficits in contextual fear conditioning. Therefore, they are particularly useful to researchers studying the molecular mechanisms underlying long-term memory formation. Research has revealed that there is reduced acetylation of specific histones in the hippo-campal neurons of these mice,[10] a finding consistent with the fact that CBP is a HAT, and with the conclusion that histone acetylation is an important part of the process of forming long-term memories.

What is truly exciting about research on these CBP-deficient mice, though, are the attempts researchers have made to influence their memories with drugs. You may recall that nature has provided a "molecular counterpart"[11] to the HATs, namely the histone deacetylases, or HDACs, which normally remove acetyl groups from histones. In a development that could have far-reaching consequences, sci-entists have discovered that some drugs inhibit the activity of HDACs, thereby having significant effects on biological and behavioral processes. For example, a compound called valproic acid that has been used since the 1960s as a drug to treat epilepsy has been found to inhibit HDAC activity.[12] These kinds of drugs are collectively known as HDAC inhibitors; they serve to *increase* histone acetylation because they work by *inhibiting* the natural acetyl-removing activity of HDACs. The following analogy should clarify the situation.

Imagine a little boy who sucks his thumb. A mother who wants to discourage this behavior can do so by attending to the child and intervening whenever he goes to suck his thumb; in this analogy, the mother is like an HDAC, because she has the effect of stopping something that would otherwise occur naturally. Now imagine what happens when the mother's phone rings and she stops attend-ing to her son: His thumb sucking is going to increase. Just as the phone inhibits the mother's intervention in her son's thumb sucking—leading to more thumb sucking—HDAC inhibitors stop HDACs from doing their job, thereby leading to increased histone acetylation. Thus, HDAC inhibitors have the same kinds of effects as HATs: They increased histone acetylation and thereby promote gene expression.

Beware of the confusion that can ensue when talking about these different kinds of molecules, each with its own acronym. HATs and HDACs are *proteins* that are synthesized naturally in our bodies; they add and remove acetyl groups to and from histones, respectively. In contrast, HDAC *inhibitors* are *drugs* that pre-vent acetyl groups from being removed from histones; they are synthesized in pharmaceutical laboratories.

In a study of genetically engineered mice with only one functional copy of the CBP gene, researchers found that if they directly injected an HDAC inhibitor into the brains of the mice 3 hours before contextual fear conditioning, this treatment led to increased histone acetylation and, importantly, an easing of their memory impairments.[13] Amazingly, this treatment helped the mutant mice perform *nor-mally*, effectively eliminating the memory deficits they ordinarily exhibit during contextual fear conditioning.[14] This finding suggests that Rubinstein-Taybi syn-drome might best be thought of as a disorder of abnormal chromatin remodeling, and that it might respond well to treatments with HDAC-inhibiting drugs.

Subsequent studies of these drugs have been equally encouraging. In particular, research on HDAC inhibitors has revealed that they enhance long-term memory formation in normal animals as they do in mutant mice.[15a–15d] One research team was especially blunt about the effects: "Increased histone-tail acetylation induced by [HDAC] inhibitors . . . facilitates learning and memory" in normal mice.[16] Likewise, after summarizing several studies on these drugs, Carey concluded, "Increased acetylation levels in the brain seem to be consistently associated with improved memory."[17]

Recovering Lost Memories: The Effects of Enriched Environments

The processes that form memories are complex enough that no one should think we are on the threshold of a brave new world in which drugs render our memories infallible, despite some recent impressive breakthroughs. Consider one big problem: Scientists currently know of at least 11 different HDACs,[18] and it is now clear that they do not all work in the same way. For instance, the HDAC known as HDAC1 is not associated with memory the way HDAC2 is.[19a–19b] Unfortunately, many HDAC inhibitor drugs affect several different HDACs, so they are relatively nonspecific. A number of biotech companies are working to create HDAC inhibitors that are more specific and therefore produce fewer side effects,[20] but observers continue to express concern that currently available HDAC inhibitors are so nonspecific[21] that their multifarious side effects make them of limited use (except in cases where someone has a lethal disease, in which case the side effects are the least of the patient's problems).[22] If a person's memory is worse than it was when she was younger but she is not suffering from severe dementia and is still relatively healthy, the memory improvements produced by HDAC inhibitors would probably not be worth the fatigue, nausea, and increased risk of infections that these drugs also cause.[23]

Getting around these difficulties will be challenging, but Li-Huei Tsai at the Massachusetts Institute of Technology has pioneered the use of some novel techniques that appear promising. As I describe it here and in the next section, this research might sound very much like science fiction, but it is not. Tsai's first step was to genetically engineer mice that develop a variety of neurological and behavioral "Alzheimer's-disease-related pathologies."[24] Doing this was no easy task, because the abnormal conditions that produce these pathologies would derail normal development if they were present from conception; people who develop Alzheimer's disease have *normal* childhoods, so a mouse "model" of this disease would need to develop normally as well, only beginning to acquire pathologies later in life.

The solution to this problem was to generate a mouse that could be *induced* to develop Alzheimer's-like pathologies in adulthood. Tsai and her colleagues therefore engineered a line of mice that could develop normally as long as they were fed a diet containing a particular chemical compound; this approach allowed the researchers to "turn on" the pathological processes whenever they wanted to, simply by switching the mice to a diet that lacked that one compound. In this way, the researchers could control exactly when and for how long the pathological processes were allowed to run.[25] When these mice are allowed to develop normally into adulthood and are then induced to develop Alzheimer's-like pathologies over a subsequent 6-week period, they end up behaving normally in terms of their activity and anxiety levels, but they show marked impairment in contextual fear conditioning and spatial memory tasks. In addition, they experience significant neurodegeneration—that is, loss of neurons (and synapses)—in their forebrains.[26]

The question Tsai has been pursuing recently is, What sorts of therapies might be able to alleviate these pathologies? One of her hypotheses was that a brain suffering from this sort of neurodegeneration might be better off if its remaining healthy neurons are supported by experiences in an enriched environment. The environment of a typical lab mouse is rather impoverished, so "enrichment" here just means providing a couple of running wheels, some Habitrail-like climbing devices, some other toys that are changed daily, and the presence of some playmates. This type of enrichment has been known for decades to improve rodents' learning abilities and to alter their brain chemistries,[27a–27b] so it was reasonable to think it could potentially help mice that had experienced the kind of neurodegeneration associated with Alzheimer's disease. And as expected, data from the Tsai lab indicate that living for a month in an enriched environment *does* facilitate learning and the formation of new memories in mice that have suffered severe neurodegeneration.[28]

But enriched environments might be even more powerful than that: It appears they can help mice recover forgotten long-term memories, a feat that would have had Sigmund Freud swooning. To demonstrate this phenomenon, Andre Fischer and his colleagues in the Tsai lab used a contextual fear conditioning paradigm in which adult mice that had not yet experienced any neurodegeneration were given a shock after three uneventful minutes in a neutral testing chamber. Because we know that in normal mice, a memory for this kind of experience is formed in the hippocampus and is then transferred after about four weeks to the cerebral cortex, Fischer sent his mice back to their home cages following the initial fear conditioning. After four normal weeks at home—during which their newly formed memories were presumably consolidated in their cerebral cortices—their diet-switch was turned on, beginning the process of neurodegeneration. After six weeks of neurodegeneration, the mice were returned to the testing chamber so their memories could be evaluated, now 10 weeks after their initial experience being shocked in the chamber. And as might be expected given their newly developed Alzheimer's-like symptoms, once they were in the chamber, they behaved like mice that had never been shocked there before; in contrast to normal, healthy mice who acted fearfully in the chamber because they remembered their experiences from 10 weeks earlier, these mice were not afraid at all. Their long-term memories of their experiences in the chamber were gone.

Or were they? Perhaps the memories were not gone, but had merely become inaccessible. To test this possibility, the research team gave a new group of mice all of the experiences just described, but rather than evaluating them immediately after 6 weeks of neurodegeneration, the team evaluated them an additional four weeks after that. Half of the mice in this study—the control mice—spent those four extra weeks in their usual cages; the other half spent them in the enriched, toy-filled environment. So to recap, here we have a group of mice that underwent contextual fear conditioning, after which they were returned to their cages where their memories were consolidated. Then, they all experienced 6 weeks of neurodegeneration, which we know is enough to cause them to have forgotten their shocking experiences 10 weeks earlier. Then, half of these mice spent 4 weeks in an enriched environment and half spent 4 weeks in their usual cages, after which their memories were evaluated.

As a result of the initial experimental steps, all of the mice—both those that experienced the enriched environment and those that did not—had similar levels of neurodegeneration. But in contrast to the control mice, the enriched-environment group behaved in the memory test as if they remembered their shocking experiences in the chamber 14 weeks earlier.[29] Thus, the researchers concluded that forgotten "long-term memories can be recovered by [environmental enrichment and] . . . that the apparent 'memory loss' is really a reflection of *inaccessible* memories . . . [similar to when patients with dementia] experience temporary time periods of apparent clarity."[30] Such results are particularly noteworthy because the memories that were recovered were formed *before* the mice experienced any neurodegeneration; environmental enrichment reestablished access to these memories "after significant brain atrophy and neuronal loss had already occurred,"[31] an outcome many researchers previously would have considered impossible.

Inhibiting HDACs with Drugs, Small RNAs, and Enriched Environments: Seeking Treatments for Symptoms of Alzheimer's Disease

Of course, the question remains: How can it be possible for mice to recover memories like this? The answer appears to be "epigenetics." In normal mice, environmental enrichment leads to the acetylation of histones in both hippocampal and cortical cells, much as the administration of HDAC inhibitors does;[32] thus, as Sweatt has pointed out, "two very different types of treatments, environmental enrichment and inhibition of HDACs" improve memory in normal rodents.[33] This observation suggests that reinstatement of "lost" memories via environmental enrichment might involve histone acetylation, a hypothesis that can be tested using HDAC inhibitors.

To examine this possibility, Fischer and colleagues exposed their genetically engineered mice to the same sequence of experiences described above, but instead of arranging for 6 weeks of neurodegeneration to be followed by 4 weeks of exposure to toys and playmates, the researchers arranged for 6 weeks of neurodegeneration to be followed by 4 weeks of daily injections of an HDAC inhibitor. As a result of the injections, the mice recovered memories of their fear conditioning experiences, memories that were lost to control mice that had similar experiences and only received daily injections of saline.[34] Thus, chronic injections of an HDAC inhibitor—like exposure to an enriched environment—led to recovery of long-term memories that were lost after neurodegeneration. These positive results led the researchers to speculate that HDAC inhibitors might also "be capable of re-establishing neural networks in human brains,"[35] much as they improve cognition in mice. And then they went one step further, arguing that if that's right, then "small molecules that target HDACs"—for instance, very small RNA molecules—could potentially be used "in patients with dementia [to] facilitate access to long-term memories."[36]

A recent study in Tsai's lab followed up on this conjecture, exploring the possibility that injecting very small RNAs into the brains of genetically engineered mice might alleviate some of their Alzheimer's-like symptoms.[37] The targeted molecule in this study was HDAC2, because HDAC2 is elevated in the hippocampus of people with Alzheimer's disease and has a causal role in producing the cognitive deficits that characterize genetically engineered mice that have experienced neurodegeneration.[38] Thus, the idea was to use small RNAs that interfere with the production of HDAC2 *alone* and thereby improve memory the way injected HDAC inhibitors do, but with fewer side effects. Motivating this study was the researchers' belief that "cognitive capacities in the neurodegenerating brain are constrained by an epigenetic blockade of gene transcription that is potentially reversible";[39] by experimentally interfering with epigenetic processes, the scientists hoped to stimulate genetic activity and thereby improve cognitive functioning.

This work revealed that preventing the accumulation of HDAC2 completely eliminated the memory impairments associated with neurodegeneration,[40] and in some cases led to the *recovery* of cognitive competences that are typically damaged by neurodegenerative diseases like Alzheimer's. These findings led the researchers to conclude that "epigenetic mechanisms substantially contribute to the cognitive decline associated with Alzheimer's disease-related neurodegeneration"[41] and that it is possible to selectively inhibit HDAC2 while leaving other HDACs functioning as normal. This was undeniably a very encouraging result. Unfortunately, getting the small RNAs into the experimental mice in the first place required the researchers to genetically alter some viruses and then inject the altered viruses into their subjects' brains, a procedure unlikely to appeal to most human patients!

Fortunately, as we have seen, HDAC-inhibitor drugs and small RNAs are not the only ways to inhibit HDACs,[42] and there is one way that is unlikely to have any unwanted side effects: environmental enrichment. In our rush to help people suffering from psychological disturbances like depression, our society has been quick to embrace medications like Prozac, drugs that work by influencing neurotransmitter systems in our brains. The effectiveness of drug treatments has reinforced our sense that these psychological disturbances are caused by biological events, and it has mislead many people into thinking that these biological events are somehow disconnected from our experiences and therefore treatable *only* with medications. In fact, depressive symptoms always *do* entail biological events, but these events often follow social events, such as divorce or the death of a loved one. Because our environments are connected to our biology like this, the biological contributions to depression can be affected by experiences like talking with a good psychotherapist. Talk therapy influences brain function much like antidepressants do.[43] Indeed, as Kandel wrote in a 2013 opinion piece in the *New York Times*, "psychotherapy is a biological treatment, a brain therapy. It produces lasting, detectable physical changes in our brain."[44] Likewise, although drugs and injected small RNAs can inhibit the effects of HDACs, it is noteworthy that enriched environments can as well. As researchers continue to work to understand memory, it is good to know that we can all help our minds stay sharp in the meantime by enriching our lives with cognitively stimulating activities,[45] exercise,[46a-46b] and other forms of physical activity.[47]

"To forgive is wisdom, to forget is genius"[48]

It is worth noting that all of this talk about the beneficial effects of HDAC inhibition should not be taken to mean that HDACs are inherently "bad." On the contrary, they perform very important functions in our bodies. As is true of genes, what matters is not so much what molecules you have in your body, but *what they are doing* (and when they are doing it). If an HDAC is affecting a DNA segment associated with the development of cancer, the HDAC is performing a very important function: silencing that cancer-promoting gene. In contrast, we would feel very differently about an HDAC that is silencing a gene that normally works to *suppress* tumor growth. A similar situation in the domain of memory led Day and Sweatt to point out that "memory formation involves both increased methylation at memory suppressor genes and decreased methylation at memory promoting genes. Thus, memory function might be driven by either hypermethylation or hypomethylation."[49] In the complex world of molecular biology, neither specific genes, specific epigenetic marks (e.g., methylation), nor specific proteins (e.g., HDACs or cortisol) can be considered "the good guys" or "the bad guys."

Likewise, although we often think of memory *loss* as a "bad" thing, it is actually not that simple. In fact, functional memory systems *need* a mechanism for forgetting. Without this kind of mechanism, we would all be in a constant state of confusion; when leaving my office on Friday, I would be faced with competing memories about where I parked my car, because I would remember *with equal clarity* having parked earlier that week on the street, in the school garage, *and* at the park "n" ride lot! When I buy a new green toothbrush to replace my old blue one, I need to *forget* the memory of my old blue toothbrush, so that I don't mistakenly use my wife's new blue one.

In a 2007 article that really drives this point home, Timothy Bredy and colleagues considered the process of *extinction* of conditioned fear, a process in which an animal forgets a previously learned association between a stimulus and an unpleasant event.[50] So far, I have been writing as if it is a *problem* when a mouse forgets the context in which he previously experienced a shock. But people with anxiety disorders sometimes continue to be fearful in safe circumstances because they can't forget about a bad—but rare—experience they previously had in those circumstances. Forgetting these earlier experiences can be a very important step toward psychological health.

The kind of forgetting Bredy and colleagues studied—the extinction of conditioned fear—turns out not to involve the *erasure* of an old memory, but rather the creation of new memories that reduce fear of previously scary stimuli. To illustrate, if the inside of a Boeing 707 induces fear in a person because he experienced a lot of turbulence the first time he was on a jet, extinction of conditioned fear would involve *learning* to *not* get anxious in that context; this new learning would normally occur with repeated exposures to the inside of a 707 during uneventful, smooth flights. Because extinction of conditioned fear is a form of learning, it should (just like any other form of learning) depend on the expression of genes that are epigenetically regulated. Accordingly, in their studies of normal adult mice, Bredy and colleagues looked at histone acetylation around promoters for the BDNF gene in prefrontal cortex cells.

The results of their study were clear. Extinction of conditioned fear was associated with increased histone acetylation in these promoters, and therefore, with increased expression of the BDNF gene in the studied cells. Interestingly, the epigenetic effects of *learning to be afraid* and *learning to no longer be afraid* were different; as these researchers put it, "acquisition and extinction of conditioned fear results in distinct histone modifications around two BDNF gene promoters in the prefrontal cortex."[51] Given the previously discussed finding that contextual fear learning and latent inhibition involve the acetylation of different histones,[52] the finding that the *extinction* of conditioned fear also produces distinctive histone modifications supports the hypothesis that there is a "histone code" for memory formation.

Bredy and colleagues understood that if histone acetylation is associated with the extinction of conditioned fear, then HDAC-inhibiting drugs might facilitate the process of *remembering to forget* outdated memories. And after testing this hypothesis, these researchers reported that the HDAC inhibitor valproic acid does improve "long-term memory for extinction"[53] because of how it increases histone acetylation. This is a particularly important finding. Anyone who has successfully fought a fear of flying knows that a single reexposure to turbulence can bring back anxiety with a vengeance; this "reinstatement" of a previously overcome fear is a bane of therapists trying to help people with anxiety disorders. Therefore, mental health professionals are justifiably excited about HDAC inhibitors; when combined with psychotherapy, such drugs might be extremely useful in the treatment of people with anxiety disorders,[54] helping them to effectively remember to forget the fears that they have learned are unwarranted.

Anxiety disorders are not the only disorders in which learning and memory play a role. Because drug addiction relies in part on learned associations between positive feelings produced by drugs and stimuli such as drug paraphernalia, many theorists have long thought that drug addiction, too, should be understood as a kind of learning and memory disorder.[55a-55b] Likewise, post-traumatic stress disorder is a condition clearly influenced by the processes that form and maintain memories.[56] Therefore, epigenetic treatments for these disorders are conceivable. In fact, the list of psychopathological conditions associated with epigenetic effects has grown rapidly in recent years, and now includes maladies such as eating disorders,[57] mood disorders,[58a-58b] schizophrenia,[59a-59b] and more. Research on the roles of epigenetic factors in these disorders has only recently gotten underway; I will consider the implications of epigenetic research for the treatment of such disorders in the chapter "Hope."

15

Nutrition

In 1989, I finished a postdoctoral fellowship and began searching for a job as a professor. One of the schools that expressed interest in my application was Pitzer College, a small college founded in the 1960s, whose primary claim to fame was membership in a consortium known as the Claremont Colleges. When I went to interview at Pitzer, most of the eight-member psychology department was nearing retirement, so it was important to me that I be impressed with the few psychologists who would continue to be around for the first part of my career. There were several reasons I ultimately took the job in Claremont, but one of them was a scientist named Alan Jones, who was at the time the youngest member of the psychology group. To all appearances, Jones was a hippie back then, a good two decades behind the times. But if you listened to him talk about his science—and if you somehow knew what the future had in store—it would have been clear that he was actually two decades ahead of his time.

Seven years earlier, Jones had published a paper in *Science* in which he and a colleague reported on studies of malnourished pregnant rats.[1] The strange thing about these studies was that even though *women* malnourished during pregnancy produce offspring who are consistently *under*weight, Jones found that pregnant rats that were malnourished for their first two trimesters produced male offspring that had normal birthweights but that began eating ravenously about 5 weeks later. Ultimately, these offspring grew up to be *heavier* than rats born to mothers who ate normally during pregnancy.

My students are always curious about where researchers get their ideas for their studies, and this experiment definitely raises that question, because it is not at all obvious why a researcher might want to underfeed a pregnant rat for two trimesters, and then suddenly start giving it access to as much food as it wants. In this case, though, Jones was modeling his work after a very specific historical event known as the Dutch Hungerwinter. In the 1980s, this heartbreaking episode at the end of World War II was relatively unknown, but it has since become recognized as an exceptionally good example of an inadvertent "experiment" on the effects of famine on developing fetuses.

In the autumn of 1944, the Nazis began a siege of western Holland, to retaliate for the activities of the Dutch resistance movement. After a few months, the blockade was so successful that daily food intake across the region had fallen to about 50% of normal. The famine was severe enough to kill over 20,000 people,[2] but some of those who survived were women in various stages of pregnancy that winter. And as abruptly as it began, the Dutch Hungerwinter came to an end with the arrival of the Allies in the spring of 1945, after which the people were again able to eat normally. The fact that the food deprivation ended abruptly meant that some fetuses were exposed to malnutrition only during their 1st trimester in utero, some were exposed to malnutrition only during their first *two* trimesters, and some were malnourished during all three trimesters. Therefore, as tragic as this story is, the individuals conceived that year have provided researchers with a valuable trove of data that has helped elucidate how prenatal experience with malnutrition influences characteristics in adulthood.

Because the brain begins developing in the first trimester of pregnancy, malnourishment in this period is associated with a variety of neurological abnormalities, including spina bifida and cerebral palsy. Researchers also discovered that embryos exposed to the Dutch famine soon after conception were twice as likely as normally nourished embryos to develop schizophrenia.[3a–3b] But Jones was interested in a more subtle and truly counterintuitive finding: Male fetuses exposed to the Dutch famine for their first two trimesters—but not their third—were more likely than normal to grow up to be obese adults.[4] This is why Jones was interested in malnourishing pregnant rats for the first two-thirds of their pregnancies. He hoped to reproduce the Hungerwinter effect in animals as a way to start figuring out how this kind of experience so soon after conception could affect a person's phenotype—a defining characteristic, in some ways—decades later in life.

By 1990, Jones had demonstrated that injecting the hormone insulin into rats when they were in their third trimester of pregnancy also contributed to the development of obesity in male offspring.[5] This experiment established how switching from famine to normal eating after two trimesters could have its physiological effects; because this kind of dietary change would *naturally* increase insulin concentrations in pregnant rats, the conclusion was that increased prenatal exposure to insulin accounted for the obesity in adulthood. Of course, the epigenetic effects of experience were not yet on anyone's radar 25 years ago, so Jones did not immediately start studying the chromatin in fetal neurons. Nonetheless, this work was clearly at the leading edge of a new way of thinking about the origins of some of our characteristics, because it suggested that a woman's food intake during pregnancy can influence her hormones in ways that can generate long-lasting effects in her children's brains.

The Developmental Origins of Health and Disease

At the end of the 20th century, the British clinical epidemiologist David Barker started synthesizing a large quantity of data into a paradigm now known as DOHaD, which stands for the "developmental origins of health and disease."[6a–6b,7] Starting with the established fact that babies born at a low birthweight grow up to be adults with "increased rates of coronary heart disease and the related disorders stroke, hypertension, and non-insulin dependent diabetes,"[8] Barker helped establish DOHaD as the discipline that studies how prenatal experiences produce long-term effects on phenotypes. At the core of the endeavor was the idea that people are malleable early in life, and responsive to their developmental environments. Barker explained why things might work this way:

> There are good reasons why it may be advantageous, in evolutionary terms, for the body to remain plastic during development. It enables the production of phenotypes that are better matched to their environment than would be possible if the same phenotype was produced in all environments... Plasticity during intra-uterine life enables animals, and humans, to receive a "weather forecast" from their mothers that prepares them for the type of world in which they will have to live. If the mother is poorly nourished she signals to her unborn baby that the environment it is about to enter is likely to be harsh. The baby responds to these signals by adaptations, such as reduced body size and altered metabolism, which help it to survive a shortage of food after birth. In this way plasticity gives a species the ability to make short-term adaptations, within one generation.[9]

Thus, just as restricting the food intake of a pregnant woman produces long-term effects in her offspring,[10] giving pregnant mammals a high fat diet[11a–11b] or even just a diet lacking certain nutrients[12a–12b] could have long-term effects as well, particularly if the environment the offspring encounters after it is born is different from the one the mother experienced while she was pregnant.[13a–13b] In that case, the fetus develops what *would* be adaptations in the environment it "expects" to encounter, but these wind up being maladaptive in the environment it *actually* encounters. This sort of "developmental mismatch"[14] between the environment present during gestation and the environment present after birth seems to characterize the experiences of the children conceived during the Dutch Hungerwinter.

A number of researchers have referred to these kinds of effects as "fetal progr amming"[15a–15c] because of how some early experiences seem to *permanently* alter how the body is structured and how it operates. As I see it, we should be wary of claims that a particular biological effect is irreversible, because as we learn more about how a system works, it is rather common to discover previously unforeseen ways of influencing it; imagine the embarrassment of any biologist who confidently proclaimed that cloning mammals would be impossible because mature cells are "permanently" differentiated! Given what we understand about epigenetics now, "programming" is almost certainly a misleading word in this domain.

Moreover, just as we shouldn't consider genetic factors to be the sole cause of complex phenotypes, we also shouldn't consider an experience like prenatal malnutrition to be the sole cause of complex phenotypes. Mark Hanson and Peter Gluckman—two of the more prolific writers currently contributing to the DOHaD literature—recently said as much in a paper on epigenetics. They wrote that environmental factors like prenatal nutrition do not *cause* diseases like heart disease and diabetes; "they merely influence the risk of disease in a later obesogenic environment,"[16] "obesogenic" referring to the cookie-and-French-fry-filled environments so many of us in the West now occupy. If you expend as many calories as you consume as an adult, you will ordinarily not become obese or develop the syndromes of obese people, regardless of what your prenatal experiences were. The phrase "fetal programming" obscures this truth.

Notwithstanding these terminological criticisms, it is clear that experiences very early in development have the potential to influence adult phenotypes, a fact that suggests a link with epigenetics. In many ways, this pattern of influence should be thought of as the very signature of epigenetics, because the processes responsible for cell differentiation—which are quintessentially epigenetic—occur very early in development and normally produce effects that persist throughout adulthood. This is one reason Gluckman and colleagues wrote in the first-ever issue of the *Journal of Developmental Origins of Health and Disease*, "The likely mechanisms that enable plasticity [of the sort that is emblematic of DOHaD] involve epigenetic processes."[17] In fact, "a growing amount of experimental data suggests that epigenetic processes explain a considerable amount of the DOHaD phenomenon."[18]

The Epigenetics of Nutrition: Beyond Overeating and "Fat Genes"

The reason our diets influence our epigenetic states is obvious once we ask where our bodies get the methyl groups that methylate our DNA: they come from our food! The most important provider of methyl groups during the DNA methylation process is a molecule called SAM. And SAM ultimately gets most of its methyl groups—the very ones it will donate during DNA methylation—from foods containing vitamins B_2, B_6, B_9 (also known as folic acid and folate), B_{12}, and choline;[19] thus, if a person's diet contains too much or too little of any of these nutrients, this can alter their supply of methyl groups.[20] The chemical constitution of these nutrients allows them to provide the raw materials necessary for several biological processes, which is why cereals are often fortified with them. This is also why women who have been pregnant are familiar with folic acid, a vitamin so essential for normal fetal development that doctors often advise women who could become pregnant to take folic acid supplements and to eat folate-rich foods like eggs, asparagus, liver, and dark green leafy vegetables like spinach. Women who consume too little folic acid in the month or so around conception are at increased risk of having a baby with major congenital abnormalities. Choline, which is present in foods like eggs, meats, wheat germ, cauliflower, and milk, is also important for normal fetal development,[21] and is an essential contributor to the process that produces SAM. And anything that adversely affects SAM production can ultimately produce epigenetic effects; not eating enough choline or folate leads to low SAM concentrations, which can lead to reduced methylation of both DNA[22] and histones.[23]

In an early experiment designed to study the effects of maternal diet on the epigenetic status of offspring, pregnant rats were fed either a normal diet, a protein-restricted diet, or a protein-restricted diet supplemented with folic acid.[24] Once the offspring were weaned, DNA from their liver cells was examined for evidence that these prenatal nutritive experiences had epigenetic effects. As expected, the offspring of mothers fed the protein-restricted diet had significantly less methylation in specific DNA segments than did the offspring of normally fed mothers. Interestingly, just supplementing the protein-restricted diet with folic acid was enough to prevent the effect; despite the reduced quantities of protein in their diets, the pregnant rats receiving this vitamin supplement had offspring with normal levels of DNA methylation in their livers. Supplementing a diet with folic acid, vitamin B_{12}, or other methyl donors can also have remarkably bold, *observable* effects on phenotypes in some mammals; the next chapter will present detailed evidence that diet can radically affect hair color in these animals via epigenetic mechanisms, while also having significant effects on the animals' health.

Perhaps surprisingly, even very subtle manipulations of a pregnant animal's diet can have significant effects on her offspring. Because major changes in DNA methylation occur normally in unfertilized eggs and in just-conceived embryos, a group of scientists in the UK thought they might be able to affect offspring by feeding mature female sheep a methyl-deficient diet for 8 weeks *before* conception and during the 1st week of pregnancy.[25] So, they fed one group of sheep a normal diet, and another group of sheep a diet that was different in only one way: It reduced the animals' access to methyl-containing nutrients. Importantly, these reductions were similar in magnitude to the reductions that occur naturally in some women who are not conscientious about their diets. Once the offspring of both groups of sheep had been conceived and allowed to develop in utero for

6 days, they were all transferred to surrogate-mother sheep that ate a nutritionally complete diet and that carried the fetuses to term. Ultimately, all of the offspring experienced the same nutritional environment for 96% of their time in utero and were born with normal birth weights, so this really was a very subtle experimental treatment.

Nevertheless, by the time they were adults, the sheep that were conceived in mothers with the methyl-deficient diet wound up fatter, resistant to insulin, and hypertensive (i.e., they had abnormally high blood pressures).[26] Furthermore, examination of the DNA in their livers when they were still fetuses revealed altered methylation patterns; most of the DNA segments affected by the dietary manipulation had reduced levels of methylation. The scientists concluded "that clinically relevant reductions in specific dietary inputs ... during the periconceptional period [i.e., both before and just after conception] can affect DNA methylation of a significant proportion of the genome in offspring, with long-term implications for adult health."[27]

This research raises the intriguing possibility that some of us have the rounder bodies we do not just because we have eaten too many calories or because we have genes that incline us to be on the heavier side. Instead, the implication of this work is that some of us might be a little plump in part because of the diets our mothers consumed before we were conceived or while we were in utero (or both). Of course, because a person's physique—like all complex phenotypes—has multiple determinants, our epigenomes alone cannot make us fat! Nonetheless, epigenetic effects of early nutritional experiences have been detected in human populations just as they have been detected in rats and sheep. Furthermore, a recent study reported that the methylation status of specific human DNA segments was able to account for about half of the variation found in the body compositions of a group of 9-year-old children.[28]

Much like altering access to B-complex vitamins, altering choline consumption during pregnancy can produce long-term effects on offspring, specifically on their behavioral and neurological characteristics.[29] Pregnant rats that eat a diet containing supplementary choline have adult offspring that perform better than control rats in specific kinds of spatial memory tasks, whereas choline-deficient diets during pregnancy ultimately impair performances of adult offspring.[30] These kinds of dietary manipulations have since been found to influence the prenatal development of the hippocampus (and other brain areas as well) in rats[31] and mice.[32] Given that a choline-deficient diet during pregnancy reduces a developing organism's access to SAM and thereby alters DNA methylation in both global and gene-specific ways,[33] it seems possible that any long-term effects of prenatal nutrition on learning and memory—like the long-term effects of prenatal nutrition on body mass—result from changes in DNA methylation.[34]

The Widespread Effects of People's Nutritional Experiences

These kinds of discoveries in rodents and sheep have led researchers to revisit people exposed to the Dutch Hungerwinter, to ascertain whether epigenetic events around the time of conception might have contributed to the disproportionate rate of obesity in this population.[35] To test this hypothesis, the researchers examined a DNA segment involved in producing a hormone that promotes prenatal growth. Compared with same-sex siblings who were not exposed to the famine before birth, those who were in utero during the famine had significantly less methylation on this DNA segment. Interestingly, people exposed to the famine late in gestation had methylation profiles similar to those of their unexposed siblings, so the effects of famine must be established earlier, closer to conception. Keep in mind, though, that by the time this study was conducted in the mid-2000s, the famine exposure had occurred 6 decades earlier; thus, the effects of an experience shortly after conception were detectable in people who were about 60 years old! The scientists who conducted the study conceded that nonnutritional stressors, such as emotional stress or exposure to cold temperatures, could have contributed to the obesity seen in this population; but even so, they concluded that their study generated "the first evidence that transient environmental conditions early in human gestation can be recorded as persistent changes in epigenetic information."[36]

A subsequent study found famine-exposed individuals to have other DNA segments, too, that were epigenetically different from the same DNA segments in their unexposed siblings.[37] In some cases, the effects depended on exposure around the time of conception, but in others, the effects depended on exposure later in gestation. In addition, the effects were somewhat different for men and women. As a result, it will take some additional work to sort out exactly how famine has the epigenetic effects it does. Nonetheless, these studies together indicate that nutritional factors in utero can influence methylation of several human genes, generating alterations that endure long after the person was exposed to famine. According to scientists active in this research area, "epigenetic alterations can no longer be ignored in evaluations of the causes of obesity and its associated disorders."[38]

Remarkably, epigenetic alterations influence a *variety* of adult phenotypes: physical conditions such as body size, metabolic conditions such as diabetes, and psychological conditions such as schizophrenia, to name a few.[39] These sorts of effects were unimaginable for a previous generation of scientists, and they have led to a new way of thinking about the origins of some diseases and about how our bodies store information related to past events. If you had asked scientists a mere 20 years ago about how our bodies store information, they would have pointed to the neural networks in our brains, which retain information collected in our lifetimes, and to our DNA, which retains information that has survived natural selection across multiple generations. But if you ask well-informed scientists the same question today, they will point to the epigenome as another information repository in our bodies.[40] The change in perspective is evident in the title of a recently published journal article: "The Epigenome: Archive of the Prenatal Environment."[41]

The discovery of a mechanism that controls gene expression and that can be influenced by dietary manipulations has opened the floodgates for researchers interested in the relationship between food and health.[42] To date, several studies have shown that dietary factors in addition to the B vitamins and choline have epigenetic effects. For example, a component of the spice turmeric—popular in Indian cuisines and a member of the ginger family—is known to inhibit the action of proteins that transfer acetyl groups onto histones (i.e., the HATs described in earlier "Zooming in" chapters). Similarly, components of some other foods (e.g., green tea) can inhibit the action of proteins that transfer methyl groups onto DNA.[43] Still other substances we consume, such as alcohol and zinc, can influence DNA methylation by affecting the number of methyl groups that are available for SAM formation.[44] These findings are likely to have important implications for us. To illustrate, the demonstration that maternally consumed alcohol can affect an embryonic mouse's epigenetic state (and ultimately the adult mouse's phenotype) could alter our understanding of how human fetuses develop fetal alcohol spectrum disorders when their mothers drink too much.[45] And research in this domain has the potential to reveal more than just the detrimental effects of stimuli like famine, alcohol, or malnutrition; it can also open our eyes to possible beneficial effects of certain diets, and inform and encourage researchers who are seeking treatments for various human ailments.

Eating Well Is the Best Revenge

An interdisciplinary field called "nutri-epigenomics"[46] has emerged in the last several years, and is devoted to exploring how nutritional factors influence gene expression.[47] Research in this domain has proceeded with some researchers seeking treatments for preexisting diseases and others exploring how dietary factors might *prevent* certain diseases by influencing epigenetic states. And while some of these studies have examined the effects of whole foods, others have examined the effects of nutritional supplements. (Another line of research similar to these has examined the effects of hormone treatments; for a particularly interesting example, see endnote number 48.)[48]

Some whole foods facilitate histone acetylation and thereby prevent gene silencing.[49] For example, a mere 3 to 6 hours after consuming broccoli sprouts, human beings were found to have increased histone acetylation in certain kinds of white blood cells,[50] a finding that could have important implications for some cardiovascular and neurological diseases, as well as for normal human aging.[51] Likewise, McGowan and colleagues have written optimistically about the utility of certain foods "as anti-inflammatory and neuroprotective agents in autoimmune diseases such as lupus and multiple sclerosis."[52] Carey has noted that other foods that have effects like broccoli include cheese and garlic, permitting the speculation that perhaps these or other foods could, "in theory . . . lower the risk of developing cancerous changes in the colon."[53]

Dietary supplements have also drawn the attention of researchers interested in nutri-epigenomics. As noted earlier, we have known for some time that enhancing pregnant women's diets with methyl supplements has positive effects on their *offspring*'s health and longevity,[54] but evidence has begun to accrue that daily consumption of SAM can have beneficial effects on adults as well. For instance, a nutritional SAM supplement marketed under the name SAM-e—and pronounced "Sammy"—appears to improve the mood of people diagnosed with clinical depression[55a–55b] and to be effective in treating the pain of degenerative arthritis.[56] These sorts of findings led McGowan and colleagues to conclude that "components of diet that influence the epigenetic machinery should be considered interventions that could affect mental as well as physical health."[57]

Of course, it might be a while before nutri-epigenomics research can yield helpful recommendations for human beings, because of how complex we are. For one thing, the foods we eat influence the availability of methyl groups throughout our bodies, so dietary treatments are unlikely to be able to target specific organs. In addition, it is important to remember that gene activation and gene silencing are not helpful in and of themselves; if the gene in question is one that has the potential to cause cancer, activating it is going to have a very different effect than activating a tumor suppressor gene (which could produce the opposite effect by preventing cells from progressing to cancer). Thus, nutritional supplements that contribute to pervasive increases in DNA methylation are unlikely to be as useful as more targeted treatments will be, once they have been discovered. Moreover, the value of dietary or other epigenetic treatments will vary depending on when in life the treatment is administered, because our brains and bodies *develop*, and thus are moving targets. So, an enormous amount of work remains to be done to determine how dietary experiences and interventions at various times influence the activity of specific genes in specific cell types.[58]

Nonetheless, the thrust of this story is already unmistakable. How our bodies appear to others, how they feel to ourselves, how we act, the nature of the emotions we experience—all of these things are affected by the nutrients we consume. And we can be fairly confident that when the data are in, they will confirm what our parents told us all along: Eat your greens and avoid the deep-fried Twinkies. But the adage that we are what we eat is only part of the story; we are also the way we are because of our parents' genetic constitutions. And what is increasingly being recognized is that we are also the way we are because of what our mothers *did* before and while they were pregnant with us. A woman who teaches her children to eat in a healthy way is giving her children an invaluable lesson, but a woman who *also* eats in a healthy way herself is giving her future children an additional head-start toward a long and healthy life.

In the last several years, it has started to look as though what future *fathers* consume can also influence their offspring's characteristics.[59a–59d] These sorts of effects strike most observers as something very different from maternal effects, because unlike fathers, mothers literally *are* the environments in which the next generation does its initial development. Thus, for many people, it is easier to imagine how a woman's behavior during pregnancy might influence her offspring than it is to imagine how a man's behavior could produce similar effects. This distinction opens the door to a broader discussion of the transmission of phenotypes across generations, that is, the question of biological and psychological inheritance. This topic is big enough and important enough to warrant its own section of this book, which will begin right after the next chapter, "Zooming in on Nutrition."

16

Zooming in on Nutrition

When I was 27 years old, I went to India with a friend. There was a major dust storm in New Delhi shortly after we arrived, but I slept right through it. I was so exhausted from both travel and jetlag that I could have slept through Armageddon. And when I finally woke up, it looked as though I had done just that; the entire city was blanketed in a fine thin layer of brown dust, making that otherwise visually explosive city look monochromatic. I was a young person in an environment unlike any I had been in before, so a lot of things I saw that day stuck with me. For example, I noticed that although almost all of the people on the street had black hair, some of them had hair that was noticeably lighter, an almost rusty color. I also noticed that although some of the people seemed to be homeless—they were bathing in the street—they still seemed happier than American homeless people, despite their poverty.

Years later, I was reading about the development of hair color when it suddenly dawned on me that the variations I saw in New Delhi that day were probably related to nutritional deficiencies and not to ethnic variations as I had initially assumed. In large swaths of the western world, it is rare to encounter people who are badly malnourished, so people in these communities typically don't have an intuitive sense that diet influences hair color; in communities where people consume adequate amounts of hair-color-relevant nutrients, it *seems* as though hair color is determined more by nature than nurture. People exposed only to well-nourished others would be less likely to notice that dietary factors influence hair color, because the importance of these nutrients only becomes apparent when they are not present in people's diets to an adequate degree.[1]

Of course, hair color is also affected in important ways by genetic factors. But as is always the case, our genes do not *determine* this phenotype independently of other factors. Our hairs have the color they do because of the amount of a chemical in them called melanin.[2] This pigment—which also colors our skin and eyes— is not a protein, so its composition is not encoded in a direct way in our genomes. Instead, melanin is *built* in a biochemical process in which specific proteins cobble together a variety of component molecules. And because some of those proteins and component molecules are only present in our bodies if we consume certain nutrients, diet influences hair color.[3] For instance, inadequate intake of copper[4] and iron[5] can interfere with the processes required to build melanin, facts that might explain why malnourished children have lighter hairs than they would otherwise have.[6] In retrospect, this is probably why some of the people I saw that day in New Delhi had rust-colored hair.

In fact, environmental factors other than diet can affect hair color in some mammals as well. Temperature, for example, influences the coloration of Himalayan rabbits, which are normally white with black extremities (i.e., ears, paws, nose, and tail). This pattern of coloration is so consistent among these rabbits that we might initially conclude that the pattern must be genetically encoded and likely to develop in just this way, regardless of any environmental factors. But it turns out that these rabbits' extremities are black because these body parts are always cooler than the body parts closer to the animal's center. How do we know that? Because if you shave the fur off of a Himalayan's back and then apply a cold pack to that area while the hair is regrowing, the new fur will come in black, not white.[7] As is the case for nutrients and human hair colors, the influence of temperature on a Himalayan rabbit's hair color is not detectable until the rabbit encounters an unusual variation in the environment (e.g., a razor and a cold pack). Thus, even if the effect of an environmental factor is hard to see in normal conditions, that doesn't mean the factor is ineffectual.

Although it is difficult in a well-nourished society to see the effects of diet on hair color, the effects of diet on some other traits are not at all subtle. Some of these obvious effects would be expected; for example, it is not surprising that malnourishing a developing brain is a recipe for psychiatric abnormality or that fetal undernutrition can affect later body weight. But some dietary effects are blatant and surprising. In a particular type of *pregnant* mice, for instance, variations in nutritionally adequate diets can have very bold effects on the offspring's coat color. And the big news here is that this dietary effect depends largely on an epigenetic mechanism.

Studies of these mice are important for a few reasons. First, one of their coat colors is associated with disease.[8] Second, these effects appear to be transmissible across generations; that is, the nutritional experiences of this kind of pregnant mouse can affect the coat colors of her grandpups,[9a–9c] an effect that has the potential to change thinking about how phenotypes are inherited. And finally, it is likely that experiments on these mice can teach us a lot about the mechanisms by which a pregnant woman's diet influences her children's metabolism, physique, and epigenetic states;[10a–10d] even if we are very different from mice in some ways, they are our mammalian kin and share about 99% of our genes,[11] so there is reason to think their molecular biology is related to our molecular biology.

The Case of the Kaleidoscopic Mice

Just as some horses are known to have coat colors unique to horses—bay, palomino, or dapple gray, for instance—some mice have coat colors associated with rodents. One such coat color is "agouti," which is the color of most wild mice. To the untrained observer, agouti looks like a medium-brown flecked with yellow; on close observation, this appearance can be seen to result from hairs that have alternating lighter and darker bands.[12a–12b]

Agouti-colored mice have a particular DNA segment that contributes to their distinctive coat color, a segment molecular biologists call "the *agouti* gene." Because this is a convenient shorthand, I will follow the biologists' lead and call this DNA segment *agouti*, but I should note up front that it is a misnomer. Although *agouti* contributes to an agouti coat color, it does not single-handedly specify that coat color, and it is known to influence a lot more than just coat color. Regardless, in most normally developing wild mice, *agouti* is switched on and off at various points while the coat is developing, thereby giving rise to the alternating bands of color that can be seen along individual hairs. Specifically, the tip of an agouti-colored hair is black because it developed when the gene was not being expressed, the middle section is yellowish because it developed when the gene was turned on, and the section closest to the body is black again, because it developed when the gene was once again silenced.[13]

Many genes (including *agouti*) come in a few alternative forms, each called an allele. In keeping with Gregor Mendel's mid-19th-century speculations, some of these alleles are considered "dominant" and others are considered "recessive." In cases where an organism inherits a dominant allele from one parent and a recessive allele from the other parent, the dominant allele is assumed to "overpower" the recessive allele, so the organism is expected to wind up with the phenotype associated with the dominant allele.[14] Mendel used uppercase letters to refer to dominant alleles and lowercase letters to refer to recessive alleles, so the dominant *agouti* allele—the one associated with the agouti coat color—is represented by the capital letter "*A*."

Several variations of *A* have been found in mammalian genomes.[15] For instance, a recessive allele represented by a lowercase "*a*" is sometimes present where we would otherwise find *A* in the genome. If both of a mouse's parents provide it with an *a* allele—in which case the mouse will be designated *a/a*—the mouse will develop a black coat, made of hairs that are black all along their lengths. Of course, because the *a* allele is recessive, if one parent provides an *A* allele and the other parent provides an *a* allele, the offspring—designated *A/a*—will have an agouti coat rather than a black one.

Another variation, a mutation that has been the subject of extensive epigenetic research, is known as the agouti viable yellow allele, symbolized by A^{vy}. As you might have surmised given the capital "A" in its symbol, the A^{vy} allele is dominant over the a allele. And as you might have surmised given its name—the "agouti viable *yellow* allele"—the presence of this allele in some mice is associated with a yellow coat;[16] in these animals, the *agouti* gene remains "on" the entire time the hairs are growing, rendering them yellow all along their lengths. *Agouti* is used to produce a protein that does different things in different cells, and its effects on coat color are due to what it does in the cells that produce hair. But because of what the protein does in *other* kinds of cells, yellow mice with an A^{vy} allele are not just abnormally colored; they are also typically obese[17] and relatively susceptible to developing diabetes[18] and cancerous tumors.[19] These mice may be "viable" in that they survive to adulthood, but they're definitely not the picture of health.

What makes mice with an A^{vy} allele exceptionally interesting is the fact that even among littermates bred to have effectively identical genomes—so called "congenic" mice—not all A^{vy} mice have the same coat color[20] (see Figure 16.1). Instead, congenic A^{vy} littermates have coat colors that fall along a continuum, varying from completely agouti, through gradations of mottled yellow-and-agouti, to completely yellow.[21] The "completely agouti" mice in such litters are actually said to be "pseudoagouti," because even though they have the exact same coat color as wild, unmutated agouti mice, they have the mutated A^{vy} allele rather than the unmutated A allele, so they are genetically different from normal agouti mice. In fact, they are genetically *the same as* their yellow siblings, but in addition to having a stunningly different coat color, they grow up to be leaner and healthier adults. Of course, this leaves us with a big question: Why the differences?

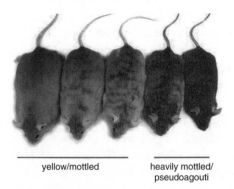

yellow/mottled   heavily mottled/
pseudoagouti

Figure 16.1 A photograph of genetically identical A^{vy} mice. These mice have a spectrum of coat colors, from yellow to pseudoagouti, with slightly mottled, half mottled, and heavily mottled coat colors in between. Reprinted with permission from Dr. Catherine Suter; original image printed in Cropley, J. E., Dang, T. H. Y., Martin, D. I. K., & Suter, C. M. (2012). The penetrance of an epigenetic trait in mice is progressively yet reversibly increased by selection and environment. *Proceedings of the Royal Society B, 279,* 2347–2353.

The differences between these genetically identical yellow and pseudoagouti mice are epigenetic. Specifically, the differences that account for their extremely different coat colors can be traced to a spot in the genome near the *agouti* gene. This spot is a kind of DNA segment known by a rather Star Trek-ish moniker—it's called a "retrotransposon" because it's a type of DNA segment that can change its position within the genome—and it contains information that can be used to create a noncoding RNA that keeps the agouti gene "turned on," thereby producing fur that is completely yellow.[22] When scientists examine the epigenetic status of this retrotransposon in congenic A^{vy} brothers and sisters, they find it to be highly methylated in pseudoagouti mice, relatively *un*methylated in their yellow siblings, and at intermediate levels of methylation in the siblings with yellow-and-agouti mottling.[23]

It makes sense that in this case, hyper- and hypomethylated retrotransposons are associated with darker and lighter fur, respectively, for the following reasons. When the retrotransposon is relatively unmethylated, the RNA that affects the *agouti* gene is *expressed*, which causes ongoing expression of the *agouti* gene; this leads the mouse to develop a yellow coat and its accompanying diseases. In contrast, a high level of methylation prevents expression of the *agouti*-activating RNA; therefore, the *agouti* gene is *not* persistently activated, allowing the mouse to develop the banded hairs that give it its normal agouti color.[24] More moderate levels of DNA methylation lead to offspring with coat colors somewhere on the spectrum between completely agouti-colored and completely yellow. Recent research has also confirmed the expected histone modifications at this retrotransposon.[25]

The observation that littermates with essentially identical genes *and* prenatal environments can nonetheless be born with varying coat colors raises an interesting question: What is responsible for the differing epigenetic states of these mice? It turns out that there is an element of randomness in epigenetics, which accounts for these observed differences.[26, 27] Although I have focused in this book on how experiences affect epigenetic marks, it is important to keep in mind that these marks can also be affected unsystematically.

You Are What You Eat: Bold Epigenetic Effects of Diet

Despite this element of randomness, DNA methylation can also be influenced by dietary factors, as described in the previous chapter. Because diet has this kind of power, Robert Waterland and Randy Jirtle, two scientists from the Duke University Medical Center in North Carolina, conducted a groundbreaking study in 2003 that involved manipulating the diets of virgin, genetically identical, black female mice that were then mated with males possessing an A^{vy} allele.[28] Specifically, half of the females were fed a normal, nutritionally adequate mouse diet throughout the study while the other half were given a special experimental diet beginning two weeks before impregnation, and continuing through pregnancy and lactation. This experimental diet was identical to the normal diet with one exception: It included supplemental methyl donors like folic acid, choline, and vitamin B_{12}. Thus, as the A^{vy} pups were developing in utero—and even after they were born and were feeding on their mothers' milk—their mothers continued to consume either the supplemented or the unsupplemented diet. The researchers' hypothesis was that the dietary manipulation might influence the coat color of the offspring in adulthood. Remember that in addition to affecting coat color, obesity, and diabetes in yellow A^{vy} mice, the *agouti* gene also contributes to cancer in these mice, so the discovery of a *nutritional* manipulation that affects this condition would indeed be something to write home about.

The results of the study were clear. The dietary supplements led to the birth of more agouti-coated offspring than found in the litters of the unsupplemented females, who produced proportionally more yellow (or mostly yellow) offspring. Furthermore, this effect lasted as the pups grew up to be adults. Thus, mice with identical genomes nonetheless developed strikingly different appearances that were influenced by the diets their mothers consumed before (and shortly after) they were born.[29]

To examine whether this effect really was related to DNA methylation as they had hypothesized, Waterland and Jirtle examined the retrotransposon near the *agouti* gene in cells taken from the supplemented offspring. As expected, the retrotransposon was hypermethylated, leading the researchers to conclude that methylation was "solely responsible for the effect of supplementation on coat color."[30] That is, the dietary supplements given to the mothers contributed to methylation of the retrotransposon in their unborn offspring, thereby *silencing* the DNA segment that contributes to the development of a yellow coat. In this way, the offspring of the supplemented mothers were more likely to have agouti coats. Moreover, Waterland and Jirtle also found epigenetic effects of dietary supplementation in *other* cells in the offspring, including liver, kidney, and brain cells. So, the maternal diet influenced more than just the offspring's coat color, contributing to these animals' lean and healthy bodies as well.[31]

Because retrotransposons are relatively common in the human genome,[32] these sorts of findings are likely to ultimately help us understand the development of people's characteristics as well. Specifically, the implication of Waterland and Jirtle's study is that nutritional supplements given to a pregnant woman can potentially influence the methylation of segments of her unborn child's DNA in such a way that the effects can last an entire lifetime. Unfortunately, the discovery that manipulations like this can have long-term effects cuts two ways. Feeding nutrients to mice pregnant with A^{vy} fetuses helped those fetuses grow up to be healthy, but accumulating evidence suggests that exposure to other substances can have long-term consequences that are detrimental.

Bisphenol A and Alcohol: Epigenetic Effects of Some Toxic Substances

As I noted in the previous chapter, maternal consumption of alcohol during pregnancy can influence the epigenetic state of mice developing in utero during the exposure;[33] presumably, this effect occurs because alcohol consumption can affect availability of the methyl donor SAM.[34] In the study that discovered this effect, some of the mice born to alcohol-consuming females developed smaller and abnormally shaped heads and faces, a pathology "reminiscent of fetal alcohol syndrome"; this led the researchers to conclude "that moderate [alcohol] exposure in utero is capable of inducing changes in the expression of genes other than A^{vy}, a conclusion supported by [a] genome-wide analysis of gene expression in these mice."[35] Scientists do not yet understand enough about how alcohol influences epigenetic states to explain the results of this study in their entirety, but the effect itself is interesting and worrisome.

Another substance of concern is bisphenol A (BPA), a chemical used in some plastics. Some studies have shown that BPA interferes with the normal functioning of mammalian hormone systems. Although legislation has restricted its use in baby bottles in countries such as Canada, Denmark, and France, BPA continues to be present in many food containers and plastic bottles around the world, in part because some studies suggest that the low levels to which most people are exposed are not harmful. Regardless of the *amounts* of BPA in the environment, most of us are exposed to it to one degree or another; a 2005 study of nearly 400 adults in the United States detected BPA in the urine of 95% of the sample.[36] Since some research suggests that BPA exposure very early in development is associated later in life with "higher body weight, increased breast and prostate cancer, and altered reproductive function,"[37] studies of the mechanism by which this substance has its effects are certainly warranted.

So far, we know that A^{vy} fetuses developing in female mice that eat BPA-contaminated food experience reduced methylation of the retrotransposon near the *agouti* gene, and are therefore at increased risk of growing up to be yellow, obese, diabetic, and cancer-plagued.[38] That is, just as a maternal diet supplemented with folic acid, choline, and vitamin B_{12} increases the likelihood of developing an agouti coat, a maternal diet mixed with BPA increases the likelihood of developing a yellow coat and an unhealthy constitution. On the upside, in the studies that produced these data, supplementing the BPA-laced diet with methyl donors like folic acid prevented the development of the unhealthy phenotypes. This finding led the researchers to conclude that "the negative effect of BPA on the epigenome was negated by supplementing the food with a mixture of methyl donors . . . Thus, food is medicine."[39] Whether or not this study warranted such an expansive conclusion, it is increasingly evident that *some* foods can help restore health, just as grandmothers have been telling their coughing, stuffy-nosed grandchildren for generations.

Research on the epigenetics of diet has yielded several interesting conclusions, but perhaps the most amazing idea to emerge from this work is the suggestion that grandparents pass on more to their descendants than just their genes and their advice. In fact, there is now experimental evidence that the effects of some prenatal experiences—such as those explored by Waterland and Jirtle[40]—can last *beyond* a lifetime, influencing the characteristics of an affected animal's descendants for at least another generation. That is, in some cases, it appears that the experiences of a pregnant female mammal can affect not just the daughter growing in her womb, but her grand-offspring as well.[41a–41c] Similar transgenerational effects of experiences have been detected in male lines, too,[42a–42d] posing what some theorists see as a challenge to traditional ways of thinking about how evolution operates.[43a–43e] The next four chapters will focus specifically on a variety of exciting discoveries related to epigenetic inheritance.

PART III

THE MEANINGS AND MECHANICS OF INHERITANCE

17

Inheritance

My brother's son turned two years old a few months ago, and he provides no end of fascination for my family. Mostly, he's just too cute for words. But there's one thing about him that stops me in my tracks sometimes. He looks like a living, breathing version of the subject of a photograph I've seen in my parents' house since *I* was a toddler. The strange thing about the photograph is that it's said to be a picture of my father when *he* was two years old, even though that's a little hard to believe: The toddler in the photograph—a blond-haired, oddly dressed cherub—doesn't look much like the masculine, dark-haired, sharply dressed father I've known my whole life. If the picture didn't provide the sepia cue that it's too old to be a current image of my little nephew, anyone would swear that it's a photograph of him rather than my father.

The question of how people come to have characteristics like those of their parents, grandparents, or older ancestors has probably always captivated people, but it took on new importance in the years after Darwin published *On the Origin of Species* in 1859. In his masterpiece, Darwin argued that the very fact that off-spring tend to resemble their parents allows for evolution and provides part of the explanation for why species differ and are so well adapted to their natural habitats. Given how important and compelling we all find the transmission of traits from generation to generation, it is somewhat surprising that as recently as 1900, no one had an inkling about how biological inheritance actually works. But the last century saw explosive growth in our understanding of these processes, shedding light on the origins of life's rich pageant and contributing to our grasp of how and why certain traits run in families.

As I have stated in previous chapters, epigenetic marks are sometimes trans-mitted across generations and play a role in the intergenerational transmission of traits. This discovery has generated controversy among biologists, because when we combine the assertion that epigenetic marks can be *inherited* with the discovery that they can be influenced by experiences, we wind up with the con-clusion that descendants can inherit attributes that their ancestors *acquired* dur-ing their lifetimes. The possibility that acquired characteristics can be inherited is a very old idea that was carefully considered by European and American biologists at the start of the 20th century, and then rejected categorically.[1] By the late 1930s, western biologists had become convinced that acquired characteristics could not be inherited. The resurrection of this idea in the context of epigenetics, then, has led some biologists to adopt a skeptical stance toward some of this work.[2a-2d]

Some care *is* warranted when considering assertions about epigenetics, and in the chapter titled "Caution" I will provide several examples of claims about epigenetics that really should be considered questionable. But there is now good evidence that some epigenetic marks can be inherited, and given particular (but perfectly reasonable) definitions of the words "acquired" and "inherited," it is also quite clear that acquired characteristics can be inherited. Consequently, recent discoveries about epigenetics are forcing biologists to reconsider some of the ideas they once held sacred.

But before moving on to inheritance, let's briefly review the conclusions we can draw from the last several chapters; even if epigenetic marks were *not* transmittable across generations, the kinds of epigenetic effects we have already encountered would be extremely important, as they highlight how experiences can influence what genes do from conception through adulthood. In rodents, the epigenetic states of fetuses are affected by the nutritional environments created by their mothers; the epigenetic states of newborn pups are affected by their mothers' caregiving behaviors; and the epigenetic states of adults are affected by the experience of learning something new. In humans or nonhuman primates, the epigenetic states of fetuses appear to be affected by experience with maternal depression, maternal diet, or domestic violence; the epigenetic states of children appear to be affected by exposure to abuse or poverty; and the epigenetic states of adults are affected by the stress of being at the bottom of a social hierarchy. And these are just the influential experiences epigeneticists have discovered to date, because they are the experiences that have been studied. At this point, it would be a reasonable bet that future studies will reveal epigenetic effects of many *other* kinds of experiences as well.

A Brief History of Modern Inheritance

The inheritance of acquired characteristics is controversial among biologists, so the discovery that some experience-induced epigenetic marks can be transmitted to descendants is controversial as well. To understand why, we need to consider what biologists mean by the words "acquired" and "inherited"; but even the definitions of these words are controversial. And because these words predate our modern conceptions, getting a handle on the controversy requires a look back at the history of these ideas.

The word "gene" was coined in 1909 by a Danish biologist named Wilhelm Johannsen.[3] Two years later, when considering exactly what biologists mean by the word "inheritance," Johannsen wrote:

> Biology has evidently borrowed the terms "heredity" and "inheritance" from every-day language, in which the meaning of these words is the "*transmission*" of money or things, rights or duties—or even ideas and knowledge—from one person to another . . . the "heirs" or "inheritors."[4]

Children tend to resemble their parents, and early biologists concluded that this reflects a kind of "inheritance"; just as material possessions can be transmitted from parents to children, biological and behavioral characteristics, likewise, were thought to be transmittable across generations. Even today, many people would accept the claim that my nephew looks like his grandfather because he *inherited* some of his grandfather's features.

But by 1911, Johannsen understood that it was naïve to think "the parent's (or ancestor's) *personal qualities*"[5] were transmitted to descendants. Darwin had thought about inheritance in this old-fashioned way, but Johannsen came to understand that this "conception of heredity represents exactly the reverse of the real facts." He continued:

> The *personal qualities* of any individual organism do not at all cause the qualities of its offspring; [instead,] the qualities of both ancestor and descendant are in quite the same manner determined by the nature of the "sexual substances"—i.e., the gametes [that is, the sperm and egg]— from which they have developed. Personal qualities are then the *reactions of the gametes* joining to form a zygote [that is, a fertilized egg]; but the nature of the gametes is not determined by the personal qualities of the parents or ancestors in question. This is the modern view of heredity.[6]

Here, Johannsen was arguing that although it looks to us as though *characteristics* are transmitted from one generation to another, the fact is that what is transmitted to the next generation is only what is contained in the sperm and egg.

According to this view, although we intuitively think my nephew looks like his grandfather because he inherited his grandfather's *features*, my nephew really inherited only raw materials provided by his mother and his father. It then fell to my nephew to *construct his own* characteristics as he developed, characteristics that—at the age of two years—are similar to the characteristics his grandfather developed by the time *he* was two. So even though we use the word "inherit" to describe the intergenerational transmission of both material possessions *and* biological traits, the two kinds of inheritance are really not much alike at all. If the inheritance of material possessions worked the way biological inheritance works, you would not be able to inherit your parents' house when they die, but instead would inherit only the lumber, granite, glass, and other raw materials required to build the house on your own.

There is another kind of biological inheritance, called *cellular* inheritance, which is very different from transgenerational inheritance. Cellular inheritance occurs when a cell divides to produce two daughter cells (as described in the chapter "Memory" and referenced in several of the preceding "Zooming in" chapters). In cellular inheritance, epigenetic marks are transmitted to daughter cells; that is, the daughter cells *inherit* the epigenetic state of their parent. This kind of epigenetic inheritance is critical for the daughter cells to be able to function like the parent cell, so this kind of inheritance is not at all controversial; there is a strong consensus among biologists that cells pass on their epigenetic characteristics to their daughters. I will not discuss cellular inheritance any further, and I mention it here only to be clear about the distinction between the two kinds of inheritance. *Cellular inheritance* occurs in an individual's body, so it takes place *within* an individual's lifetime. In contrast, *transgenerational inheritance* is the process by which individual organisms come to look and act like their parents, so it takes place across more than one generation.

Weismann Crushes Lamarck: Vanquishing the Inheritance of Acquired Characteristics

More than a century before Johannsen wrote about "the modern view of heredity," a French biologist named Jean-Baptiste Lamarck—the man some credit with coining the word "biology"—had published his own thoughts about biological inheritance. Lamarck should probably be celebrated as the man who gave the world the first-ever theory of evolution that actually attempted to explain *how* evolution might work.[7] However, he is mostly denigrated as the man who hypothesized that evolution entails the inheritance of acquired characteristics. Although this idea was rejected in the 20th century, most 19th-century thinkers considered Lamarck's hypothesis reasonable; a half-century after Lamarck published his ideas, Darwin even incorporated them into his own theory of evolution. When he wrote *On the Origin of Species*, Darwin believed the inheritance of acquired characteristics was compatible with natural selection, and in later editions of the *Origin*, he seemed increasingly convinced that Lamarck's mechanisms play a significant role in evolution.[8] It is quite clear that Darwin, like Lamarck, thought characteristics acquired through use or disuse could be transmitted to descendants.[9]

Everyone knows that we acquire some of our characteristics through the use or disuse of our bodies; for example, when we use our muscles, they get bigger, and when we don't, they shrink. A central proposition in Lamarck's theory was that such characteristics could be inherited. Lamarck thought this could explain the existence of animals like blind cave fish,[10] who normally spend their lives in darkness and who begin developing eyes as embryos but then grow up to be sightless as adults.[11] Specifically, he imagined that once upon a time, sighted fish lost their vision because they did not *use* that sense, and that their descendants then simply inherited their ancestors' blindness (remember, Lamarck was writing over 100 years before Johannsen figured out that organisms don't actually inherit characteristics per se from their ancestors). Likewise, a prototypical Lamarckian explanation asserts that giraffes have their long necks because of how ancestral giraffes *used* their necks, stretching them to reach the otherwise unreachable twigs and leaves high up in trees. Lamarck thought this neck stretching could have led to longer necks that were then inherited by offspring.

Neither Lamarck nor Darwin understood *how* characteristics are transmitted across generations. But because they both just wanted to make the case that species evolve, the insight that mattered was that evolution is possible whenever offspring resemble parents, *regardless* of how characteristics might be inherited. Of course, the question of *how* inheritance works is important, but it was a question that could have been answered with any of several hypotheses at the time, and any of those hypotheses would have been consistent with the general claim that living things evolve.

Lamarck's theory was generally held in high regard into the 1880s, when a German biologist named August Weismann started raising questions about *how* inheritance might work. In an 1889 essay, Weismann specifically addressed the question of the inheritance of acquired characteristics and its role in evolution. After calling Darwin out as a Lamarckist, Weismann wrote:

> Darwin was not only an original genius, but also an extraordinarily unbiassed [*sic*] and careful investigator. Whatever he expressed as his opinion had been carefully tested and considered. The impression is gained by every one who has studied Darwin's writings, and perhaps it in part explains the fact that doubts as to the correctness of the Lamarckian principle adopted by him have only arisen during the last few years. These doubts have, however, culminated in the decided denial of the assumption that changes acquired by the body can be transmitted. I for one frankly admit that I was in this respect under the influence of Darwin for a long time, and that only by approaching the subject from an entirely different direction was I led to doubt the transmission of acquired characters [i.e., characteristics]. In the course of further investigations I gradually gained a more decided conviction that such transmission has no existence in fact.[12]

To defend his newly won conviction, Weismann then describes experiments in which he first cut off the tails of mice, and then let the tail-less mice breed. The offspring—all with normal-length tails—were then similarly mutilated and allowed to breed. This next generation had normal tails too, so Weismann cut them off and let this generation breed as well. After five generations of this sort of treatment, none of the offspring were ever found to have a tail any different than the tails of their ancestors. Weismann acknowledged that his experiments did not *prove* that mutilations cannot be transmitted, because such a process might require more than just five generations. But as supporting evidence, he observed that cultural practices like circumcision have been carried out on well over a hundred successive generations of male Jewish babies without such practices ever resulting in foreskin-free newborns. So as far as Weismann was concerned, the experiences we have during our lifetimes do not affect the characteristics of our offspring, and the central mechanism proposed in Lamarck's theory of evolution had to be dead wrong.

Weismann's arguments were eventually enshrined in modern biology in a concept known as the Weismann barrier, a hypothetical boundary between germ cells—that is, sperm or eggs—and the rest of the cells that make up a body, the so-called somatic cells. This barricade is said to prevent alterations in somatic cells from having effects on the other side of the barrier, in the germ cells; this ensures that acquired characteristics cannot be inherited, because—remembering Johannsen's insight—offspring inherit only what is in the germ cells. From this perspective, to count as an example of "inheritance of an acquired characteristic," exercise-induced growth in a weightlifter's *muscle* cells would need to affect his *sperm* cells in a way that would make his son's muscles big *regardless of the son's experiences*. As Weismann saw it, if experience-induced effects on a person's somatic cells (e.g., muscle cells) cannot affect that person's germ cells, then the inheritance of acquired characteristics must be impossible.

Modern biology has confirmed that within two weeks of conception, some of the not-yet-differentiated cells in human embryos are induced to become "primordial germ cells" that will ultimately develop into sperm or eggs. Biologists refer to this process as the "segregation of the germline,"[13] a phrase that commendably captures their belief that once these cells differentiate from the somatic cells, they are "protected" from the influence of experience. And in fact, just as Weismann argued, segregation of the germline prevents experience-induced effects on somatic cells from affecting germ cells. In this way, if your great grandfather, your grandfather, and your father were all born with six fingers on each hand (but were otherwise normal), you are likely to be born with a sixth finger on each hand too, even if all three of these ancestors had their extra digits surgically removed in childhood.

This idea—that the hereditary material cannot be affected by experiential factors[14]—is known as "hard" inheritance, and it is responsible for the widespread belief in genetic determinism, the idea that phenotypes can be determined strictly by genes.[15] It is also a central tenet of the so-called modern synthesis,[16a–16c] the collection of concepts biologists cobbled together in the first half of the 20th century when they combined Darwinian ideas about evolution with emerging ideas about genetics. The modern synthesis (which is also known as the neo-Darwinian synthesis) is still accepted orthodoxy among most biologists today;[17a–17b] thus, genes alone are seen as being the drivers of evolutionary change[18] and the experiences we have in our lifetimes are understood to have no effect on our offspring.

This is why it is controversial to claim that epigenetic effects of experience might be inheritable.[19] Remember, for example, that the epigenetic effects of licking and grooming on newborn rats are found in the *brain cells* of the offspring; regardless of how interesting this finding might be, the inability of these effects to breach Weismann's barrier means that the offspring's germ cells cannot be affected. So, given traditional thinking in biology about "hard" inheritance, the effects of attentive mothering on a rat's stress reactions should not be transmittable to subsequent generations. As it happens, there are now a few well-studied cases of epigenetic effects that *are* transmitted through the germline[20a–20c]—that is, cases in which experiences alter epigenetic marks in sperm or eggs—but these might be exceptions. Thus, according to traditional thinking in biology, even if additional research reveals ubiquitous effects of experiences on the epigenetic states of *somatic* cells, we do not need to worry (nor, in some cases, can we hope) that these effects are going to be transmitted to our children's great-great-grandchildren.

Inheriting the Environment

There is just one problem with the neo-Darwinian assumption that "hard" inheritance is the only good explanation for the transgenerational transmission of phenotypes: It is hopelessly simplistic. Genetic determinism is a faulty idea, because genes do not operate in a vacuum; phenotypes develop when genes interact with nongenetic factors in their local environments, factors that are affected by the broader environment.[21a–21n] As the developmental biologist Scott Gilbert has put it, "The normal regulation of phenotype production by the environment should be considered a normal component of development."[22] Therefore, if a parent survived because she developed a particular characteristic and her offspring need to develop that same characteristic to survive as well, the offspring are going to need to inherit more than just their parent's genes; they will also need to "inherit" the nongenetic factors that helped their parent develop the adaptive characteristic in the first place.

Organisms always develop in specific contexts, and organisms that survive and reproduce will normally conceive the next generation in contexts like those in which *they* developed. In this way, individuals of the next generation are typically born into environments that are, in many ways, much like the environments their parents were born into; as a result, they then have similar experiences. And having inherited their parents' DNA *and* (in a sense) their parents' developmental environments, the offspring then typically develop the characteristics that helped their parents survive, doing so in the same way their parents did.

There is nothing particularly surprising about this claim; it follows merely from recognizing that, for instance, dolphins develop and then bear their offspring in the water whereas elephants develop and then bear their offspring on the land.[23] Because the development of adaptive traits always occurs in particular kinds of contexts, natural selection cannot "select" specific genes independently of their contexts. Instead, nature selects gene-environment *combinations* that together produce mature animals capable of surviving until they reproduce.[24] Because of the dawning awareness that natural selection works like this, scientists have increasingly accepted the idea that genes *coevolve* with their environments, an insight that has fostered a boom in research on the coevolution of genes and culture[25] and on the coevolution of genes and the microorganisms that live inside of us.[26]

This perspective on natural selection is representative of a school of thought known as developmental systems theory, or DST,[27] first proposed by the psychologist Susan Oyama in 1985 and later elaborated by the philosopher of science Paul Griffiths and the psychologist Russell Gray.[28] In conveying one of the theory's central ideas, Griffiths and Gray wrote, "species-typical traits are constructed by a structured set of species-typical developmental resources . . . Some of these developmental resources are genetic, others, from the cytoplasmic machinery of the zygote to the social events required for human psychological development, are nongenetic."[29] Thus, Johannsen was right; rather than inheriting *characteristics*, each new generation must *construct* those characteristics using raw materials— developmental resources—that their ancestors bequeathed to them. But whereas most of Johannsen's followers considered those raw materials to be chromosomes alone, Griffiths and Gray's focus on the context-dependent nature of development helped them see that the resources required for development include more than just DNA. The developmental resources we use to build our traits include our genes, of course, but they also include a variety of nongenetic factors.[30]

Simply by virtue of being conceived when and where they are, offspring effectively "inherit" several types of developmental resources, many of which are *required* to survive and reproduce. These include parent-provided resources such as cytoplasm in a mother's egg, a female mammal's ready-for-pregnancy uterus, and (of course) DNA. In addition, some animals provide their offspring with nutrition and shelter, and some even provide things like communication systems (among other resources). Other vital resources are provided independently of parents. These include resources that exist because of the cooperative actions of a group of individuals;[31] a community well is a good example, because although a pair of parents might not have helped dig the well, it still supports the survival of their offspring. Yet other resources are features of the natural environment, such as air, gravity, or wild blueberries; these factors are not provided by anyone in particular, but they still play important roles in phenotype development, and they are still effectively passed from generation to generation, ensuring that new organisms develop in environments like those that fostered their parents.

Because factors like gravity, a community well, a safe home, and a particular genome all influence how a person develops, all such factors are important developmental resources, regardless of their source (parents, other members of the community, or nature). From Griffiths and Gray's perspective, what matters is that offspring invariably develop in a context that has been provided to them and that affects the development of their phenotypes. And crucially, when these offspring grow up and reproduce, they too will raise their offspring in the same kinds of contexts that contributed to their own successful development. This understanding of the transgenerational transmission of the environment will help explain how some epigenetic effects of experience can be reliably passed down from one generation to the next.

The Demise of "Hard" Inheritance: Reopening the Door to Lamarckism

Adaptive characteristics develop only in certain circumstances, but they still normally reappear reliably in each descendant generation, reflecting the transgenerational transmission of *both* genetic and nongenetic factors;[32] in this way, the reliable reproduction of a phenotype in successive generations is tantamount to the transgenerational transmission of that phenotype. Consider, for example, our linguistic abilities, which are adaptive because they undoubtedly help us survive and reproduce. These abilities develop only in the context of other communicative people; their development depends on experience, as is evident from the tragic cases of feral children who fail to develop linguistic competence because they grow up in communicative isolation.[33a–33b] But in ordinary circumstances, linguistic abilities reappear reliably in generation after generation, because normal children are always raised in social contexts that provide linguistic interactions; linguistic abilities emerge during human development because each succeeding generation is normally provided with both the DNA and the social factors required to develop these abilities. Because of this reliable reappearance across generations, our linguistic abilities are just as transgenerationally transmittable as are any other adaptive characteristics.

This kind of transmission is different from the kind that most 20th-century biologists had in mind when they spoke of "hard inheritance," a phrase that implied inheritance *independent of experience*, that is, genetically determined inheritance. Does this mean we should consider the transmission of characteristics that *depend on experience* to be a kind of "soft" inheritance?

Awkwardly, this usage would be inconsistent with the original definition of "soft inheritance" developed by the renowned evolutionary biologist Ernst Mayr. Mayr coined the phrase "soft inheritance" to refer to a hypothetical kind of inheritance—actually, a Lamarckian kind of inheritance—in which experiences modify "the genetic basis of characters [i.e., characteristics]."[34] Of course, we now know that ordinary experiences never alter the sequence information in DNA, so given Mayr's definition, there can be no such thing as "soft" inheritance. In fact, this has been the established position of evolutionary biologists for some time: All inheritance is "hard," because ordinary experiences do not alter DNA sequence information. (I am using the word "ordinary" here because there are some *exceptional* experiences, such as being exposed to ionizing radiation or carcinogens, that can cause alterations in a DNA sequence.)

But look again at Mayr's definition. It *presumed* that some characteristics have a "genetic basis." This turned out to be an ill-founded presumption, because *all* characteristics develop from gene-environment interactions; none have a strictly "genetic basis."[35] In fact, nongenetic factors—and in some cases, experiences—can and do play critical roles in the development of the adaptive characteristics we "inherit" from our parents, from our linguistic abilities to some of the structural and organizational features of our brains. So although this kind of inheritance is not "soft" (because the experiences do not actually change DNA sequences), it is not "hard" either (because it is not genetically determined, or otherwise context-independent).

Mayr's distinction between "hard" and "soft" inheritance is no longer useful, because no one disputes the fact that DNA sequence information is impervious to ordinary experience. Nonetheless, some researchers have continued to refer to "soft inheritance" in some recent scientific works,[36a-36c] particularly in articles about epigenetics. In these articles, however, the definition of "soft" inheritance has been changed in a subtle, but important, way: It is no longer taken to imply changes in DNA sequence information. For instance, some writers consider the inheritance of epigenetic marks to be "soft," because even though DNA sequence information is not modified by normal experience, epigenetic marks that can be transmitted through the germline *can* be modified by experience.[37] Others have written that "soft inheritance has now been reborn: the demonstration of developmental epigenetic processes provides a solid molecular basis for understanding how environmental influences can affect the phenotype of the next generation."[38] However, because the phrase "soft inheritance" means different things to different people, I find it to be potentially confusing, so I will not use the hard/soft distinction in subsequent chapters.

Instead, I will proceed with the understanding that contextual factors influence the development of *all* of our characteristics, including physical traits like our body weights, our brain structures, and our skin colors, as well as psychological traits like our IQs, our religious beliefs, and our linguistic competences. None of our characteristics have a "genetic basis" alone, so the idea of "hard" inheritance as something distinct from some other kind of inheritance is a bankrupt notion. *There is only one kind of inheritance*, and it requires the transmission of both genetic and nongenetic developmental resources.[39] As Darwin recognized, if a characteristic is reliably reproduced from generation to generation—however it happens—that characteristic can be the object of natural selection and can be evolutionarily important. Such a characteristic is "inheritable" even though its development depends on nongenetic factors.

When considered from this perspective, there is a very real sense in which *all* characteristics are "acquired characteristics," because they are not present in zygotes and therefore have to be *acquired* during development. In this sense, then, we should not be surprised to find that children can "inherit" characteristics "acquired" by their parents, particularly when the developmental events experienced by offspring are similar to the developmental events experienced by their parents; this sort of thing happens all the time—literally![40] Thus, Lamarck's ideas were not as silly as Weismann—and most 20th-century biologists—would have had us believe.[41]

In fact, there are several ways children come to resemble their parents, and epigenetic marks can play important roles in these processes. As I have noted, there is good evidence that in some cases, epigenetic effects can be transmitted through the germline.[42a–42c] But Meaney-style epigenetic effects are different; by the time rats are born, their germ cells were long ago segregated away from their somatic cells, so the epigenetic effect of neonatal licking and grooming—which influences DNA in the (somatic) cells of their brains—cannot be transmitted through their sperm or eggs. And yet, studies I will describe in the next chapter indicate that the relevant DNA in the brains of rats licked and groomed as infants actually *is* epigenetically similar to the relevant DNA in their mothers' brains; thus, epigenetic effects can be "inherited" *even if the epigenetic marks are not transmitted through the germline*. What matters in evolution is that characteristics be transmitted from generation to generation, regardless of *how* that happens; from this perspective, then, it does not matter whether experiences produce epigenetic effects that are transmitted via the germline, or whether the epigenetic effects are transmitted some other way. Regardless of exactly how it works, it is now clear that some epigenetic effects can be passed from generation to generation.

18

Multiplicity

The idea that there are creatures living inside of us is the stuff of horror movies. When people watching *Alien* see the antagonist's spawn bursting out of Executive Officer Kane's chest, the horror comes from seeing a man die in an explosion of blood and guts, but it is heightened by the realization that the slimy, toothy alien has been growing inside of him ever since its mother attached herself to Kane's face. Parasites are probably extra creepy for us because we know such things are not fictional at all. The idea of a worm up to 10 meters long—that's over 32 feet!—living inside of a person's small intestine seems like an urban legend born around a boy scout campfire, but such tapeworms are real, and actually somewhat common among beef-eaters in many of the poorer parts of the world. Nonhuman organisms can and do live inside of us, so the willies are warranted.

Because of the bad press parasites receive, it might come as a surprise to learn that perfectly *healthy* human bodies host nonhuman organisms as well. In fact, this is the typical state of a healthy human body, because some of these organisms actually contribute to our health in the first place. Some of the microorganisms in our gut, for instance, synthesize vitamins that keep us healthy, regulate how we store fat, or allow us to break down components of vegetables we would otherwise be unable to digest;[1] others are thought to produce chemicals that help restore health after we have been ill.[2] Since these kinds of bacteria help us, we don't call them parasites; we call them "symbionts," a name that reflects the fact that we have a symbiotic relationship with them, meaning the relationship is not harmful to either party and could very well be of benefit to both. One of the crazy things about the symbionts in our intestines is that by the time we're adults, we have about 10 times as many of them living inside of us as we have cells of our own bodies![3] These organisms represent as many as 40,000 different species,[4] and together, they contain millions of genes, far more than the 20,000 or so genes contained in *our* cells.[5] That's right: There's at least as much microorganism DNA in your body as there is *human* DNA in your body.[6] The journal *Nature Reviews Microbiology* published an article about our resident microbes in which an editor put it bluntly: "To say that you are outnumbered is a massive understatement."[7]

Our guests may not be as cinematic as the *Alien* was, but they're clearly a force to be reckoned with, and they're unquestionably nonhuman organisms that make a home of our bodies.

These stowaways do more than just influence physiological functioning. It is now clear that the foreign organisms residing within us are *required* for the normal development of our digestive systems.[8a–8b] In fact, our microorganisms and our intestines appear to have coevolved with each other so that our bacterial symbionts are actually capable of causing the expression of *our* genes within some of our intestinal cells, thereby contributing to the normal postnatal development of our intestines.[9a–9b] Thus, the effects of our microbes must be considered "epigenetic" in the broad sense of that word, even if they do not methylate our DNA or modify our histones. But this is not why I am beginning this chapter by discussing symbionts. My question here is related to inheritance: If these organisms are required for normal development, how does nature ensure that they are passed down from parents to their new offspring?

Despite the crucial roles that bacteria play in the development of the human gut, they are not transmitted to offspring through the germline. And yet, they are already present in all normal newborn babies. As Scott Gilbert has explained, "We never lack these microbial components; we pick them up from the reproductive tract of our mother as soon as the amnion bursts."[10] That is, just after a mother's "water breaks," her about-to-be-born daughter's environment is suddenly flooded with these organisms that will then enter and live inside of her, helping her digestive tract develop normally. And when the daughter grows up and gets pregnant herself, she will pass these beneficial microbes on to her children in the same way. Even though this mechanism of transmission does not involve the germline at all, it certainly seems as though it should qualify as a kind of "inheritance," and it highlights the message of this chapter: There are multiple ways to "inherit" characteristics like those of our parents.

In a genuine scientific tour de force—a book titled *Evolution in Four Dimensions*[11]—Eva Jablonka and Marion Lamb catalogued a variety of ways in which developmental resources can be reliably transmitted from individuals to their offspring. Developmental resources can be transmitted to offspring through the germline, as happens when a sperm and egg provide the DNA during the formation of a zygote, or through other channels, as happens when developmentally essential gut microbes are passed from a mother to her children. It is also the case that *epi*genetic features can be passed through the germline, so nongenetic information (i.e., information not represented in the DNA sequence) can nonetheless pass through the channel that ordinarily carries genetic information (thereby complicating our understanding to some extent). In the end, Jablonka and Lamb described four types of systems that contribute to the transmission of information across generations: genetic, epigenetic, behavioral, and symbolic.

Relatively simple organisms transmit information across generations by using both the genetic and epigenetic inheritance systems; more complex animals have access to other systems as well. As Jablonka and Lamb put it, "every living organism depends on both genetic and epigenetic inheritance, many animals transmit information behaviorally, and humans have an additional route of information transfer through symbol-mediated communication."[12] After presenting in the next section some of the more interesting ways phenotypes can be reproduced in successive generations, I will focus in the following section on a particular kind of inheritance, a kind that allows epigenetic effects like those produced in the Meaney lab to be transmitted to offspring even though such effects are produced in an animal's brain cells long after its germline has been segregated from the other cells of its body.

Inheritance Systems: A Few of the Many Ways to Transmit a Phenotype

Among the processes that allow individuals in a new generation to acquire characteristics like their ancestors' are those that involve observation and imitation. Jablonka and Lamb recognized these as forms of "socially mediated learning," which they defined as "a change in behavior that is the result of social interactions"[13] with other community members, be they parents, other family members, or strangers. Socially mediated learning is evident in people but also occurs in, for example, birds and whales that learn to sing specific songs by imitating what they hear.[14]

Another good example of socially mediated learning has been provided by a troop of Japanese monkeys. Specific behaviors typical of this troop originated with an especially innovative female in the 1950s and then propagated through the troop (or, in some cases, through the innovator's family). One of the innovations involved forsaking the practice of eating individual grains of wheat picked up from the beach, and instead collecting handfuls of sand-and-wheat and then throwing them into the water, whereupon the sand would sink and the wheat grains would be left floating on the surface where they could easily be collected into a satisfying mouthful. First observed by Japanese researchers in 1956, this behavior was seen in 13 out of 15 monkeys in the innovator's family by 1962.[15]

This behavior—and others learned by troop members, such as sweet-potato washing—were then clearly reproduced across successive generations. In the end, the researchers wrote:

A total of more than 450 monkeys were recorded from 1952 until 1999. None of the monkeys who experienced the emergence of these . . .

behaviors is alive now, but their descendants are still dipping sweet potatoes into the sea, throwing grains of wheat into the water, and bathing in
the sea. These behaviors have been transmitted over the generations . . .
the sixth generation descendants of the monkeys in the initial study periods are still engaging in sweet-potato washing.[16]

In a very real sense, then, behaviors can be reliably transmitted from one generation to the next—inherited—via a socially mediated mechanism.

Unlike these sorts of observable behaviors, some kinds of developmental
resources can be supplied only by an individual's parents. For instance, DNA
sequence information and other information conveyed through the germline is
always transmitted from parents, of course. But as is evident from how we inherit
our normal gut symbionts, parents also transmit developmental resources through
nongermline channels. A behavioral example of nongermline transmission of an
influential developmental factor can be found in individual female butterflies.
These insects prefer laying eggs on specific kinds of plants, and this behavior can
then produce effects that reverberate across generations. As Jablonka and another
colleague describe it, in some cases,

> when caterpillars are fed on a new species of plant . . . they later tend to
> prefer the new host plant. Moreover, the feeding preferences of young
> [caterpillars] and egg-laying preferences of adults [i.e., butterflies] are
> often related, because females lay their eggs on the same species [of
> plant] as that on which they fed as caterpillars.[17]

In this way, a given female might develop a food preference that she will pass on
to her descendants; because she will lay her eggs on the plant she has come to
prefer to eat, her offspring will develop the same food preference because they
will grow up eating that same kind of plant. And because the female offspring will
then ultimately lay eggs on that same plant, the effect can be transmitted across
multiple generations.

A pregnant woman's behavior, too, can influence the later-appearing characteristics of her children. When we are fetuses, we live in an environment constructed by our mothers' bodies, and this environment is influenced by our
mothers' behaviors. For example, a pregnant woman's diet influences the chemistry of the amniotic fluid in her womb, and because fetuses swallow amniotic fluid,
their early experiences with particular flavors can affect their later food preferences. In fact, babies whose mothers drank carrot juice regularly in their final trimester of pregnancy were more tolerant of carrot-flavored cereal when they were
5.5 months old than were babies whose mothers did not consume any carrot juice
in this time period. Similarly, babies born to women who drank water throughout

their pregnancy but who drank carrot juice while breastfeeding were also more tolerant of carrot-flavored cereal,[18] presumably because the breast milk they consumed gave them experience with this flavor. Thus, human food preferences can be transmitted across generations via substances that an embryo, fetus, or infant detects in its mother's womb or breast milk, or that an infant detects in either parent's saliva or scent.[19a–19b] This is how early experiences with particular flavors could contribute to the perpetuation across generations of different ethnic and cultural cuisine preferences.[20]

Because the intrauterine environment is altered by more than just the flavor of a mother's diet, this mechanism of information transfer has the potential to be very influential. In fact, because a woman's hormonal state can be influenced by factors such as stress or malnutrition, these experiences too can potentially influence her embryo or fetus. As we have seen, women who experienced the Dutch famine during pregnancy were more likely to have children who developed schizophrenia[21] or obesity[22] by adulthood. Fetuses can also hear maternal speech while they are in utero, and this experience produces a preference for the mother's voice that is present at birth.[23a–23b] Of course, not all early-life experiences produce effects that will be detectable in multiple descendant generations, but some do. And regardless, it is clear that mothers (and in some cases, fathers) bring stimuli into the local environments of their offspring, stimuli that affect the offspring's development and that in some cases lead the offspring to have phenotypes like their parents' phenotypes.

Inheriting Epigenetic States via Behavior

A particularly interesting example of parent-to-offspring transmission demonstrates how the *epigenetic* effects of experience might be "inheritable" even if those effects do not influence germ cell DNA. As we saw in the chapter "Experience," female rats that lick and groom their offspring a lot (i.e., high LG mothers) raise daughters that grow up to be high LG mothers themselves,[24] and this is true regardless of whether the daughters are being raised by their own mothers or by foster mothers; that is, the effect is due to the daughters' *experiences* with high LG caregivers. Thus, the transgenerational transmission of this mothering style entails a behavioral mechanism.[25] More recent research[26] has revealed that in this kind of inheritance, an epigenetic state influences a parent's behaviors, and these behaviors then cause the offspring to end up in that same epigenetic state,[27] a situation that sets up a pattern able to sustain itself across multiple generations.

To explore this phenomenon, a research team led by Frances Champagne studied estrogen receptors in the brains of female rats that had been cross-fostered to high- or low-LG mothers.[28] Estrogen receptors are an essential element in the system that allows estrogens—the primary female sex hormones—to perform their functions, including the stimulation of maternal behavior in many mammals.[29] Because estrogens and LG both affect maternal behavior, Champagne's group hypothesized that LG might affect the production of estrogen receptors. As expected, they found that female rats exposed to high LG produced more estrogen receptors, because the DNA used to produce those receptors in the highly groomed rats was relatively unmethylated in the brain area studied.[30a–30b] Thus, licking and grooming produces an epigenetic effect in female rat pups that increases the number of estrogen receptors in their brains, and this increase normally causes the females—once they are adults with their own litters—to lick and groom *their* offspring a lot, effectively transmitting the high LG phenotype to the next generation.[31] Because maternal behavior influences methylation of a DNA segment that plays a role in maternal behavior, the behavior is maintained across generations (see Figure 18.1). This is an example of a transgenerational epigenetic effect that depends on offspring *experiences*,[32] because the daughters end up with methylation patterns and behavioral patterns like their mothers even though the germline is never affected.

Just as this epigenetic mechanism can reproduce high LG mothering in successive generations, *low* levels of LG can likewise be perpetuated, because relatively neglected pups end up with *fewer* estrogen receptors in their brains and therefore grow up to be low LG mothers. This sort of inheritance-via-behavior does not occur only in cases of maternal neglect; unfortunately, active maltreatment also appears to be transgenerationally transmittable. In one informative study that I described in "Zooming in on Experience," researchers exposed newborn

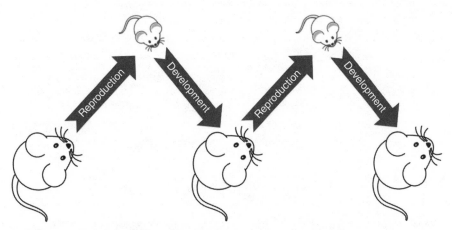

Figure 18.1 A schematic diagram representing nongenomic transmission across generations of both an epigenetic state (reduced DNA methylation) and an associated behavioral phenotype (maternal licking and grooming). Maternal behavior in the adult generation affects DNA methylation in the offspring. This DNA methylation then affects maternal behavior when the offspring develop into adulthood.

rats to mothers that were so stressed that they treated their pups abusively, dropping them, handling them roughly, dragging them, and stepping on them.[33] Pups exposed to this kind of ill-treatment for 30 minutes per day on each of the first 7 days of their lives grew up to be adults with more methylation on specific genes in their prefrontal cortex cells, genes that are vital for neuron survival. And in an effect with important implications for inheritance, when the abused female offspring grew up and reproduced, *their* 8-day-old offspring had increased methylation of *the same genes in the same brain areas* that were affected in their mothers.[34] As in the Champagne team's study, this effect did not involve the germline. Instead, it appears to reflect the fact that the mothers that were abused as newborns grew up to be abnormally anxious, and likely to abuse *their* offspring in turn.[35]

Crucially, these sorts of effects might underlie similar kinds of transgenerational phenomena in human beings.[36, 37] For instance, Champagne has pointed out that "up to 70% of abusive parents were themselves abused . . . [and that] 20–30% of abused infants are likely to become abusers. [Likewise,] a mother's own attachment to her mother is a good predictor of her infant's attachment."[38] The possibility that these sorts of patterns reflect epigenetic effects is particularly exciting because epigenetic effects are potentially reversible, either through interventions with specific drugs[39] or treatment programs that provide other kinds of experiences.[40a–40b] Additional study of the epigenetic effects of abusive parenting could illuminate the mechanisms responsible for transgenerational cycles of violence and point the way toward effective treatments for the pathologies caused by abuse. As Champagne sees it, "intervention within the lifespan of an individual is possible and may disrupt the continuity of the effects of adversity across generations."[41]

As fascinating as it is that behavior can play a critical role in the transmission of some phenotypes across generations, this phenomenon is no more (or less) important than the transmission of developmental resources through the germline. If an experience influences the epigenetic marks in an ancestral individual's *germ* cells—and if epigenetic marks can be passed on to descendants—then the effects of that experience could be reproduced reliably in multiple subsequent generations, even if intervening generations never have the kind of influential experience the ancestor had. This is one reason biologists are particularly interested in the transmission of developmental resources through the germline.

Erasing Epigenetic Endowments

Several kinds of factors in addition to DNA are transmitted through the germline,[42] and like DNA, these factors contribute to the reliable reproduction of phenotypes in successive generations. Mammals' eggs, for example, contain several different kinds of nongenetic structures and molecules that are essential for normal development after conception,[43] and these are transmitted along with DNA through the germline.[44] All of these factors have effects that are "epigenetic" in the broad sense, and they are all inherited from the previous generation.

In addition, there is now strong evidence that epigenetic marks like methyl groups can, in some cases, be transmitted through the germline. The Australian molecular biologists Lucia Daxinger and Emma Whitelaw have dubbed this kind of inheritance "transgenerational epigenetic inheritance via the gametes,"[45] an unwieldy name that nonetheless captures the nature of the occurrence. The first evidence that transgenerational epigenetic inheritance via the gametes can occur in mammals appeared in 1997,[46] when a group of researchers discovered that certain manipulations of mouse embryos produce epigenetic effects that can be inherited. These researchers wrote that they observed such inheritance even though "epigenetic modifications, such as DNA methylation . . . are not normally thought to be inherited through the germline."[47]

Biologists at the time had been convinced that such effects were impossible, because normally, epigenetic marks are "erased" between generations; as DNA makes its voyage from parents to offspring, epigenetic marks are typically "cleared" twice (see Figure 18.2). For the sake of illustration, think about your own mother. Immediately after she was conceived, the epigenetic marks on her newly constituted genome were removed in a process known as epigenetic "reprogramming." When you think about it, this makes a lot of sense. After all, we know that mature, differentiated cells have distinguishing epigenetic marks that make them the kinds of cells they are, and this is true of mature sperm and egg cells as well. In contrast, newly formed embryos are composed of undifferentiated *stem* cells, so they must *not* have the distinguishing epigenetic marks of the sperm and

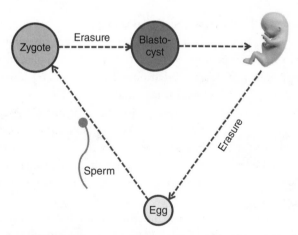

Figure 18.2 A schematic diagram of the "life cycle" of methylation. DNA methylation is "erased" once shortly after a new organism is conceived (a zygote is a newly conceived organism, and a blastocyst is an early embryo), and once more in the primordial germ cells that will become that new organism's sperm or egg cells.

egg that created them! Thus, almost all of the epigenetic marks on the DNA provided by your grandparents had to be removed from your mother's genome very soon after she was conceived, in order to render her cells pluripotent,[48] that is, able to develop into any of the very different kinds of cells that make up a body.

Then, within the next 2 weeks, some of the cells in your embryonic mother began the process of differentiating into the primordial germ cells that ultimately gave rise to her eggs, one of which developed into you. The creation of primordial germ cells initially entails adding some epigenetic marks, but ultimately the DNA in these cells is stripped of *all* of its epigenetic marks.[49] Thus, as DNA travels from one generation to the next, it goes through a two-part resetting process; first, it loses most of its epigenetic marks shortly after it is involved in the conception of a new individual, and then, it is wiped completely "clean" of its epigenetic marks— however briefly—when that individual is beginning to form his or her own new sperm or egg cells.

Thirty years ago, the following was "common knowledge" among biologists: (1) epigenetic marks are completely "erased" between generations, making transgenerational epigenetic inheritance impossible; (2) only DNA sequence information can be transmitted from parents to offspring; and (3) "hard" inheritance is, therefore, the only game in town. This understanding nicely preserved Weismann's disbelief in Lamarckism: Parents cannot pass on to their children the effects of their lived experiences. But within years of the 1997 discovery of epigenetic inheritance through the mouse germline,[50] this story required major revision.

Resurrecting Lamarck

The next chapter will focus specifically on transgenerational epigenetic inheritance via the gametes. As we will see, additional research on epigenetic inheritance has provided compelling evidence that DNA methylation can survive each of the two stages of "erasure" that normally occur between generations.[51] Researchers are still trying to determine if methylated DNA can somehow completely escape normal epigenetic reprogramming, or if non-DNA factors in the germline (e.g., perhaps RNA) might somehow be able to *reestablish* previously existing methylation after it has been erased in the normal process.[52a–52b] But regardless of how it happens, DNA methylation patterns do sometimes elude epigenetic reprogramming and can therefore be transmitted to descendants directly through the germline.

Although DNA methylation *can* be inherited through the germline, there continues to be debate about how often this occurs. To date, it still seems that most epigenetic marks are erased as DNA moves from parents to offspring; in a recent review of the evidence for this kind of inheritance in mammals, Daxinger and Whitelaw concluded, "Transgenerational epigenetic inheritance via the gametes is likely to be rare."[53] This should not surprise us, because the clearing of epigenetic marks between generations is extremely important; such a process restores pluripotency, ensuring that all stem cells have access to all of the genetic information they might need as development unfolds. Epigenetic marks transmitted through the germline would have the potential to affect *all* cell types in a descendant, which is unlikely to be a good thing, since different cell types need different epigenetic patterns.

Nevertheless, Jablonka and Lamb have predicted that transgenerational epigenetic inheritance via the gametes will ultimately prove to be more common than many biologists now anticipate. In 2005, they wrote:

> From basic biological principles and by extrapolation from what has already been found, we believe that it is highly likely that there is much more epigenetic inheritance than has so far been identified. People have hardly started looking for it. We predict that many more cases will be found, especially in plants and simple organisms, but not only there . . . [Consider the cases scientists have already discovered]—they are probably just the tip of an iceberg. We are convinced that now that . . . people are beginning to look at methylation and other aspects of chromatin structure, they will find a lot of variation . . . epigenetic variants exist, and are known to underlie the inheritance of phenotypic traits.[54]

When we consider direct, germline transmission of epigenetic marks *and* indirect mechanisms of epigenetic inheritance such as the varieties that depend on animals' behaviors and experiences, we can understand why Jablonka and a colleague concluded four years later that "epigenetic inheritance is ubiquitous."[55]

Because DNA methylation can be influenced by experience[56] *and* can be transmitted through the germline,[57a–57b] it is time to revisit Lamarck's idea that acquired characteristics can be inherited.[58a–58b] Like most evolutionary biologists, Richard Dawkins has emphatically denied the possibility that acquired characteristics can be inherited, writing "all evidence suggests that this idea is simply false."[59] And if we define "acquired" as referring specifically to mutilations like the sort Weismann inflicted on the tails of mice, then Dawkins is right; there is no reason to think mutilations experienced by one generation will reappear in the next generation (unless the descendants have the same kinds of experiences their ancestors did). But it should be apparent by now that there is not just one way to define the words "acquired" and "inherited,"[60] and that different definitions will lead to different conclusions. If we adopt a broad definition of inheritance—a definition that calls a phenotype "inherited" as long as it is reproduced reliably in successive generations—then a variety of experiences contribute to inheritable phenotypes. And in fact, a broad definition is *required* to understand some kinds of inheritance, such as the sort that causes the daughters of high LG rats to become high LG mothers themselves, or the sort that provides humans with the health-promoting bacteria in our guts; defining inheritance in a narrow way would interfere with our ability to understand how characteristics like these run in families.

But even if we adopt a narrow definition of inheritance that necessarily involves the *germline*, we still need to accept that acquired characteristics might be inheritable, because—as we will see in the next chapter—some phenotypes are transmitted to descendants *even when the descendants do not have the experiences that contributed to those phenotypes in their ancestors.* Categorically denying the inheritance of acquired characteristics requires defining "acquired" and "inherited" in *extremely* narrow ways,[61a–61b] and frankly, definitions this narrow are downright unhelpful, because they render so many transgenerational effects incomprehensible. Contemporary theorists disagree about the extent to which 21st-century biologists will need to revise their thinking about inheritance in general,[62a–62d] but for anyone committed to the idea that only genetically determined characteristics can be inherited, a major upheaval is looming.

‖ 19 ‖

Evidence

With age, I have become more interested in history. When I was younger, the years before I was born seemed inconsequential to me, and even now, the 1950s strike me as kind of otherworldly, because they were over before I was born. What little I know of the 1950s, I've picked up by watching movies and consuming other media from that era, but I've done the same with the 1920s, so for me, the 1920s and the 1950s are equally enigmatic. In contrast to the late 1950s, some of my memories from the late 1960s remain fresh; I'm still in touch with my friend from 3rd grade, and when we're together, 3rd grade doesn't seem that long ago. I recognize how odd this is now, because the 1980s occupy a similar place in my mind as the 1990s, but I know that these two decades are as qualitatively different for my current undergraduates as the 1950s and 1960s are for me; for my students, the 1990s might be a little fuzzy, but the 1980s really feel like a black hole.

My parents were born in the mid-1930s, twenty-five years before I was conceived. So it is hard to believe that events in that dark decade had repercussions that affected me biologically. The Great Depression and the rise of the Nazis obviously left psychological scars that have influenced later generations in several ways,[1] but if Weismann and the neo-Darwinists are right, events my parents experienced as children in the 1930s could not have influenced the *biological* materials they transmitted to me when I was conceived. Surely my *grandparents' experiences* should not be relevant in understanding my biological endowment. The idea that events in my maternal grandmother's life might have affected this endowment back in 1936—before my mother was even a fetus—seems virtually nonsensical.

And yet such effects are possible. Studies of epigenetic inheritance per se have shown that epigenetic marks can sometimes be transmitted through the germline. Furthermore, studies of the inheritance of acquired characteristics suggest that epigenetic marks *that have been influenced by experiences* can be transmitted through the germline. Not long ago, biologists would have insisted that events like this are impossible.

Transgenerational Epigenetic Inheritance via the Gametes

Some of the strongest evidence of transgenerational epigenetic inheritance has come from experiments on a particular kind of mouse I described in "Zooming in on Nutrition," a mouse that carries a gene known as A^{vy}. To review briefly for readers who skipped that chapter, this DNA segment can affect both the mouse's coat color and some of its other characteristics. Some of these so-called A^{vy} mice have yellowish coats; yellow A^{vy} mice tend to be obese and relatively likely to develop diabetes and/or cancer. Other A^{vy} mice have the *exact same genome* as their yellow siblings, but they have a brownish coat and are typically lean and healthy; the coat color of these mice is said to be pseudoagouti. (This odd name reflects the fact that the coat color of normal brownish mice is called "agouti." Lean A^{vy} mice have the exact same coat color and healthy disposition, but because they're genetically different from normal mice, they're called *pseudo*agouti.)

The differences between yellow and pseudoagouti A^{vy} mice are epigenetic. Specifically, a DNA region near A^{vy} is highly methylated in pseudoagouti A^{vy} mice and relatively unmethylated in yellow A^{vy} mice. To some extent, the amount of methylation at this location is influenced by random processes, but experimental studies have also revealed that a pregnant mouse's diet can affect the methylation of her offspring's DNA at this spot.[2]

In the late 1990s, researchers already knew that coat color in A^{vy} mouse pups was somehow related to their mothers' coloration.[3] Specifically, when fat, yellow A^{vy} mice get pregnant, they are more likely than their leaner, pseudoagouti twin-sisters to bear pups with yellow coats; in fact, in marked contrast to pseudoagouti mothers that pass on their A^{vy} gene, yellow mothers that pass on their A^{vy} gene always have offspring with some yellow in their coats.[4] Because all A^{vy} mice are genetically identical, the transgenerational transmission of coat color was understood to entail a nongenetic mechanism. And because biologists in the 1990s were confident that epigenetic marks are wiped "clean" in sperm and eggs, they reasoned that there was only one possible explanation for the transgenerational effect: Something about the prenatal environment—that is, the mother—had to be responsible for the family resemblance.[5]

There is only one problem with this assumption: It's wrong. In a beautifully designed test of the prenatal environment hypothesis in 1999, a team of researchers led by Emma Whitelaw took newly fertilized eggs from yellow, biological mothers and transplanted them into the uteruses of black foster mothers, where they were allowed to develop free of all the factors that characterize the wombs of yellow mothers.[6] Surprisingly, the researchers found that "transfer between different intrauterine environments does not affect the phenotypes of offspring;"[7] that is, the coat colors of the offspring were related to the coat colors of their biological mothers regardless of the uterine environment in which they developed. So, neither genes nor the prenatal environment could explain why offspring looked like their mothers. But if this transgenerational effect isn't related to either genes *or* environment—and if you're a 20th-century researcher operating under the assumption that epigenetic marks can't be inherited—what other kind of factor could there be?

One possible answer is that the cytoplasm in a yellow mother's egg is responsible for the effect. However, in studies of mice that inherited the A^{vy} gene from their father rather than from their yellow mother, some of the offspring are born with the brownish pseudoagouti coat. This means there cannot be anything in the cytoplasm of a yellow mother's egg that *precludes* the development of a pseudoagouti mouse.[8] So why is it that when a yellow *mother* provides the A^{vy} gene—containing the exact same sequence information as a father-provided A^{vy} gene—the offspring are never strictly pseudoagouti?

Whitelaw and colleagues ultimately concluded that the conventional wisdom about epigenetic marks being completely "erased" between generations had to be mistaken. Instead, they wrote, the best explanation for the transgenerational effect in A^{vy} mice is "the inheritance of an epigenetic mark causing silencing" of DNA near the A^{vy} gene.[9] Because A^{vy} genes provided by mothers and fathers do not generate the same kinds of effects, it appears that epigenetic marks in this vicinity are completely erased during sperm development but not during egg development. Therefore, when a pseudoagouti mouse gets pregnant, the methylation near her A^{vy} gene might not be erased in her eggs, giving her offspring a greater likelihood of developing the pseudoagouti coloration themselves.

Since this discovery, it has become clear that the A^{vy} gene is not unique. Another gene associated with epigenetic inheritance is called *Axin-fused*. *Axin-fused* is a DNA segment involved in the development of a kinked tail in mice. However, not all mice with the *Axin-fused* gene develop a kinked tail; mice with relatively unmethylated *Axin-fused* genes typically develop kinked tails, but their genetically identical relatives can have normal tails if their *Axin-fused* genes are highly methylated.[10] In both cases, mothers or fathers can pass on their epigenetic state to their offspring, thereby influencing the tail types seen in the next generation.

There are two reasons why the inheritability of this kinked-tail phenotype is important. First, it indicates that the inheritability of the *pseudoagouti* phenotype is not the only phenomenon of its kind, so it cannot be easily dismissed as a freakish exception. Second, unlike the pseudoagouti phenotype, the kinked-tail phenotype can be transmitted through the paternal line, so it cannot be caused by cytoplasmic factors. As the authors of the seminal study on this phenomenon noted, "Unlike the egg, the sperm contributes very little (if any) cytoplasm to the zygote, and therefore paternal inheritance . . . argues against the possibility that the effects are due to cytoplasmic or metabolic influences."[11] Instead, when a father mouse passes on his kinked-tail to his pups, it is because his *Axin-fused* gene has avoided the epigenetic reprogramming that normally happens when sperm are produced. Transmission through the *male* line in these studies makes it clear that similar tails across generations reflect genuine transgenerational epigenetic inheritance via the gametes.

Russian Nesting Dolls: Recognizing Direct Effects of Experience

Clearly, DNA methylation can be transmitted from parents to offspring via the gametes.[12a-12b] Taking this fact together with the fact that experiences can influence DNA methylation,[13] it seems that some *acquired* epigenetic information might be inheritable through the germline. And because such epigenetic marks influence phenotypes, it has started to look like Lamarck and Darwin may have been right all along about the inheritance of acquired characteristics. But have any scientists explicitly tried to influence an animal's epigenetic state and then looked to see whether the effects of that experience can be transmitted to the next generation?

We have seen that a pregnant mouse's diet can affect her offspring's DNA methylation and coat-color,[14] and this might seem to address the question, because in this case, a mother has an experience that can be detected in her offspring. But a closer look reveals that this effect need not involve inheritance at all. Instead, the effect in the offspring might have been produced *directly* by the dietary manipulation; this is because when you manipulate a pregnant mouse's diet, you also alter the nutritional experiences of the fetuses growing inside of her. To sidestep this experimental problem, some researchers have started investigating transgenerational effects of experiences in male lines only, a strategy that takes advantage of the fact that a mammalian father's experiences are not also experienced directly by his offspring.

In these paternal-line studies, any effects of an experience must be transmitted to offspring via the father's sperm, because male mammals do not carry fetuses (and, therefore, do not provide fetuses' prenatal environments).[15a-15b] Several such investigations have been conducted. In one study, for example, experimenters deprived male mice of some food in the month *before* they mated; this manipulation led to offspring with abnormally low blood sugar levels, a finding that suggests that a father's nutritional experiences can influence epigenetic reprogramming in sperm and influence offspring *independently of the offspring's fetal environment.*[16] Similarly, male rats fed a high fat diet have female offspring that develop into adults with abnormal insulin secretion,[17] and male mice fed a low protein diet produce offspring with altered cholesterol and fat metabolism, at least some of which reflects altered DNA methylation in the offspring's liver cells.[18] At first glance, these studies might seem like they reveal a Lamarckian kind of inheritance, since the nutritional experiences of a father are influencing his offspring.

But here too, there is an important difference: The offspring in these studies are *affected* by the experiences their fathers had before they were conceived, but they do not necessarily *inherit* phenotypes like the phenotypes their fathers acquired as a result of those experiences.

A 2006 study by Jennifer Cropley and colleagues came closer to demonstrating a Lamarckian effect.[19] These researchers fed a methyl-supplemented diet to a group of pregnant pseudoagouti A^{vy} mice, but only in the middle of their pregnancies. After being born, the offspring were fed a normal, nonsupplemented diet. As expected, the offspring of mice that ate the supplemented diet were more likely to have pseudoagouti coats than were the offspring of similar mice that ate a nonsupplemented diet. But the real question is: What happens when the female pseudoagouti offspring grow up and get pregnant, especially if they continue to eat a nonsupplemented diet throughout *their* pregnancies?

In a result that would surprise anyone convinced that acquired characteristics can never be inherited, the *grand*pups of the mice that were fed the supplemented diet were more likely to retain the brownish coats of their grandmothers than were the descendants of the grandmothers that were fed a normal diet (see Figure 19.1). So, supplementing the maternal diet produced effects in the fetuses that were exposed to that diet, but *also* in the *next* generation, that is, in pups that were *not* exposed to a methyl-supplemented diet.[20] As Cropley and colleagues described it,

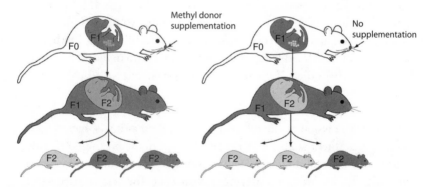

Figure 19.1 A schematic diagram illustrating the effect of methyl donor supplementation in the germ line. Epigenetic changes to the A^{vy} gene in primordial germ cells that have been exposed to methyl donors during differentiation (Left) are maintained throughout the production of new sperm or egg cells, and throughout the production of new embryos. Thus, pseudoagouti F_1 mice that are genetically and phenotypically identical but were subject to different diets in utero (Left vs. Right) can produce phenotypically different populations of F_2 offspring. Reprinted with permission from Dr. Catherine Suter; original image printed in Cropley, J. E., Suter, C. M., Beckman, K. B., & Martin, D. I. I. (2006). Germ-line epigenetic modification of the murine A^{vy} allele by nutritional supplementation. *Proceedings of the National Academy of Sciences of the USA, 103,* 17308–17312.

a pregnant pseudoagouti mouse that was only exposed to the supplemented diet *when she was a fetus* gives birth to "phenotypically different offspring than does an otherwise (genetically and phenotypically) identical female who had no exposure to methyl donor supplementation; this grandparental effect is directly attributable to the epigenetic state" of the DNA near the A^{vy} gene.[21] Thus, here we have a situation where an animal's prenatal experience alters its phenotype, and that experience-influenced phenotype is then passed on to the next generation, even if the next generation never has the kind of experience that affected its ancestor. Put succinctly, "the result suggests that a pregnant mother's diet may have an influence on the phenotypes of her grandchildren, independent of the diet consumed by her children or grandchildren."[22, 23]

This sort of "grandmother effect" is undoubtedly fascinating and important. Nevertheless, some theorists remain skeptical that this kind of effect reflects genuine Lamarckian inheritance, for the following reason: When a grandmother's experience influences her grand-offspring's characteristics, the experience still has the potential to affect the grand-offspring *directly*. Even if it is not immediately obvious, the fact is that physical material that is used to create the *grand*-offspring is present in the grandmother's body when she is pregnant with her own offspring. This is important because the diet consumed by a pregnant mammal has the potential to affect *all* of the cells developing in her embryo, including the cells that will ultimately become that embryo's eggs. Therefore, the diet of the *first* generation has the potential to affect that individual herself (obviously), her daughter (because the daughter is growing as an embryo inside of her mother), and her granddaughter (because the egg that will be fertilized one day to produce the granddaughter is already present in a primordial form in the embryo exposed to the grandmother's diet). Two neurobiologists have offered a strong argument to this effect:

> While transmission to the offspring of perturbed animals may suggest epigenetic rather than environmental factors, it does not completely rule out environmental influence, because the cells that ultimately generate the offspring are present at the time of treatment. Thus, transmission to a subsequent third generation is important to demonstrate that the phenotype is indeed transgenerational, germline-dependent, and is not a direct effect of the treatment itself.[24]

As a result, a number of researchers have started studying if the effects of experience might persist in *great*-grand-offspring, because such descendants cannot possibly be influenced *directly* by their great-grandparents' experiences.

Before considering studies of inheritance across additional generations, we should stop and consider the surprising implications of the Cropley team's work. Even if these sorts of "grandmother effects" reflect not inheritance but a direct effect of a dietary manipulation on grand-offspring, the phenomenon is still amazing. Viewed from this perspective, my grandmother's early-20th-century experiences could potentially have influenced my 21st-century body, as far-fetched as that might sound. Although there is no sense in which I existed in the 1930s—I wasn't conceived until the end of 1959—the fact is that the egg I grew from originated in 1936 as a primordial germ cell in the embryo that ultimately developed into my mother. Therefore, any experiences my pregnant grandmother had that influenced the epigenetic state of that primordial germ cell would have had the potential to influence my development, *if* that cell (once it was fertilized in 1959) somehow escaped the epigenetic reprogramming that normally occurs just after conception. This Russian-doll-like person-in-a-person-in-a-person situation can be enough to make one's head spin, but studies I will describe in the next chapter have made it clear that these sorts of effects actually might be detectable in human beings.

Experiences That Keep on Giving: The Inheritance of Acquired Characteristics

To explore the possibility that an experience can affect an animal's *great*-grand-offspring, researchers have manipulated the diets of rodents and looked for effects of those manipulations in the so-called F_3 generation (where F_0 represents the animals that are fed the altered diet, F_1 represents the offspring of those animals, F_2 represents the grand-offspring, and so on). At least two experiments have indicated that nutritional experiences can produce inheritable effects that cannot be *direct* effects of the diet. One study revealed that pregnant rats fed low protein diets had great-grand-offspring with abnormal glucose metabolism, even though the great-grand-offspring, their mothers, and their grandmothers all ate nutritionally adequate diets.[25] Another study found that feeding female mice a high fat diet for 6 weeks before conception produced detectable effects in some of their F_3 descendants.[26] Specifically, great-grand-daughters born to *males* of the F^2 generation had abnormally large bodies, so the researchers concluded that their results evidenced "a stable germline-based transgenerational mode of inheritance."[27] In both of these studies, then, an experience produced effects that were detectable in descendant generations, even though those generations could not possibly have been directly affected by the experience.

Another study that reached similar conclusions examined how mice are affected by the experience of being separated from their mothers in an unpredictable—and therefore, stressful—way.[28] We've already seen that mice separated from their mothers grow up to be hyperresponsive to stress as adults, and that the experience of early separation affects DNA methylation in their hypothalamic cells.[29] Likewise, mice that experience unpredictable separations exhibit "depressive-like behaviors" as adults.[30] But in a striking discovery, males separated from their mothers in this way developed *sperm* cells that had abnormal methylation patterns, and these males ultimately produced some descendants that exhibited depressive-like behaviors akin to those seen in their ancestor, *even if the descendants experienced normal parenting.* Thus, a stressful experience early in life altered DNA methylation in the sperm of the stressed mice, and the alteration was detectable in the next generation's brain and sperm cells as well.[31] Because the behaviors observed in this study were transmitted from *male* mice to their descendants, the effects on the descendants (i.e., the F_2 generation) cannot have been caused *directly* by the stressful separations that their fathers experienced; likewise, these effects cannot reflect the influence of maternal care for the F_2 generation (or the influence of any other environmental factors, including factors in the cytoplasm). Instead, the finding of experience-induced epigenetic changes in germ cells supports the Lamarckian conclusion that in this case, the descendant generations actually did inherit behavioral characteristics originally *acquired* by their ancestor.[32]

Regardless of how it occurs, inheritance is significant because it is an essential feature of evolution by natural selection.[33] Accordingly, if acquired characteristics can be inherited, experiences can potentially influence evolution (even if most 20th-century biologists denied this possibility). This state of affairs has led some researchers to investigate whether transgenerational epigenetic inheritance via the gametes might have evolutionary consequences.

For example, Cropley and colleagues[34] selected male pseudoagouti mice born to methyl-supplemented mothers, and raised them on a supplemented diet. At maturity, these mice were mated with black females, and any male pseudoagouti offspring were selected to receive the exact same experiences as their fathers—they were raised on a supplemented diet and then mated with black females. The Cropley team followed this procedure for five generations, each time combining ongoing dietary supplementation with selective breeding of the pseudoagouti mice. Neither supplementation nor selective breeding alone has been found to change the proportion of pseudoagouti pups born in descendant generations, but by *combining* the experience of dietary supplementation with selective breeding, the Cropley group was able to produce descendant generations made up of increasing proportions of pseudoagouti pups. Thus, this study has implications for how we think about evolution, because the typical phenotype seen in the descendant population was different from the typical phenotype seen in the ancestral population, even though the genomes of these animals never changed.

Once the fifth-generation descendants were born in this study, the researchers stopped supplementing their diets; the goal was to see if the pseudoagouti phenotype would still appear disproportionately in the sixth generation even in the absence of the dietary experiences that influenced the ancestors. Keep in mind that the mice observed in this study were all male, so none of the descendants could have been influenced *directly* by the supplemented diets that were fed to their fathers. Amazingly, the proportion of pseudoagouti pups born to the fifth-generation, *non*supplemented mice was still high. Without continued supplementation, the seventh and later generations reverted to the original proportions of yellow and pseudoagouti offspring; nonetheless, Cropley and colleagues concluded that the results of their study mean that "multi-generational exposure to a dietary stimulus coupled with selection for a phenotype can progressively increase the prevalence of that phenotype in the population ... [and that this effect is] due solely to the interaction of environment and epigenotype, demonstrating that purely epigenetic traits can provide a substrate for selection."[35] Thus, natural selection should be able to operate on "inheritable" phenotypes that depend on *epigenetic* factors just as surely as it operates on phenotypes that depend on genetic factors. If this statement is correct, then experience-induced epigenetic processes could very well have significant effects on evolution.

Poisoned Environments, Perturbed Evolution

Research on the transgenerational transmission of epigenetic information has generated some rather frightening data on the effects of environmental toxins. In 2005, a group of researchers led by the American biochemist Michael Skinner reported that exposing pregnant rats to a chemical called vinclozolin can produce specific abnormalities detectable in the exposed animals' great-great-grand-offspring (the F_4 generation).[36] Unfortunately, vinclozolin is commonly used in vineyards to kill molds—and on farms to kill fungi that might otherwise infect peaches, lettuce, or strawberries, for example—so although the rats in Skinner's study were exposed to more of this pesticide than people ordinarily encounter, this is not a substance that is absent from our environments.

Vinclozolin interferes with the normal functioning of male hormones including testosterone, and when it is injected into a female rat's body early in pregnancy, her male offspring will grow up to have abnormally low numbers of sperm and an increased incidence of infertility. However, these specific abnormalities appear in otherwise normal rats, so vinclozolin does not simply have a general toxic effect on the development of these animals;[37] its effects are more targeted. When a fetus is exposed to vinclozolin during the development of its gonads, its germline is affected, so the consequences of the encounter can be detected for generations. If an F_1 rat is exposed in the 2nd week of gestation, its descendants in the F_2, F_3, and F_4 generations will be abnormal even if they are never exposed to the pesticide themselves.[38]

Among the abnormalities detected in the descendants of vinclozolin-exposed rats were 15 abnormally methylated DNA segments in their sperm cells.[39] Although the rats exposed to vinclozolin in the Skinner study were female, their male offspring were abnormal and the male offspring of *those* males were abnormal (and so on). Thus, the transgenerational epigenetic effect was detected in the male line, providing yet another example in which an experience affected inheritance through the germline.[40]

In a thought-provoking follow-up to this study, female rats were able to tell the difference between male rats whose ancestors were never exposed to vinclozolin and male rats whose parents and grandparents were similarly *un*exposed, but whose paternal *great*-grandmother *was* exposed to vinclozolin.[41] Even though the exposure had occurred generations before, the descendants of exposed rats were relatively unattractive to females, who generally preferred mating with males whose ancestors were never exposed to the pesticide. Skinner and his team concluded that their findings constituted "direct experimental evidence for a role of epigenetics as a determinant factor in evolution,"[42] because they show that "an environmental factor can promote a transgenerational alteration in the epigenome that influences sexual selection and could impact the viability of a population and evolution of the species."[43] As might be expected, some researchers were skeptical about these results,[44] but they have since been replicated in Skinner's lab;[45] if this proves to be a reliable phenomenon, the implications of this work would be far-reaching.

There have also been reports of transgenerational effects of environmental toxins on people, but because these data have not come from controlled experiments, additional work is needed before we can be confident such effects are detectable in human lineages. Still, the research literature already contains some ominous accounts of the effects of a drug called DES (diethylstilbestrol), a drug prescribed to millions of women in the 1970s who were at risk of a miscarriage. Tragically, although DES did help prevent miscarriages, many of the women who took it gave birth to children who now suffer from abnormalities, including an increased likelihood of developing certain kinds of cancers. Even worse, this increased risk now appears to be a trangenerational effect, with more maternal granddaughters than would be expected by chance ending up with ovarian cancer.[46, 47] The possibility of such transgenerational effects should certainly give pause to regulatory agents charged with protecting us from potentially dangerous engineered chemicals, be they drugs, pesticides, or food additives.

There have also been reports of transgenerational effects of diet in human populations; these will be the subject of the next chapter. And although these studies, too, have been merely correlational, the data are beginning to pile up in support of the idea that our ancestors' experiences influence the characteristics we develop.

Even if the specific effects I will describe next are not genuinely Lamarckian—that is, even if ancestral experiences do not affect ancestors' phenotypes in ways that cause their descendants to develop those *same* phenotypes—they are almost certainly epigenetic, and they suggest that the experiences of one generation can influence the biological endowment passed to subsequent generations.

Grandparents

Famine has been a threat throughout human history and has not yet been eradicated, even though the earth generates enough crops to provide food security for all of us.[1] The last famine in Europe was the Dutch Hungerwinter in 1944, but every subsequent decade has brought famine to at least one unfortunate population. (The following list was selected to illustrate the spatial and temporal extent of the problem: the Great Leap Forward famine began in China in 1958, the Biafran famine in what is now Nigeria began in 1967, Pol Pot's Khmer Rouge brought famine to Cambodia in the wake of their 1975 coup, a two-year famine in Ethiopia began in 1983, the Arduous March famine began in North Korea in 1994 after apocalyptic flooding, the Niger food crisis affected over 2 million people in 2005 and 2006, and the Maplecroft Food Security Risk Index has listed Afghanistan as being at extreme risk for food insecurity every year of the current decade to date.) In fact, the Secretary-General of the United Nations, Ban Ki-moon, announced at the end of 2009 that 6 million children die of hunger around the world each year, a staggering death rate of 1 child every 5 seconds. Tragically, these kinds of events seem likely to continue plaguing people for the foreseeable future.

Famine affects more than the hungry children and adults exposed to it. As scientists knew by the end of the 20th century, the not-yet-born offspring of pregnant women who are exposed to famine are also at risk. As we have seen, individuals exposed to the Dutch Hungerwinter shortly after they were conceived were at increased risk of developing severe neurological and psychological abnormalities,[2a–2c] and a disproportionate number grew up to be obese adults[3] in danger of developing heart disease and diabetes.[4a–4b] Exposure to the Dutch famine before birth has also been associated with epigenetic effects, including reduced methylation of a gene used to produce a prenatal growth-promoting hormone[5] and increased methylation of a variety of other genes.[6] These effects were detected in blood cells taken from famine-exposed individuals nearly 6 decades after the famine ended.[7] Prenatal undernutrition could very well have produced these effects directly, so there is no reason to assume that methylation patterns were transmitted across generations in these cases.

In the early 1990s, reports began to surface that suggested that famine can affect generations beyond those actually exposed to it. Two studies reported significant effects on the birthweights of *grandchildren* of women who were pregnant during the Dutch famine;[8a–8b] these effects seemed to be transgenerational, because they were detected in grandchildren (i.e., the F_2 generation) who were adequately nourished for their entire lives, starting at conception.[9] Likewise, a more recent study found that the grandchildren of women exposed to the Dutch famine during pregnancy were significantly shorter and significantly leaner than the grandchildren of women never exposed to the famine.[10]

These kinds of findings suggest that undernutrition produces effects across multiple generations, but it is not yet clear whether this interpretation is warranted. Remember, when such effects occur in maternal lines, the F_2 generation could be affected directly by the grandmother's experiences during her pregnancy, because the primordial germ cells that will become that generation are actually present inside of the embryo that is developing inside of the grandmother. Therefore, effects in the F_2 generation might or might not reflect transmission across generations; it will be interesting to learn what we can from the *great*-grandchildren of women who were pregnant during the Dutch Hungerwinter, after studies of these individuals have been completed. At present, we are left with the conclusion of a recent comprehensive review of studies on the effects of famine in the F_2 generation: When all of the available and relevant data are considered in the aggregate, these studies have yielded results that are "inconclusive."[11]

Even if we become more confident that these kinds of studies reveal genuine transgenerational effects of famine, it remains unclear what roles, if any, epigenetic marks play in producing the effects. No data are currently available regarding the transgenerational transmission of epigenetic marks in human beings. Nonetheless, a few relatively recent studies—which have all been described in the *European Journal of Human Genetics (EJHG)*—have discovered some transgenerational effects of dietary experiences, effects that were unthinkable a mere 15 years ago. None of the *EJHG* studies explicitly looked at DNA methylation or histone modification, but there is widespread speculation that the mechanisms underlying the observed effects are most likely epigenetic.[12a–12c] And regardless of *how* these effects occur, they constitute some of the strongest evidence yet obtained that a person's *experiences* might influence his or her grandchildren's characteristics via materials transmitted through the germline.

A Surprise in Sweden

The *EJHG* data were all collected in Sweden, for good reasons that will become clear. Most Americans know little of Sweden, certainly not the parts of the country beyond Stockholm, the only Swedish city with close to a million residents (the next largest city in Sweden has about half that population). Thanks to film versions of Stieg Larsson's bestselling book *The Girl with the Dragon Tattoo*, many people have seen what parts of Sweden can look like in the winter. But these films were shot on location in the southern half of the country; as cold and isolated as these locations appeared on film, they did not capture the reality of life hundreds of miles further north. One of the scientists involved with the *EJHG* studies is Lars Olov Bygren, a man who grew up in the northernmost reaches of the country, in a remote village called Överkalix. Bygren describes Överkalix as "a small forest area, very beautiful . . . cold; my home . . . was 10 miles north of the polar circle,"[13] a latitude that makes Anchorage, Alaska, seem tropical by comparison! However, although Överkalix has always been relatively inaccessible, the community there has kept meticulous records since 1799 regarding both community members and annual crop yields; good records were instrumental in allowing the king to collect the taxes he felt were rightfully his.[14] This remarkably rich data set has also allowed Bygren—along with other researchers such as Gunnar Kaati and Marcus Pembrey—to do innovative epidemiological studies of how the amount of food available to a given generation is related to the characteristics of that generation's descendants.

An unfortunate circumstance that has made these data even more valuable is the fact that for much of the 19th century, the harvests in Överkalix were extremely variable. Kaati and colleagues "classified the harvests of the years 1800, 1812, 1821, and 1829 [and also of 1831–36, 1851, and 1856] as total crop failures."[15] In striking contrast, good years could bring bumper crops; in Överkalix, "a surfeit of food was available after the harvest in 1799, 1801, 1813–15, 1822, 1825–26, 1828, 1841, 1844, 1846, 1853" and several other years.[16] Although these data do not tell us about the food that individuals in Överkalix actually consumed in these years, it seems a safe bet that the population was undernourished in some periods and very well fed in others, because in good years, two or three times more food could be available than was available in lean years.[17] We know for sure that the people living in Överkalix in the 19th century could not import additional food supplies in the years when the crops failed, because they were effectively cut off from the rest of the world during their long cold winters; as Kaati and Bygren's group noted, "there were no railways or roads, and in the winter the frozen Baltic Sea prevented any transport over water."[18] However, in spite of the diminished food supplies in some years, the mortality rates across the years were not particularly variable, so although some years saw crop failures, these events did not generally cause people to starve to death; instead, the people just tried to hang on, hungry, through the winter.

To examine the effects of food availability in one generation on characteristics of later generations, Kaati and colleagues considered data from 239 people born in either 1890, 1905, or 1920; specifically, they looked to see whether these people's risk of death from cardiovascular disease or diabetes was related to the amounts of food available to either their parents or grandparents.[19] The researchers were specifically concerned with ancestors' nutritional environments at a particular point in development, namely the so-called slow growth period that normally occurs just before the adolescent growth spurt; the team defined this phase as occurring between 9 and 12 years of age for boys and between 8 and 10 years of age for girls.[20] Although this is a period in which the rapid physical growth experienced by children slows down considerably, it is also the period in which boys experience important developments in cells that will ultimately become mature sperm.

The initial results of this research[21] were quite a revelation. They indicated that if insufficient food was available when a particular male was in his slow growth period, his future son was less likely to die from complications of cardiovascular disease. Similarly, his future *grand*children were less likely to die from complications of diabetes. In shocking contrast, the risk of death from diabetes-related causes increased *fourfold* among the *grand*children of men whose slow growth period occurred when there was an excess of food. A follow-up study with better controls confirmed these effects, and revealed that for fathers, too, experiencing an overabundance of food during the slow growth period was associated with an increased risk of mortality for their sons.[22] Thus, if a boy falls on lean times during his slow growth period, his future descendants will be healthier than if he always lived through times of plenty.

Importantly, these effects were transmitted through the fathers and the grandfathers, so the grandchildren were not present in any way—as embryos or even as primordial germ cells—when the feasts or famines were ongoing. Therefore, the effects were transmitted through the germline. And because Kaati and colleagues "found no evidence of intense [natural] selection,"[23] it is unlikely that the differences between the grandchildren reflected differences in their genes (i.e., their DNA sequence information). As a result, scientists working in this domain generally agree that the mechanism of transmission could very well involve epigenetics.[24a-24d] Pembrey argued explicitly in favor of this interpretation of the Överkalix data when he wrote that the slow growth period in boys is "associated with the emergence of the first viable pools of [cells that will give rise to mature sperm] and the beginning of re-programming of methylation imprints, just the kind of dynamic state in which a nutrition-sensing mechanism could operate."[25]

The Long Reach of Ancestors' Experiences

Pembrey and colleagues followed up this work by looking at a different population and at an experiential event other than food consumption.[26] Specifically, using data from the Avon Longitudinal Study of Parents and Children—a study of contemporary British families—the Pembrey team examined the effects on children of a father's decision to begin smoking cigarettes early in life. This study, too, detected a transgenerational effect through the paternal line; the age at which a boy began smoking cigarettes was positively related to his future son's body mass index (a rough measure of body fat percentage).

Because this effect was specific to offspring of a particular sex,[27] Pembrey and colleagues then returned to the Överkalix data to examine whether the effects of food availability were transmitted to grandchildren in a sex-dependent way.[28] Sure enough, a statistical reanalysis of these data confirmed the same kind of sex-specificity seen in the Avon data. In particular, when a paternal grand*father* in Överkalix experienced hunger during his slow growth period, his grand*sons* enjoyed a significantly reduced risk of mortality, perhaps adding as many as 30 years to their life spans.[29] In contrast, when it was the paternal grand*mother* in Överkalix who experienced hunger during her slow growth period, her grand-*daughters* enjoyed a significantly reduced risk of mortality. On the downside, if grandparents lived through years of abundant food supplies while in their slow growth periods, this had dire consequences for their grandchildren; if it was a grandfather having this experience, his grandsons were at increased risk of mortality, whereas if it was a grandmother having this experience, her granddaughters were at *twice* the risk of dying at a given age compared with control females.

There are three important things to note about these findings. First, even though some of these effects involved women, they were all transmitted to the youngest generation through the male line, that is, through the fathers. For instance, when grandmothers' experiences affected their granddaughters, it was via the grandmothers' *sons*. Said another way, these effects always involved the *paternal* grandparents; the amount of food available to the maternal grandparents had no detectable effects on their grandchildren's mortality. Second, the experiences of a man's father were related to the fate of his sons (but not his daughters), and the experiences of *that same man*'s mother were related to the fate of his daughters (but not his sons). Because the observed effects were transmitted across generations *through the same fathers*,[30] social or economic variables cannot account for the findings.[31] Finally, food availability during the grandparents' *puberty* was not related at all to the fates of their grandchildren; in the grandfathers, the only time in their lives that was important (in terms of how food availability affected their descendants) was their slow growth period. In contrast, in the grandmothers, their slow growth period was important too, but an even *more* important time was between when the grandmother was conceived and when she was three years old. This makes sense, given that this is when a female's eggs are formed;[32] the importance of nutrient exposures in this time period is to be expected, given the studies described in the previous chapter on dietary effects in rodents.

Based on these data, Pembrey and colleagues concluded that "a sex specific, male-line transgenerational response system exists in humans."[33] Their confidence in this conclusion was bolstered by the fact that the Avon and the Överkalix studies found the exact same pattern of data "in terms of the exposure-sensitive periods and sex specificity," a result that "supports the hypothesis that there is a general mechanism for transmitting information about the ancestral environment down the male line."[34] When Bygren was asked in a 2012 interview to offer some speculation about this mechanism,[35] he acknowledged that we really still have no firm idea about how it all might work, but that somehow—likely through events involving DNA methylation, histone modifications, or RNA activity—the experience of gluttony, starvation, or exposure to cigarette smoke produces an epigenetically "marked" genome, which is then transmitted to subsequent generations.

Meanwhile, Halfway Around the World . . .

One additional study has provided support for the idea that a father's experiences can influence the characteristics of his not-yet-conceived offspring. Many people across Southeast and South Asia are in the habit of chewing a psychoactive product made from a combination of the leaves of a plant in the pepper family and the seeds from a particular kind of palm tree; because the plant is called the betel vine and the seeds are called areca nuts, the product is sometimes called betel nut, although it is also known by other names including betel-quid or paan. A euphoria-inducing stimulant, betel nut is both carcinogenic and addictive; the World Health Organization identified it as "the fourth most common habit" in the world after "consumption of tobacco, alcohol and caffeine-containing beverages," with 600 million people estimated to be using it in 2001, which was about 10% of the world's population at that time.[36] The lips, gums, and teeth of betel nut chewers are stained a vivid red that was rather startling to me when, as a relatively naïve 27-year-old, I first encountered betel-quid addicts on the streets of New Delhi. But from a scientific perspective, the tooth-staining property of the areca nut has been useful; skulls containing betel-stained teeth have been excavated from a Vietnamese archeological site, allowing scientists to infer that people have been chewing betel-quid since the bronze age, hundreds of years BCE.[37]

A 2006 study of Taiwanese men[38] examined the possibility that a father's betel-quid chewing might be associated with an early onset in his offspring of the so-called metabolic syndrome, a condition characterized by obesity, insulin resistance, and increased risk of diabetes and cardiovascular disease.[39] After controlling for betel nut chewing among the offspring, the children of betel nut chewers were more than twice as likely as the children of nonchewers to develop the metabolic syndrome early in life. In addition, the more betel nut the fathers chewed before the birth of their children, the higher the risk to the children; as the authors of the study reported, "significant dose-response relations were found between the risk of early [metabolic syndrome] and the quantity and duration of paternal exposure to betel quids."[40] Finally, among children whose *parents* did *not* have metabolic syndrome, those whose fathers chewed betel nut before they were conceived were approximately two-and-a-half times more likely to develop metabolic syndrome relatively early in life,[41] even if the children never chewed any betel nut themselves.

Because this is an effect seen in the male line, the offspring cannot have been directly affected by the betel nut exposure. And because it mirrors a transgenerational effect of betel nut exposure in male mice,[42a–42b] the phenomenon is likely to be reliable. Nonetheless, it is not yet clear what causes the effect. The authors of the study pointed out that exposure to betel nut can damage DNA itself, but that "epigenetic phenomena . . . could also account" for the findings.[43] What is clear is that there are likely several sorts of experiences a father-to-be can have—exposure to tobacco, to betel nut, to an excess of food resources—that will have transgenerational effects on his descendants.

Epigenetics, Experience, and Inheritance

It is now apparent that in addition to carrying DNA, the germline can also carry some phenotypically relevant epigenetic marks.[44] Thus, DNA sequence information does not have exclusive access to this channel of transgenerational transmission. But once all of these germline materials have been transmitted to a new generation, they still need to interact with nongenetic factors to develop the new organism's behavioral and biological phenotypes. Germline materials and other developmental resources both play critical roles in phenotype development, so "inheritance via the germline" is no more special than any other kind of inheritance.

As interesting, important, and surprising as it might be that some of the effects of *experience* can be transmitted through the germline, we should keep in mind that experiential effects can also be transmitted in other ways; biologists are particularly interested in inheritance via the germline, but inheritance that depends on the transmission of other factors can be just as consequential. Abusive parenting behaviors, for example, are transmitted across generations in both monkeys[45] and human beings[46] via the transmission of specific experiences rather than via the transmission of specific information in the germline. Nonetheless, this phenomenon clearly warrants scientific attention. Once we understand that all of our behavioral and biological characteristics *develop* and that materials transmitted through the germline cannot single-handedly determine our characteristics, the special status that some theorists have granted to the germline starts to look less deserved.

In general, we should remember that an individual's experiences can affect his or her descendants whether the germline is affected or not. As we saw in the previous chapter, I might have been *directly* affected by my maternal grandmother's nutritional experiences in 1936; the effects of those experiences would be just as significant for me as any effects of the epigenetic information I might have received through the germline from my paternal grandfather. Regardless of the *mechanism* that produces the effects, the fact remains that some of our characteristics are better understood by not losing sight of our ancestors' experiences.

Is it interesting that a father's betel nut consumption, for instance, can influence his not-yet-conceived children's characteristics? Of course it is, and it would be interesting (and helpful) to know whether this effect involves the transgenerational transmission of epigenetic marks. But we have always known that a father's actions have the potential to influence the characteristics of his children and subsequent descendants, so in some ways, these kinds of findings should not seem revolutionary. If Barack Obama's *father* had not taken advantage of a scholarship in 1959 that took him from his home in Kenya to the University of Hawaii, President Obama would probably not have acquired the multicultural perspective that, in very important ways, defines him. Similarly, it is unlikely that the president's daughters—the grandchildren of that peripatetic Kenyan—would have been students at the excellent University of Chicago Laboratory Schools, where their brain structures and functions were altered through mechanisms that allow teachers everywhere to influence their students' minds. Because our psychological and biological characteristics are profoundly affected by the contexts in which we grow up, it should be obvious that what happens to grandparents reverberates through the ages to affect their descendants. In this way, there is nothing particularly special about how one generation's experiences affect later generations. The molecular discoveries we have been discussing are fascinating and important, but they do not fundamentally change a simple fact: What you do—and what happens to you—affects your descendants.

Even when we consider evolution, it should not matter whether a phenotype's development depends on information transmitted through the germline. For instance, there is little reason to consider the germline when trying to understand how Japanese monkeys inherit potato-washing behaviors from their ancestors. But a behavior like this that is transmitted via social learning can nonetheless have evolutionary consequences;[47a–47b] monkeys that wash their potatoes are more familiar with the ocean, they eat more (and more varied) marine organisms in their diets,[48] and they are more likely to take up activities like swimming, a behavior that could allow a subpopulation to colonize a previously uninhabited island and embark on a new life away from their troop, which would produce the kind of reproductive isolation known to have evolutionary consequences.[49a–49b] Because novel behaviors that can be learned from parents and grandparents have the potential to drive evolutionary changes just as novel genetic mutations do, there is an important sense in which understanding evolution does not require knowledge of the *mechanisms* responsible for the transgenerational transmission of phenotypes. In retrospect, we should have expected this; Darwin knew nothing of DNA or its mechanistic role in inheritance, but despite this ignorance, he still got the story of evolution right.

On the other hand, for anyone interested in *influencing* a characteristic, it matters very much how the characteristic develops. If we want to help a healthy young adult avoid the obesity that claimed the lives of his parents or if we want to stop the transgenerational transmission of abusive parenting, we need to understand *how* behaviors in ancestors are reproduced in their descendants. To discover ways to help people suffering from detrimental biological or psychological conditions, scientists need to remain focused on the *mechanisms* responsible for the development of these conditions; only an understanding at this level of detail will permit helpful intervention in development. It is probably obvious that I think we should support further research on epigenetics (not to mention genetics, psychology, and all the levels of analysis in between). But scientists' focus should be on how knowledge about this kind of molecular information can facilitate the helpful manipulation of development; we should remain skeptical of the idea that anything about our bodies or minds is single-handedly *determined* by molecular information transmitted through the germline, whether it be DNA sequence information or epigenetic information that has been altered as a result of our ancestors' experiences.

Armed with all of this information about how our experiences can influence our epigenetic states, how our epigenetic states can influence our phenotypes, and how those phenotypes can effectively be transmitted across generations, we are now in a position to ask some important questions. What does all of this mean for us? What kinds of lessons can we take away from the emerging science of behavioral epigenetics? How will this new information affect how we live our lives? These intriguing questions and several others will be addressed in the next three concluding chapters.

PART IV

IMPLICATIONS

‖ 21 ‖

Caution

As I was writing this book, I received an e-mail from one of my students. The note contained a link to a website that turned out to be a blog designed to advertise a forthcoming book. Because my student knew that I have spent my 25-year career studying infants, he thought I would be interested in this webpage, because it discussed the epigenetic effects of diet, stress, and toxins on developing babies. The link in the e-mail steered me to a blog post about epigenetics and autism; I read it with enthusiasm, hoping to learn something of value.

The post started off well, pointing out that autism is still a poorly understood disorder, that its diagnosis is on the rise, and that it is probably best thought of as a syndrome affecting more than just the nervous system. The author pointed out the very interesting finding that a large proportion of children diagnosed with autism also have gastrointestinal complications, and then made the accurate statement that dietary factors can influence gene expression. But he continued, stating that by feeding your child in particular ways you can reduce their risk of autism by turning off "autism genes," a claim that is unsubstantiated at best.

In the long run, our understanding of epigenetics will probably change how doctors practice medicine, how politicians regulate industry, and how the rest of us live our lives. Virtually everyone will feel the implications of this new knowledge. But today, we remain very far from being able to apply information about epigenetics in a practical way. The gap between the future that many people foresee and the reality of the present has been a source of some trouble, as epigenetics enthusiasts like this autism blogger have rushed in with bold speculations that are almost certainly ill-considered.

Although research on epigenetics will ultimately yield revolutionary insights, this research has not yet produced many—or, some would say, any—novel, concrete, trustworthy recommendations. Specifically, no dietary manipulations have been discovered that target genes associated with autism. In fact, the genetics of autism is still extremely unclear[1] and few genes have been found that contribute to the development of the disorder in a major way;[2] the mere existence of "autism genes" remains very controversial.[3]

And because epigenetic treatments for any condition would need to target specific cell types—since every cell type has a different epigenetic state—the suggestion that we currently know how diet affects autism via epigenetics is absurd. The evidence available to us strongly suggests that our diets have significant effects on the functioning of our genes, but we are still a long way from being able to prescribe diets that will protect babies from neurological conditions like autism. Unfortunately, no one currently knows how we might be able to use the results of epigenetics research to help us raise happy, healthy babies.

This example of questionable speculation is, unfortunately, not at all exceptional; a lot of similar speculation has already appeared in various digital and print media. Therefore, it seems advisable to briefly delay consideration of the implications of behavioral epigenetics research and to take note here of some claims about epigenetics that should be considered with a large dose of skepticism.

The Dangers of Determinism

Many writers have written about how behavioral epigenetics strikes at the heart of genetic determinism, and, in fact, the discovery that epigenetic states can be influenced by experiences *is* antithetical to genetic determinism. Several articles in the popular press have focused on this implication, as evidenced by titles like "Why Your DNA Isn't Destiny"[4] which appeared in *Time Magazine,* or "Victory over the Genes"[5] which appeared (as "Der sieg über die gene") in the popular German news magazine, *Der Spiegel.* By the end of the 20th century, it was already apparent that genes do not operate deterministically,[6a-6c] and with the discovery that genes can be silenced or activated by experiences, everyone has now come to the same conclusion.

Unfortunately, it is possible to embrace epigenetics in a way that, perhaps inadvertently, fosters *other* forms of determinism. For instance, because several of the more compelling findings regarding behavioral epigenetics have emerged from labs studying the long-term effects of early life experiences, several writers have implied that babies' early experiences necessarily have permanent effects on their characteristics. But in general, we should be wary of claims that treating babies in particular ways will "inoculate" them against future afflictions, because although nutritious diets and enriched environments are obviously important, human development is not a deterministic process, so our mature characteristics are no more determined by our epigenetics than they are by our genetics. Actually, any of the developmental resources that contribute to our phenotypes, including, for example, epigenetic marks, nutritional factors, DNA sequence information, and specific experiences, can mistakenly be thought to determine developmental outcomes. Thus, *epi*genetic determinism—the idea that an organism's *epi*genetic state invariably leads to a particular phenotype—is still a form of determinism, and as such, it is only marginally less perilous than genetic determinism. Both perspectives are equally unfounded, as they both erroneously assume that our fate is somehow sealed early in life, even before significant developmental events have taken place.

Journalists in particular have shown a tendency to slip into epigenetic determinism by suggesting that environmental factors can switch genes on and off and thereby single-handedly *cause* phenotypes such as a specific disease state or a short stature. This kind of writing has the potential to perpetuate the same error as the "gene *for* a phenotype" error that has plagued biology for decades, an error that incorrectly presumes that there are genes that *dictate* particular phenotypes; the only difference is that this kind of writing replaces the "gene" with the more epigenetically flavored "gene switch." But diseases—and certainly phenotypes like height—are not caused by single factors like genes *or* gene switches; they develop through interactions involving many of the components in a very complex system.[7] Thus, epigenetic abnormalities ought not be thought of as single-handedly causing diseases, let alone phenotypes more generally; the development of phenotypes depends on the contexts in which epigenetic marks (and other developmentally relevant factors, of course) are embedded.

In the chapter "Experience," I hinted at my concern about replacing genetic determinism with epigenetic determinism; there, I noted that the Meaney team's use of the phrase "epigenetic programming"[8] unnecessarily implies that a rat's early experience of maternal neglect *inevitably* causes it to be a fearful adult. In fact, several subsequent studies have revealed that the effects of early experiences are reversible,[9a–9c] so it remains true that phenotypes are not predetermined in a rigid way. Instead, an animal with a given phenotype at one point in time might have a different phenotype later on, depending on the experiences it has as its life unfolds.

This is a double-edged sword. On one hand, it means that even if a harrowing experience in childhood contributes to a person having a post-traumatic stress disorder today, the person will not necessarily remain symptomatic in the future; treatments for these symptoms exist, and continue to be refined.[10] On the other hand, it means that there is no pre- or perinatal program of epigenetic manipulation that can ever *ensure* smart, happy, healthy offspring, because intelligence, contentment, and healthiness are characteristics that *develop* over many years of postnatal life. Expectant mothers who carefully monitor their diet and stress throughout gestation and infancy, but who then pay no attention as their children enter a wider world containing Cheetos, Big Macs, and Ring Dings are probably more likely to end up with obese teenagers than are mothers who are less conscientious during pregnancy, but who then carefully teach their preteen children how to eat in healthy ways and how to be self-disciplined. As much as we would like to believe that maternal behavior can "inoculate" fetuses or babies to ensure health and intelligence later in childhood, it just doesn't work this way; raising happy, healthy people is an endeavor that takes years.

Biological determinism of any sort is bad news, and not just because it can delude us into believing that we have placed a child permanently on the right track and can therefore now safely pay less attention to her development. Another risk comes from the detrimental effects of believing that, for instance, a particular child is "never going to amount to anything" or is otherwise predictably destined for some unfavorable fate; telling a child what he will never be capable of can profoundly influence what he is ultimately incapable of! And biological determinism can have consequences that are negative for adults, as well; a woman who believes it is imperative to "bond" with a newborn within moments of delivery—lest the baby inevitably grow up to have "attachment issues"—is likely to be distraught if she is hospitalized following delivery and therefore unable to spend this time with her baby. Fortunately, despite some evidence that maternal separation can be stressful for newborn *mice*,[11] there is no evidence that a newborn *baby's* first experiences have permanent effects on its relationship with its mother;[12] but a woman who believes she has forevermore missed her chance to forge a normal attachment relationship with her baby could be harmed by her misunderstanding.

Even in situations where we know that certain prenatal experiences *can* have very long-term effects, determinism is still an inappropriate framework for thinking about human development. For example, no one today doubts that drinking alcohol during pregnancy is bad for a fetus, but in the hundreds of years before scientists established this relationship, innumerable fetuses exposed to some alcohol nonetheless grew up to be healthy, normal adults. This does not mean pregnant women should drink alcohol freely, of course, but it does mean that developmental outcomes are not as easy to predict as we sometimes think. Therefore, it is probably always a bad idea to apply a deterministic worldview to a human being. Like DNA segments, epigenetic marks should not be considered destiny. And like epigenetic marks, early experiences should not be considered destiny. How a given child will develop after an isolated trauma, for example, depends on a lot more than simply the experience of the trauma itself.

Healthy Lifestyles, Healthy Skepticism

The first chapter of this book contained the following quotation: "Epigenetics ... has decisive power for inducing cancer."[13] Like the fact that human development is not a deterministic process, the discovery that epigenetic factors play important roles in the development of some diseases is a double-edged sword. On one hand, this discovery holds out the possibility that epigenetic treatments for these diseases will be forthcoming. On the other hand, it can leave some people with the impression that our health is more controllable than it is. Actually, some self-help books have explicitly stated that discoveries about epigenetics mean that individuals afflicted with pathological conditions should be able to consciously restore themselves to health by engaging epigenetic processes through changes in cognition or attitude. Although our thoughts and attitudes do influence how our bodies function, it is almost certainly an overinterpretation of existing epigenetics data to claim that people can purposefully influence their epigenetic functioning in ways that can cure cancer or other serious diseases.

There are at least two reasons for thinking this idea is potentially dangerous. Although our thoughts *can* influence our body's stress responses, I am not aware of any evidence that we can *consciously* control the epigenetic activity in our cells. I am strongly in favor of an open-minded approach to healthcare that seeks treatments that *work*, for whatever reason; I am very happy for anyone who beats cancer using any technique whatsoever. But claims that visualization or other meditative techniques *will* cure cancer through epigenetic mechanisms are misleading; such assertions have not yet been studied—let alone confirmed—and they imply that anyone who succumbs to their ill health is in some way complicit with that outcome (e.g., "if you're sick, it must be because you haven't taken care of yourself properly or haven't treated the illness by altering your lifestyle in the proper holistic way"). I appreciate that the authors of self-help books are trying to convey a positive message to the world, but the subtext in some of these books is actually offensive in cases where ailments cannot simply be treated with lifestyle changes. There are certainly pathological conditions that *can* be treated with lifestyle changes, but there are other conditions that are not so easily managed, and the discovery that experiences alter gene expression has not immediately provided us with the tools to cure these conditions.

There is another reason to be concerned about the suggestion that we can heal ourselves through the powers of epigenetics and positive thinking. It is possible that such claims could taint epigenetics by associating it with pseudoscientific ideas like astrology, rebirthing therapy, or the healing powers of crystals or therapeutic touch. This should concern all of us, because our emerging understanding of epigenetics is extremely important, and if there are a lot of writers using "epigenetics" as a buzzword to sell snake-oil-like products, there is a risk that this legitimate line of research will lose respect. Scientists still have very little understanding of how epigenetic factors are related to most pathological conditions, and at present, we will all be best served by acknowledging that fact. Of course, it is perfectly reasonable to praise healthy lifestyles, because consuming a nutritious diet, exercising, avoiding tobacco products, and otherwise engaging in positive behaviors can have positive effects on our minds and bodies. But even if we know, for instance, that your diet can affect the epigenetic state of your genes, we still have little idea of which genes in which cells are affected by which foods (or why), so making specific claims about the effects of specific diets (or other lifestyle factors) on pathologies that we do not yet understand is probably a very bad idea.

Forging Ahead

In September 2012, Judith Shulevitz, the science editor for the *New Republic* magazine, published an opinion piece in the *New York Times* in which she wrote, "In the past decade or so, the study of epigenetics has become so popular it's practically a fad."[14] Two years later, there can be no doubt that curiosity about epigenetics is still on the rise. Consider Figure 21.1, generated by Google Books Ngram Viewer, which plots how frequently a word—in this case, "Epigenetics"—appeared in books each year. Clearly, epigenetics is "trending." Given the likelihood that increasing numbers of people will be using this word in everyday conversation in the coming years, it is important to think about how to best understand this new science.

Research in behavioral epigenetics is likely to generate some exciting applications in the near future, and in the next chapter, I will present recent findings that support this kind of optimism. But this is a new science, and there is still very little that we can be confident about. In the final chapter of this book, I will discuss some well-founded conclusions we can draw from behavioral epigenetics, but for now, it is important to be clear about its *limits*. As we have seen, epigenetic factors cannot single-handedly determine future developmental pathways or outcomes, so epigenetics is not a mechanism by which we can instill in babies an unalterable propensity for health or intelligence. Another limitation worth mentioning is that epigenetics is unlikely to be a conduit to the psychological memories of our ancestors, notwithstanding some writers' speculations to that effect,[15a–15b] or a recent intriguing scientific report about the transgenerational transmission of memories.[16] Even though our cognitive-behavioral memory systems (i.e., normal memory) might have co-opted epigenetic *cellular* memory,[17] there is little reason to believe epigenetic marks can transmit genuine *cognitive* memories across generations. Epigenetic marks reflect *aspects* of the histories of our ancestors

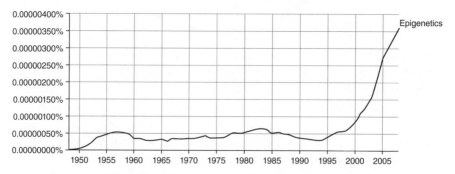

Figure 21.1 A display generated by Google Books Ngram Viewer. This graph plots how frequently the word "Epigenetics" has appeared in books each year between 1945 and 2008.

(e.g., epigenetic marks might record *how much* our ancestors ate at particular times in their lives), but it is hard to believe that our genomes carry specific memories of our ancestors' experiences (e.g., there is no evidence that epigenetic marks serve as a record of *what* our ancestors ate—or otherwise experienced subjectively— at particular times in their lives). Given what neuroscientists understand about memory and development, we can be fairly confident that people cannot experience "past lives," so the idea that epigenetic marks might give us access to our ancestors' memories seems rather implausible.

As the age of epigenetics dawns, it is as if we are opening a new door in a castle we've been inhabiting for years, and although there is no light in the space behind the door, our torch is providing a partial view of what appears to be a truly enormous, previously unknown area right here in our own castle, a space that is at least as big as the space we've been living in for many decades. There's a lot of new terrain to explore, but to just run into the darkness as if we've found paradise would be a mistake. The discovery that genetic activity can be influenced by our experiences does not mean we can simply wish away our ills. Likewise, cowering in the doorway, afraid to look around because the unknown seems mysterious would be an error as well. The reality is that we now need to do a lot of careful research to help us understand what to do with what we've found so far, and to open more doors in our castle.

22

Hope

Last summer, my wife and I met a man in Juneau, Alaska who had recently relocated there from Kansas. When we asked him if he had traveled around Alaska before settling in Juneau, he confirmed that he had, but that he had decided to stay in Juneau because it was so "secluded." After we asked him if he liked it there, he began telling us about how difficult the long, dark winter months had been and about how high suicide rates are in Alaska. But then he told us that he had found something "better than any drug," not knowing that I would be aware of this common treatment for seasonal affective disorder; in the winter, he said, he would sit in front of a bright white light and it made him feel better.

That night at dinner, I mentioned to my wife that I was writing about two of these issues in my book: The influence of light on the functioning of DNA in some of our neurons, and the influence of reduced social contact on gene expression in white blood cells. To a person writing a book about research on epigenetics, the potential implications of this work are everywhere. It will still be a while before we all feel the effects of scientists' emerging understanding of epigenetics, but it is reasonable to assume that this new understanding will be a game changer in many domains. How doctors practice medicine, how mental health professionals treat people with psychopathology, how public health experts encourage wholesome lifestyles, and how the Environmental Protection Agency evaluates the effects of environmental toxins[1a-1b]—all of these will be transformed by the emerging science of epigenetics.

In fact, the repercussions of this science could be felt even farther afield. For instance, research on epigenetics could change how our courts interpret statutes of limitations, because of the possibility that offspring can inherit epigenetic changes originally acquired when their ancestors were exposed to environmental toxins. It could change how ethicists and legislators evaluate the competing interests of fertile women and employers, because employers might not hire fertile women in a paternalistic attempt to protect future offspring from detrimental epigenetic effects of particular workplace substances. It could change how insurance companies evaluate the risk of underwriting policies for individuals with particular epigenetic profiles. And it could change how the US Food and Drug Administration (FDA) tests the effects—and evaluates the risk—of drugs, nutritional supplements, or foods (e.g., derived from cloned animals, perhaps).[2] Because our epigenomes are as central to human nature as are our genomes, we can expect research on epigenetics to have wide-ranging consequences.

Many of these consequences will already be evident from the preceding chapters. Because epigenetic processes are responsible for the differentiation that turns embryonic stem cells into mature cells, a good understanding of epigenetics could help researchers "dedifferentiate" cells and thereby grow replacement tissues for people with degenerative diseases. Because memory utilizes epigenetic processes, epigenetic treatments could help ease some of the symptoms of people suffering from dementia or milder forms of memory impairment. Because early exposure to neglect, abuse, or poverty has epigenetic consequences—and because the epigenetic effects of poor parenting in rodents can be alleviated with drug treatments that could ultimately be effective in people, too—research on these effects has the potential to improve many lives. Because the results of research on epigenetics will likely illuminate how diet contributes to diabetes, heart disease, hypertension, obesity, and stroke, this knowledge could reduce the incidence of these conditions. And because some epigenetic marks seem to be inheritable, studies of this occurrence might spur overdue changes to the neo-Darwinian understanding of evolutionary processes. Any one of these ramifications of epigenetics research could be considered extremely important. Together, they should be recognized as monumental.

Widening the Perspective: The Role of Epigenetics in Pathology

Many of the implications of epigenetics apply to all of us, because we all form memories, experience circadian rhythms, deal with life's stresses, and begin life as children exposed to parenting of one quality or another. Because these are universal experiences, this book has focused on epigenetic effects in these domains and has mostly ignored the development of abnormal conditions. But epigenetic contributions to various disorders are extremely important, even if cancer, psychopathology, and other diseases with epigenetic components affect only some of us. Because scientists have invested countless hours and research dollars exploring the epigenetics of pathological conditions, many of the implications of epigenetics research can be seen in these areas.

Recently, epigeneticists have generated a blizzard of research data, and in these pages I have only considered the tip of the resulting snowdrift. In part, this narrow focus reflects my concern with *behavioral* epigenetics, the branch of the field that asks how epigenetic factors affect behavior or other psychological processes;[3] if we use epigenetics to explain why we are fearful in unfamiliar situations, why we fall asleep at 8 p.m. when we fly thousands of miles from home, or why we react as we do when we find ourselves in a situation we have learned is dangerous, we are explaining how our epigenetic states affect our behaviors. But just as interesting is the converse, that is, how our behaviors affect our epigenetic states. If our behaviors provide us with experiences that change our epigenetics, this is a topic behavioral epigeneticists would find worthy of consideration as well.[4] And because many medical conditions are influenced by lifestyle—lung cancer is related to smoking cigarettes, for example, and heart disease is related to certain diets—it can be worthwhile to ask about the role of epigenetics in these relationships.

At present, we know relatively little about exactly how our behaviors alter our epigenetic states in ways that contribute to pathology. But it is clear that our epigenetic states are related to certain kinds of pathologies, that certain kinds of pathologies are related to our experiences, and that our experiences are related to our epigenetic states (see Figure 22.1). So all of the pieces of the puzzle are present; we just need to figure out how they fit together.

Although I have hardly mentioned it so far, the most salient topic in epigenetics today is probably cancer.[5] This is because scientists now know that cancer cells typically have DNA that is less methylated than the DNA in normal cells. A decade ago, studies with mice revealed that abnormally low levels of DNA methylation are involved in causing tumors,[6] and, according to Andrew Feinberg, subsequent studies suggested "that epigenetic disruption of stem cells is a common unifying theme" that explains cancer origins, and that changes to the methylation of our genomes "occur early and ubiquitously in cancer."[7] It might seem counterintuitive that cancer is associated with DNA *hypo*methylation, because we know that licking and grooming leads rats to have hypomethylated GR genes, an epigenetic state associated with *healthier*, less fearful rats. But as mentioned earlier, methylation per se is neither good nor bad; what matters is *which* DNA segments are methylated. In the case of cancer, our cells contain genes that can cause uncontrollable cell proliferation when the genes are overexpressed; therefore, demethylation of these genes can contribute to the development of malignant tumors.

Somewhat surprisingly, although global hypomethylation leads to tumor formation, cancer has also been associated with the *hyper*methylation of *particular*

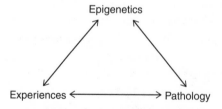

Figure 22.1 Experiences, epigenetics, and pathology mutually influence one another.

genes.[8] This is not as unreasonable as it initially sounds, because in addition to containing genes that contribute to cell proliferation, normal cells contain so-called tumor-suppressor genes that ordinarily help produce cancer-deterring proteins. Suppressing a tumor-suppressor is like damaging a car's brakes—it can speed up a dangerous process. So, when tumor *suppressor* genes are *hyper*methylated and therefore go unexpressed, tumor development is more likely. Because epigenetic alterations play critical early roles in the development of cancer,[9] at least one writer has actually *defined* a cancer-causing agent as "something that alters epigenetic regulation."[10]

Emerging insights about the epigenetic nature of cancer have already yielded some effective treatments that I will discuss below. But we are still largely ignorant about how all of this works,[11] so it remains to be seen how epigenetics research will change how we treat cancer and seek to prevent it. Nonetheless, these efforts will almost certainly yield specific recommendations eventually, because at least 90% of cancer cases are associated with lifestyle or environmental factors,[12] so how we behave can reduce our risk of succumbing to this scourge.

Seeking Immortality in the Epigenetics of Aging

Changes in DNA methylation are not found only in cancer patients. As we age, the extent to which our genomes are methylated changes, and the amount of DNA methylation found in some individuals undergoes strikingly extensive changes in as little as 10–15 years.[13] In addition to helping explain why many common diseases first appear when we get older,[14] this finding could potentially help us understand aging itself as an epigenetic phenomenon. Although people have traditionally thought of aging as a normal process—because we all go through it—some scientists have speculated that aging should perhaps be considered a disease,[15] one that can potentially be cured.[16] So far, the data we have on the relationship between epigenetic changes and human aging is strictly correlational, meaning we do not yet have conclusive evidence that epigenetic changes *cause* aging.[17] Nonetheless, it is clear that a detailed understanding of epigenetic processes has the potential to modify the once-certain belief that the changes we associate with old age are inevitable.

We currently know little about how epigenetics and aging are related—for instance, we don't know if aging causes epigenetic changes or vice versa—but some exciting new data suggest that it could be the epigenetic changes that are running the show.[18a–18c] The epigenetic effects revealed in these data occur at the tail ends of chromosomes, where there are DNA segments known as *telomeres*. Telomeres effectively serve as chromosome "caps" that function like the plastic pieces at the ends of shoelaces, which keep the laces from unraveling.[19] These "caps" are related to aging because every time a cell divides, its chromosomes' telomeres get a little bit shorter. Once the telomeres in a cell have reached a critically short length, that cell can no longer divide, at which point the cell becomes inactive (or dead), having entered old age. The fact that most of our cells can divide only a fixed number of times before their telomeres are too short to permit further duplication limits the life span of a body.[20] This discovery has led some scientists to believe there could be a way to extend our life spans to previously unthinkable lengths,[21] if only we can find a way to keep telomeres functioning as they do in younger cells.

Telomeres cannot be methylated[22] because of how they are constituted, but the histones they are wrapped around *can* be modified through the addition or removal of acetyl groups.[23] In this way, telomere functioning can be influenced by epigenetic events. Scientists have discovered a protein called sirtuin-6 that is present in mammalian cells and that can remove acetyl groups from histones, and this action appears to have important effects on how telomeres function.

Sirtuin-6 (SIRT6) is not the only protein that can remove acetyl groups from other molecules; there is a whole class of proteins that do this, and collectively they're known as deacetylases. But most deacetylases strip acetyl groups somewhat indiscriminately from histones *and* other kinds of molecules.[24] The special talent of SIRT6 is that it specifically deacetylates histones that are associated with telomeres. Moreover, SIRT6 deacetylates these histones in a way that allows telomeres to function normally. We know this because human cells experimentally depleted of SIRT6 eventually develop damaged telomeres.[25] Thus, by virtue of its epigenetic activities, SIRT6 might be involved in regulating life span.

Experimental studies have revealed that genetically engineered mice that are deficient in SIRT6—but that are otherwise normal—develop early symptoms of aging,[26] a finding that could mean SIRT6 has some youth-conferring properties. And in a truly sensational development, a group of Israeli scientists recently created some genetically engineered mice that *overexpress* SIRT6, and sure enough, male mice engineered in this way have a significantly longer life span than normal mice. These researchers concluded, "The regulation of mammalian lifespan by [SIRT6] . . . has important therapeutic implications for age-related diseases."[27, 28] Clearly, this is *very* exciting research. And because SIRT6 activity has also been linked to a syndrome in which *humans* age prematurely,[29] this work could apply to people in the same way that it applies to mice. Centuries-long life spans might sound like the stuff of science fiction, but research in this domain suggests that some fantastic breakthroughs in life-extension might be possible in the future. The potential antiaging implications of epigenetics research can, perhaps, best highlight how genuinely transformative this science might turn out to be.

Moving beyond general age-related infirmities, epigenetics research has also changed conventional thinking about some specific diseases, such as type II diabetes and cardiovascular diseases (e.g., stroke and coronary artery disease). Research on the mechanisms responsible for these kinds of conditions has confirmed that experiences very early in development—perhaps even before birth or early in infancy—can have long-term effects on health. Ongoing work in this area could one day reveal epigenetic marks that would permit early predictions about the later development of these disorders.[30a–30b] Finding such marks would be an important breakthrough, because for these kinds of diseases, screening and interventions should take place very early in development.[31] Of course, we still have a way to go before we understand how to *prevent* these kinds of diseases, but as Peter Gluckman and colleagues have written, "if epigenetic biomarkers at or soon after birth do prove to be good indicators of the developmental trajectory and of subsequent risk of disease, then we will be able to use them to identify optimal strategies for supporting health before and during pregnancy."[32]

Memory Disorders: Addiction, Alzheimers, and Post-Traumatic Stress Disorder

As interesting and important as discoveries about cancer, aging, and cardiovascular or metabolic diseases might be, people fascinated by the human psyche will also be intrigued by epigenetic data related to abnormal behaviors, thoughts, or emotions. There is an almost palpable excitement about epigenetics these days among mental health professionals,[33] and it's understandable; epigenetic states seem to be associated with psychological states, and there is reason to hope that epigenetics research will help us finally learn what causes—and how to best treat—specific psychopathologies. Evidence of the widespread interest in these questions was available in the first issue of the 2013 volume of the journal *Neuropsychopharmacology*,[34] which contained a special section comprising 15 articles on epigenetic mechanisms in psychiatry, including papers on memory impairment, post-traumatic stress disorder, cocaine use, depression, schizophrenia, stroke, and epilepsy. Even more recent papers have reported correlations between epigenetic profiles and behavioral abnormalities as diverse as bulimia[35] and chronic physical aggression in childhood.[36a–36c]

Psychopathologists are excited about epigenetics because of the growing quantity of circumstantial evidence linking epigenetic variations to psychological variations.[37] (In addition, there is enthusiasm about the "novel" insight from epigenetics that explaining pathology requires references to more than just "genetic" or "environmental" factors; endnote number 38 considers this idea further, and why it isn't actually novel.)[38] It is important to note, however, that much of what has been written about the role of epigenetics in psychopathology remains speculative. In fact, there is still scant—if any—direct evidence that epigenetic factors *cause* psychiatric disorders.[39] Nonetheless, the evidence that *is* available is certainly suggestive, and there is a lot of it, some of which we have already encountered. For instance, I have already described studies that found different DNA methylation profiles in the brains of suicidal versus nonsuicidal people.[40a–40b] Likewise, I have already described the contribution of epigenetic factors to the formation[41a–41e] and retrieval[42] of long-term memories. Discoveries about the roles of epigenetic factors in memory have obvious implications for memory-related disorders such as Alzheimer's disease,[43] and they also have implications for other kinds of memory-related psychopathology.

One such pathology is post-traumatic stress disorder (PTSD). As a team of researchers who study *memory* in animals pointed out recently, epigenetic mechanisms are involved in learning that is relevant to post-traumatic stress, so "these mechanisms may contribute to [PTSD] in humans."[44] Likewise, a pair of researchers studying PTSD per se have written that although there is no evidence of "epigenetic modifications that are specific" to PTSD, many empirical observations from recent studies are "compatible with epigenetic explanations" of PTSD.[45] Additional knowledge about the epigenetics of learning has the potential to improve our understanding and treatment of PTSD.

Another psychological condition associated with memory is addiction, and like recent work on PTSD, research on addiction has started to focus on epigenetics.[46a–46c] Among the addictive substances that have been associated with epigenetic effects are alcohol,[47] tobacco,[48] cocaine,[49a–49b] amphetamines,[50] and morphine.[51] Because addiction relies in part on learned associations between the subjective effects of drugs and the contexts in which drugs are consumed (including the paraphernalia used during drug consumption), some addiction theorists consider the mechanisms that support long-term associative memory to be central contributors to addictive behavior;[52a–52b] these include epigenetic mechanisms. As Carey has put it, "addiction to stimulants such as cocaine [or amphetamines] is a classic example of inappropriate adaptations by memory and reward circuits in the brain. These maladaptations are regulated by long-lasting changes in gene expression. Changes in DNA methylation . . . underpin this addiction."[53]

Studies of addiction in mice have revealed that cocaine induces a number of epigenetic effects.[54a–54b] For example, one research team has identified "a crucial role for histone methylation in the long-term actions of cocaine."[55] In summarizing the current state of research on the epigenetics of addiction, a pair of neuroscientists wrote that this is "an exciting new area of research with potential therapeutic benefits. The ability to reverse the epigenetic landscape controlling the addicted state offers an approach that may aid in the development of more effective treatments for addiction."[56] As is true for all of the conditions discussed in this chapter, scientists still have only a weak understanding of how epigenetic factors contribute to drug addiction, but there are good reasons to believe that additional research on these mechanisms will bear fruit.[57]

Psychotic Disorders: Schizophrenia and Bipolar Disorder

The major psychotic disorders—schizophrenia and bipolar disorder—are also starting to share their secrets with epigenetics researchers. After spending several futile decades searching for the presumed genetic causes of these conditions, researchers have finally begun to focus on factors other than DNA sequence information.[58a-58d] Many researchers now view epigenetics as a promising field that's likely to shed light on the origins of psychiatric diseases.[59] This optimism stems from two sources.

The first reason researchers believe epigenetics will help explain psychiatric diseases is the insight that *normal* psychological processes like learning and memory depend on epigenetic regulation; therefore, if something is awry in a person's behaviors, thoughts, or emotions, epigenetic factors could be the culprit. The second reason psychiatric researchers are optimistic about epigenetics is based on the fact that monozygotic (MZ, or "identical") twins do not always share the same diagnosis.[60] For example, if one twin of an MZ pair is diagnosed with schizophrenia, the likelihood that the other twin will develop the disorder is still less than 50%,[61] even though MZ twins share identical DNA sequence information; the analogous number for MZ twins at risk of *bipolar* disorder is even lower, at about 30%.[62] Because the nongenetic factors that *must* account for this sort of discordance have to somehow produce *physical* effects in twins' brains, psychiatric researchers have started to think that epigenetic differences between twins could be the key to understanding these conditions.[63] This hypothesis has received important empirical support, notably in a recent study of MZ twins who were discordant for major psychosis. The scientists who conducted this study found DNA methylation differences that were associated with the twins' phenotypic differences,[64] a finding consistent with the idea that epigenetic factors contribute to schizophrenia and bipolar disorder. Similarly, other studies have found abnormal histone acetylation patterns in the brains of people with major psychosis, patterns that likely increase the risk of developing psychotic disorders by altering gene expression.[65]

Despite researchers' enthusiasm for studies of epigenetic contributions to major psychosis, this line of scientific inquiry is still in its infancy.[66] Many people anticipate important breakthroughs in the coming years, because the idea that differential gene *expression* is what accounts for discordance among MZ twins makes so much sense. But as the psychiatric researchers Bart Rutten and Jonathan Mill wrote in 2009, "while it is easy to theorize about the role of epigenetic processes in mediating susceptibility to psychiatric disorders, actually investigating these modifications at a molecular level is not so straightforward."[67] This reality led Rutten and Mill to point out that "direct evidence for epigenetic dysfunction in both schizophrenia and bipolar disorder is still limited,"[68] and unfortunately, this remains true.[69] Even the data that *are* currently available are of limited value, because they merely reflect correlations between epigenetic and psychological states, and do not help us understand whether the epigenetic factors play a causal role in psychopathology. As one team of researchers noted in 2012, "Most reports that associate epigenetic abnormalities with psychiatric disease do not ascertain whether the association is causal, or if it is a consequence of disease, its treatment, or other disease-related confounds (i.e., recreational drug use)."[70] Nonetheless, researchers working to characterize the relationship between epigenetic abnormalities and the major psychoses continue to be hopeful about the promise of epigenetics, and activity in this research area remains lively.

Autism is another behavioral disorder that has started to draw the attention of epigenetics researchers. As with the major psychoses, the fact that MZ twins can be discordant for autism has suggested to researchers that epigenetic factors might contribute to this condition.[71] As early as 2006, some researchers had taken notice of evidence that "epigenetic factors can have a role in ASD [autism spectrum disorder] susceptibility,"[72] but the picture has not become much clearer since then. There is now evidence that different DNA segments are transcribed in the brains of individuals with and without ASD diagnoses,[73] but to the best of my knowledge, we do not yet know what kinds of epigenetic processes produce these differences or why these processes occur.

One thing that seems apparent is that until we really understand the causes of autism, some writers will remain willing to offer rank speculation about how to prevent this disorder. As we saw in the last chapter, authors writing books for the general public might be particularly vulnerable to this temptation,[74] but some scientists seem willing to overinterpret the available data as well. For example, a 2012 publication on "epigenetics in autism" contained the following alarming (and grammatically perplexing) statement: "Adequate intake of folic acid [i.e., vitamin B_9] will ensure proper DNA methylation status and prevent from [*sic*] aberrant genomic change in neurons and malnutrition possibly induce [*sic*] hypomethylation, which leads to genomic changes in neurons, resulting in mental diseases including autism."[75] In fact, researchers currently know of no single cause of autism,[76] so we can be relatively confident that adequate intake of a vitamin will not single-handedly prevent it. We can hope that in the future, we will understand what combinations of genetic, epigenetic, and environmental factors lead to the development of autism when those factors and their products come together in specific locations in a body at specific times. But at the moment, autism remains poorly understood.

Mood Disorders: Major Depression

The final psychopathology I will discuss here is depression. The fact that suicidal and nonsuicidal people have brains containing DNA that is methylated in different ways[77a-77b] immediately suggests a possible connection between epigenetics and depression. Likewise, because abused or neglected children are at risk of becoming depressed adults,[78] and because such individuals also have abnormal DNA methylation patterns in their brains,[79a-79d] we should not be surprised to find depression associated with epigenetic effects.

Conveniently, depression is a condition for which researchers have managed to create so-called animal models—animals with humanlike abnormalities—to use in their studies. Animal models allow researchers to conduct experiments that can actually reveal something about the *causes* of pathology. These sorts of experiments have revealed that experiences that produce depression-like symptoms in animals also have epigenetic effects, and that drug treatments that interfere with those epigenetic effects are able to alleviate the depression-like symptoms. Such results have left researchers thinking that the association between depression and epigenetics is not merely a coincidence.

For example, exposing mice to what is known as "chronic social defeat stress" creates a very important animal model of depression.[80a-80b] Although it might be cruel to expose innocent mice to the sort of bullying that this procedure entails, this line of research has been extremely valuable in helping scientists learn how chronic stress can produce depression-associated changes in the brain. And just as important, this work has started to clarify exactly how it is that antidepressant medications have the effects they do.

The chronic social defeat stress protocol entails exposing a male test mouse to a highly aggressive mouse, from which the test mouse typically tries to escape. When the test mouse discovers that he is unable to flee, he will ordinarily cry out and become submissive. After 10 minutes in the company of the aggressor, an experimenter places the test mouse in a different compartment of the cage, where he is separated from the bully by nothing more than a clear plastic divider with holes in it; for the next 24 hours, the test mouse is left in a state of chronic stress because he can see, hear, and smell his threatening tormenter in the next compartment. The next day, the entire process is repeated, but with a new bully... and then repeated again on each of the next ten consecutive days. This protocol produces a "defeated" animal that mimics several of the symptoms that characterize *human* depression.[81]

In a landmark study using this procedure, Nadia Tsankova and a team of researchers in Dallas, Texas, examined hippocampi taken from defeated mice 4 weeks after their harrowing experiences. The team discovered that the chromatin in this tissue contained more methyl groups at specific locations on specific histones associated with specific genes, lending support to the idea that social experiences can have long-lasting epigenetic effects in mammalian brains. In their discussion of these results, the researchers wrote, "Our findings suggest that histone hypermethylation may represent a stable stress-induced molecular scar in the hippocampus . . . and that the search for newer antidepressant agents will identify those that are more effective in demethylating histones at repressed genes."[82]

A more recent study by Evan Elliott and a team of neurobiologists in Israel found that this same depression-inducing protocol caused social avoidance in only *some* of the intimidated mice;[83] others were relatively resilient even after experiencing 10 days of social stress. Importantly, in the mice that became socially avoidant—and only in those mice—being bullied produced long-term demethylation of a DNA segment used in the brain to build a stress-causing hormone.[84] Thus, chronic social stress produced depression-like symptoms in these mice, and it appeared to do it by epigenetically up-regulating production of this hormone. As a result, the researchers concluded that their findings implicated "epigenetics as a primary regulator of behavior."[85]

Both the Tsankova team and the Elliott team also reported that if the traumatized mice were treated with an antidepressant drug every day for at least a few weeks following their stressful experiences, they behaved like normal mice. These findings were expected, because antidepressants are known to normalize the behaviors of depressed animals; this is why they are called antidepressants! But in a particularly informative finding, both sets of researchers found that repeated antidepressant treatments had epigenetic effects as well, effectively reversing the effects of the social defeat stress.[86a-86b] Elliott and colleagues concluded that antidepressant medications can influence DNA methylation in a way that is correlated with both stress hormone production and social behavior,[87] and Tsankova and colleagues concluded that their "experiments underscore an important role for histone remodeling in the [development] and treatment of depression."[88] Because social defeat stress produces a number of other epigenetic effects in adult mice as well,[89a-89b] it is possible—and perhaps even likely—that research on the epigenetics of depression will ultimately yield a detailed understanding of *how* bad experiences can make us depressed, and of *how* existing psychiatric medications can make us feel better.

First-Generation Epigenetic Medicine: Treating Cancer

Knowing what causes depression, cancer, schizophrenia, and heart disease is valuable for several reasons, perhaps the most important being that it opens the door to developing better treatments for these conditions. Scientists have only just begun the research that will allow epigenetic medicine to come into its own, but this work has already generated some successes, and it is now easy to imagine a future in which epigenetic treatments are common. We should be cautious with our conjectures, of course, because the sheer complexity of the molecular systems within us[90a–90b] means there are plenty of things that could go wrong when doctors start prescribing epigenetic treatments. But there is definitely reason to be optimistic.

As I noted at the end of the chapter "Memory," scientists have experimentally improved the memories of both normal and impaired lab animals,[91a–91c] and in "Zooming in on Memory," I provided details about how they accomplished this feat with drugs. Readers who missed those details might appreciate the following two-paragraph summary of how some epigenetic treatments work.

In general, there are two classes of epigenetic drugs I will discuss here. The first class contains drugs that interfere with DNA methylation. These drugs work by inhibiting the activity of proteins that normally methylate DNA, proteins called *DNA methyltransferases*, or DNMTs; drugs that inhibit DNMTs are known as DNMT-inhibitors. By interfering with DNA methylation, DNMT-inhibitors leave DNA strands *less* methylated. And because hypomethylated DNA can be "read" by cellular transcription machinery, DNMT-inhibitors are drugs that increase gene expression.

The second class of epigenetic medications contains drugs that inhibit the activity of deacetylases. As I noted above when introducing SIRT6, deacetylases remove acetyl groups from other molecules; when they remove acetyl groups from histones (as SIRT6 does), they are called *histone deacetylases*, or HDACs; drugs that inhibit HDACs are known as HDAC-inhibitors. By interfering with the *de*acetylation of histones, HDAC-inhibitors leave histones *more* acetylated. And because histone acetylation is associated with gene activation, HDAC-inhibitors are drugs that increase gene expression. Thus, both DNMT-inhibitors and HDAC-inhibitors are drugs that increase gene expression.

The FDA has sanctioned a very small number of drugs that specifically target epigenetic marks, although several others are currently undergoing clinical trials.[92] Two of the first generation of epigenetic drugs are HDAC-inhibitors approved for the treatment of a particular type of cancer; two others are DNMT-inhibitors approved for the treatment of a group of blood disorders that often develop into leukemia. HDAC-inhibitors are thought to fight cancer by increasing the activity of tumor suppressor genes. Unfortunately, they have been somewhat disappointing, because they have proven relatively ineffective against tumors that grow in localized organs; instead, they work best on so-called liquid tumors that circulate throughout the body, such as blood cancers like leukemia or lymphoma.[93] Still, the discovery of epigenetic drugs that can bring *any* cancers under control has certainly encouraged scientists who are working to develop such medications.

Newer research in this domain has sought to improve the weapons in our anticancer arsenal by developing epigenetic drugs that produce more focused effects than do currently available drugs. One problem with first-generation HDAC-inhibitors is that they are nonselective; they affect histones in a relatively indiscriminate way and are therefore toxic at high doses.[94a–94b] Likewise, first-generation DNMT-inhibitors affect virtually any DNA segment they can access, regardless of what those segments do. But as we know, *which* DNA segments are activated or silenced matters very much—activation of some genes can lead to cancer whereas activation of tumor-suppressor genes has the opposite effect—so drugs that increase gene expression *in general* are of limited value because they can affect untargeted genes and thereby produce undesirable consequences.[95]

Fortunately, researchers have discovered some compounds that are more selective than first-generation epigenetic drugs—these recently discovered chemicals modify very specific *histone methylation* marks[96]—and pharmaceutical companies are working feverishly to develop more of these drugs, in part because successful epigenetic medications will probably be worth billions of dollars.[97] But even compounds that affect specific components of specific histones would still not necessarily target particular DNA segments; like HDAC-inhibitors and DNMT-inhibitors, drugs that influence histone methylation are still likely to work in a genomewide manner and therefore not be very precise. Consequently, other researchers are working to target specific genes through the use of molecules that interfere with the production of histone-acetylating proteins.[98] Because there are so many different avenues currently being explored, making specific predictions about what the future holds for epigenetic medicine would probably be foolhardy. But the hope is that additional work in this domain will eventually produce epigenetic therapies that can be fine-tuned to address specific disorders.

The Future of Epigenetic Medicine: Treating Memory Disorders

Treating psychopathology with epigenetic drugs is probably even more difficult than fighting cancer with such medications.[99] Not only are available epigenetic drugs nonselective with respect to the genome; currently, we do not even know the extent to which they differentially affect specific human brain regions, so psychiatrists will not be able to prescribe them until a lot of additional testing has been completed.[100] Moreover, although a person with a fatal blood disorder might be willing to suffer through the unpleasant side-effects of a DNMT-inhibitor (for example) if the drug is keeping them alive, this drug would never be prescribed for a less deadly condition because of the possibility that the drug itself could render some cell types cancerous.[101] But these kinds of obstacles have not prevented researchers from studying the effects of epigenetic drugs on *rodents'* behaviors, and some of the discoveries these researchers have reported are amazing. And because efforts are ongoing to find ways to more selectively target epigenetic marks, this research might ultimately lead to treatments that can help people with their memories, their anxieties, their mood disorders, or their addictions.

In the domain of memory, HDAC-inhibitors have effects in mice that would be therapeutically valuable if they prove to be reproducible in human beings.[102] Memory seems to be better in brains with higher levels of histone acetylation in general, and HDAC-inhibitors seem to consistently improve memory in normal,[103] disordered,[104] and aged[105] mice. As an example of how remarkable some of this research is, consider the following study that compared young adult mice with mice well past middle age.

All of the mice in this study first went through contextual fear conditioning, but the oldest mice exhibited impaired learning, much as elderly people often do. In addition, after conditioning, the oldest mice had less hippocampal histone acetylation than did their younger counterparts. So, the researchers then assembled a new set of aged mice and injected an HDAC-inhibitor called SAHA directly into their hippocampi, to see if the increased acetylation produced by the drug might help them better remember their experiences. These elderly mice—along with some elderly control mice that were *not* exposed to SAHA—were then subjected to contextual fear conditioning. And voilà: compared with the untreated mice, those injected with SAHA now had hippocampal histone acetylation like their younger counterparts. Most importantly, their ability to remember their conditioning experience was restored to its former level.[106]

Such findings have obvious implications for people with diminished memories, including those with Alzheimer's disease as well as those with ordinary age-related memory impairments. But the application of this kind of discovery could be much broader, since memory plays important roles in human psychopathologies like anxiety disorders[107] and drug addictions.[108] For example, it is possible that memory-improving drugs could also help prevent *relapse* in individuals who have successfully overcome an addiction or an anxiety disorder.

The Future of Epigenetic Therapies: Treating Depression and Anxiety

Scientists studying stress reactions and depression have also reported extraordinary effects of epigenetic drugs. For example, Meaney and colleagues[109a–109b] investigated whether an HDAC-inhibitor could reverse the epigenetic and behavioral effects of depriving young rat pups of licking and grooming. After experiencing low-LG mothering shortly after birth, neglected rats grew up to be relatively fearful in adulthood, as expected. But after these rats had an HDAC-inhibitor called trichostatin A (TSA) injected directly into their brains, they began to behave as fearlessly as their untreated counterparts who had been reared by *high* LG mothers. Such findings suggest that TSA effectively undid the effect of inattentive mothering on fearful behaviors in adulthood.[110] It is important to remember that licking and grooming affects *DNA methylation*; thus, since TSA—which has its effects on *histone acetylation*—reversed the effects of neglectful mothering, HDAC-inhibitors like TSA can likely alter DNA methylation, even though DNA methylation was once thought to be extremely stable.[111] The implications of these results are far ranging, of course. If researchers are able to develop ways to use epigenetic drugs safely and precisely in human beings, it is conceivable that treatment with these drugs could diminish the depression and anxiety that normally results from childhood neglect or abuse.

Epigenetic drugs also effectively treat mice that have depression-like symptoms caused by stress exposure. In one study of social defeat stress, infusion of HDAC-inhibitors directly into a specific brain region produced strong antidepressant-like effects;[112] in some cases, the drugs produced effects on gene expression patterns that were remarkably similar to the effects of a well-known antidepressant drug, Prozac.[113] In another study of mice,[114] exposure to milder forms of stress—for instance, weeks of staying in a tilted, soiled, small, or perpetually lighted cage—robbed mice of their interest in social interactions and other pleasurable stimuli like tasty treats (this symptom, called anhedonia, is common in human depression). As in the study of social defeat stress, the depressive symptoms caused by *mild* stress were relieved by treatment with an HDAC-inhibitor, SAHA; in addition, the depressive symptoms caused by mild stress were relieved by treatment with the first of the modern antidepressant drugs, imipramine. Importantly, in addition to alleviating the behavioral symptoms of depression, both SAHA and imipramine had significant effects on histone deacetylases and histone modifications.

These findings about imipramine are important because they suggest that the antidepressants currently dispensed by psychiatrists might actually relieve depression by influencing epigenetic activity, even if no one previously understood that this is how they work. The results of the studies just described are consistent with the idea that antidepressants work via epigenetic effects.[115a-115d] More support for this idea comes from Catherine Dulac's observation that "repeated electroconvulsive treatment, one of the most effective treatments for major depression, triggers histone modifications," thereby altering the expression of several genes in a sustained way.[116] Because depression treatments as disparate as drug therapy and electroconvulsive therapy both produce epigenetic alterations, it could be that *all* current treatments for depression will one day be understood to work via epigenetics; in fact, it is already the case that numerous psychotropic drugs have been found to produce epigenetic changes in the brain.[117] But regardless of whether sweeping statements about antidepressant therapies turn out to be warranted, there can be little doubt that ongoing work on epigenetics and mood disorders could ultimately generate new approaches for treating conditions like anxiety disorders or major depression.[118]

The benefits of epigenetics research will ultimately accrue to more than just pharmaceutical companies and the people who use their drugs. As we have seen, dietary manipulations can affect epigenetic states, too, and sometimes in profound ways.[119a-119b] Unfortunately, some of the problems associated with epigenetic drugs also plague dietary manipulations, as there are currently no ways to target specific genes, histones, organs, or brain structures with such manipulations. Thus, consuming methyl-rich foods or supplements might increase DNA methylation in a nonspecific manner, in which case it would be difficult to predict the effects of such actions. For example, although providing depressed people with methyl groups (e.g., in the form of the dietary supplement SAM-e) produces antidepressant effects,[120a-120b] providing healthy adult rats with methyl groups (e.g., in the form of a methyl-containing compound infused directly into their brains) *increases* their fearful behaviors.[121a-121b] So, the effects of methyl supplementation might, in some cases, be antithetical to one another. Of course, if a particular diet or supplement has been shown to have desirable effects, it can be recommended even if we do not yet understand how it works. But additional research on the epigenetic effects of dietary manipulations will almost certainly clarify our understanding, and thereby provide more effective treatments in the future.

Epigenetic treatments need not be limited to those involving drugs or diet; other experiences, too, have epigenetic effects that could one day be employed therapeutically. For example, although HDAC-inhibitors improve memory in mice, similar effects have been found by giving mice experiences in enriched environments.[122] And whether memory is improved by drugs *or* by experience with an engaging environment, the effect appears to depend on histone acetylation.[123] Unfortunately, the nonspecificity of current dietary and drug treatments might be a problem for experiential treatments as well; we do not yet know the extent to which experiences in enriched environments increase histone acetylation in gene-specific ways. Nevertheless, additional research on the epigenetic effects of enriched environments, too, is likely to yield valuable insights.

Some Legal and Ethical Implications of Behavioral Epigenetics

Beyond the implications of epigenetics research for what we decide to eat, for how we choose to structure our environments, or for the ways in which doctors practice medicine, there are likely to be legal and ethical implications of these new discoveries. In a pioneering article, the law professor Mark Rothstein and his colleagues[124] concentrated on these issues explicitly. Among the concerns they addressed were some related to the fact that several metals and hormone-disrupting chemicals that are present in contemporary environments have epigenetic effects.

This raises the issue of how lawmakers and the courts will handle regulation of these substances; the fact that some of these effects can influence development in the *descendants* of people originally exposed to the substance makes this a complicated legal issue. American courts to date have maintained that manufacturers are liable for injury caused by their products, but only if the injured person was actually exposed to the product, either in utero or later in life. Thus, the courts have been unwilling to hold corporations liable for injury to a *grandchild* of a person exposed to a harmful product, perhaps in part because such a ruling would enable contemporary corporate leaders to be sanctioned for the unwitting mistakes of an earlier generation of leaders, and in part because it would render it significantly more expensive and challenging for regulatory agencies like the FDA to test the effects of drugs, as it would require testing across multiple generations. In addition, because toxins capable of producing epigenetic effects are more likely to affect poor or otherwise vulnerable members of society, the epigenetic effects of such toxins raise questions about environmental justice.[125]

Worries like these led Rothstein and colleagues to the following conclusion:

> Numerous legal and ethical issues are raised by epigenetics, especially regarding individual and societal responsibilities to prevent hazardous exposures, monitor health status, and provide care. Epigenetics . . . adds a multigenerational dimension to environmentally-caused adverse health effects. Epigenetics serves to highlight the effects of inequality in living and working conditions, as well as a range of disparities in access to health care and other societal opportunities . . . [126]

Clearly, additional research on epigenetics will stoke further ethical and legal debate over such issues, and in fact, such debate has already begun.[127]

At present, we still know relatively little about epigenetics, so there is not much that can be said for certain about the implications of research on this biological system. But the studies conducted to date have been provocative, so life scientists and social scientists continue to be excited about how epigenetics research might eventually help us understand and ameliorate the human condition. Some of what I have written in this chapter has been, by necessity, speculation. Nonetheless, it is an extremely interesting time to pay attention to molecular biology, and there are many reasons to think the next few decades of epigenetics research will reveal some of Mother Nature's very important secrets.

23

Conclusions

Much can be said about the science of epigenetics, but it should be apparent from the previous chapter that a lot of what can be said is conjecture. What happens when we leave behind the future-oriented guesswork? Is there anything we can take away from behavioral epigenetics research that we can feel confident about today?

Waddington chose the word "epigenetics" to characterize the developmental events that produce our phenotypes, so epigenetics is really all about development. And focusing on the *development* of characteristics—whether we are talking about physical characteristics like height or eye color, or psychological characteristics like temperament or intelligence—can lead to insights that other perspectives might miss. The firm, overarching conclusions we can draw from behavioral epigenetics research are actually no different from the conclusions we can draw from a broader understanding of development. The research on epigenetics that I've been describing merely helps drive these points home. But the points are so valuable and often overlooked that even if the takeaway lessons of behavioral epigenetics are the same as the lessons provided by 20th-century developmental science, they are worth rediscovering in the context of new data.

Lesson 1: Multiple Factors Collaborate to Build Traits; DNA Alone Does Not Determine Them.

Our characteristics develop because of the mutual activities of a variety of genetic, epigenetic, and environmental factors *that operate as an integrated system*. Our traits are not predetermined by any single factor; we are more than our biological endowments. Developmental scientists have understood for decades that genetic determinism does not capture the reality of development. Instead, we are as we are because of the interactions that occur during development between the various resources we inherit from our ancestors, several of which constitute the *contexts* in which development takes place. These contexts include the nongenetic, biological factors that we receive from our parents around the time of conception (and from our mothers during prenatal development), and also the cultures and physical environments in which we live out our lives. This is an important message, because it can help us resist the illusion that we have no control over who and how we are. What we do matters.

The findings of behavioral epigenetics make this point loud and clear: Genes are responsive to their environments, so the genes we are born with can never be the whole story. This means that an infant's aptitude for accomplishment cannot be predicted with anything close to certainty. Twentieth-century molecular biology left many people with the mistaken belief that it is possible for a person to be conceived with a certain innate potential, such as a specific IQ range, a sexual orientation, or a likelihood of an early death from heart disease. But because all of these phenotypes *develop* over time in particular influential contexts, this view is incompatible with what we now know about biology.[1] The insight that our characteristics are not predetermined flows from a developmental perspective, so it is not new;[2] recent work on epigenetics has merely made it easier to *see* how impossible it is for our genes to specify our destiny. If we want to know whether a baby is going to be exceptionally bright as an adult, we're going to have to wait and find out.

It might seem that recent discoveries about epigenetics can be incorporated into existing dichotomous understandings of nature and nurture. In other words, perhaps these discoveries only move the boundary between a person and the environment from the surface of the skin to a spot deeper inside. But even though epigenetics research shows our environments penetrating so deeply inside of us that they can be imagined sitting side by side with our genes, it would be a mistake to think that a principled distinction can be drawn between the molecules that are "us" and the molecules that are "the environment." To give just one example of why such an idea should be rejected, consider the fact that sections of a person's chromatin are made of DNA *bonded with* methyl groups that might have come from that person's breakfast, and that those methylated sections of DNA are going to do what they do because of their properties considered as a whole. As a result of this state of affairs, it makes little sense to imagine a well-defined line between DNA and environmental factors. Many people have understood for a long time that our environments get inside of us and are literally incorporated into our bodies; the study of epigenetics has merely helped us see *how* that can happen in a way that influences gene expression, and this has encouraged some scientists to shift their attention from studying the genetic determination of traits to studying the gene-environment *co-construction* of traits.

The insight that our characteristics are collaboratively constructed during development obviously precludes any sort of environmental or epigenetic determinism just as surely as it precludes genetic determinism. Of course, there are cases where early experiences *do* have long-term effects, and as we have seen, some early experiences produce epigenetic effects that are detectable years later;[3]

Meaney's discovery that postnatal mothering can epigenetically influence rats' stress reactivity in adulthood certainly *seems* to warrant the label "epigenetic programming."[4] But because these sorts of effects can also be reversed,[5a-5c] such early experiences do not dictate the future. Although we know relatively little about what sorts of experiences can change early-established epigenetic marks, we currently know of both pharmaceutical manipulations[6a-6b] and environmental manipulations[7a-7b] (e.g., social or physical "enrichment" of the environment) that can alter adult mammals' epigenetic states and thereby alleviate symptoms. Therefore, epigenetic marks can be altered by events later in life, so we do not have to be overly pessimistic about the long-term effects of bad early-life experiences. As Champagne has noted, "The neurobiological plasticity within both parents and offspring demonstrated in laboratory studies also suggest that, when adversity is experienced early in development, the quality of the later life environment can compensate or shift development in such a way that deficits can be ameliorated."[8]

Development continues throughout the life span, so early experience does not need to be considered "destiny" any more than a genetic endowment does. Who we are in the future depends on our current internal state *and* on the context in which we find ourselves. So even though genetic and nongenetic factors in our pasts contribute to our current states and thereby influence our paths forward, there will always be other factors in our present environments that can steer development in a new direction.

Lesson 2: The Neo-Darwinian Synthesis Needs Revising.

A second lesson from research on epigenetics is that the neo-Darwinian theory of evolution—a theory that *defines* evolution strictly in terms of changing gene frequencies—does not suffice as a unified theory of biology, because it disregards the role of development in producing adaptive traits.[9] There are two *very* important points to keep in mind at this juncture. The first point is that the required revisions do not validate creationist viewpoints, despite the claims of some intelligent-design theorists.[10] Epigenetics research provides no support for the discredited idea that people are unrelated to other primates,[11] and it provides no support for the discredited idea that biological systems are "irreducibly complex"[12] and therefore inexplicable in Darwinian terms. The second point is that the needed revisions to neo-Darwinism will actually bring us back in line with Darwin's original ideas. When the architects of the neo-Darwinian synthesis tried to integrate Darwin's ideas with classical genetics some 80 years after Darwin published *On the Origin of Species*, they defined evolution in terms of genes alone, and thereby ignored the thorny problem of development.[13a-13b] But because the emergence of all of our adaptive characteristics *depends* on development (i.e., these characteristics are not predetermined by our genes), this move has turned out to be problematic. The neo-Darwinian attempt to explain evolution with a nondevelopmental theory of genes relied on the assumption that "acquired" characteristics cannot be "inherited," but as we have seen, a sharp distinction between "inherited" and "acquired" characteristics is not warranted. Therefore, a return to Darwin's original perspective seems reasonable, since it was clear in the *Origin of Species* that Darwin was comfortable with the idea that some acquired characteristics might be reliably transmitted across generations.

The idea that the neo-Darwinian synthesis must be revised to reflect the importance of development predates the recent spate of evidence on epigenetics; this evidence merely reinforces the conclusion that the neo-Darwinian synthesis needs revising. Eva Jablonka and Marion Lamb captured the situation with some cogent reasoning:

> Epigenetic inheritance . . . introduces new and, from the point of view of present day neo-Darwinism, subversive considerations into evolutionary theory. It is easy to see why if we think first about culture, rather than epigenetics. Human symbolic culture is undoubtedly undergoing evolutionary change . . . Even in a world of genetically identical individuals, we can imagine evolutionary processes that would lead to many different cultures. Cultural variation is, to some extent at least, decoupled from DNA variation; and to understand cultural evolution, we need to study this autonomous aspect of variation. The same is true for epigenetic variation. Heritable epigenetic variation is decoupled from genetic variation *by definition*. Hence, there are selectable epigenetic variations that are independent of DNA variations, and evolutionary change on the epigenetic axis is inevitable.[14]

As a result, a theory of evolution that has nothing to say about epigenetic contributions to evolution is necessarily incomplete and in need of modification. Jablonka and Lamb concluded their paper on the evolutionary implications of epigenetics with the following summary:

> Epigenetics requires a broadening of the concept of heredity and the recognition that natural selection acts on several different types of heritable variation. Although the current gene-centered version of Darwinism— neo-Darwinism—is incompatible with Lamarckism, Darwinism is not. In the past, Lamarckism and Darwinism were not always seen as alternatives: they were recognized as being perfectly compatible and complementary. In the light of epigenetics, they still are. Recognizing the role of epigenetic systems in evolution will allow a more comprehensive and powerful Darwinian theory to be constructed, one that integrates development and evolution more closely.[15]

Lesson 3: Our Epigenetic States Are Dynamic and Reflect Our Experiences.

The discovery that our epigenetic states are dynamic and not influenced solely by biology[16] really is news, because scientists have long considered epigenetic phenomena like DNA methylation to be exceptionally stable across the life span.[17] But it is now clear that a wide variety of experiences can influence epigenetic marks, from exposure to certain chemicals or diets to interaction with a nurturing mother or a stimulating physical environment.

Numerous theorists have made this point succinctly. To share just a few examples, Tania Roth, a behavioral epigeneticist at the University of Delaware, wrote, "The susceptibility of the genome to epigenetic modifications provides a layer of genetic regulation that is sensitive to a lifetime of experiential and environmental factors."[18] Marinus van IJzendoorn, a developmental scientist at Leiden University in the Netherlands, wrote with his colleagues, "Epigenetic studies make clear that the environment penetrates the genome at its core, and influences the expression or nonexpression of genes."[19] And Michael Meaney wrote with one of his colleagues, "The environment regulates the cellular signals that control the operation of the genome"[20] by *physically remodeling it;*[21] "thus the operation of the genome is dependent upon context."[22]

Randy Jirtle and Michael Skinner made the same point with a bit more elaboration:

> The word "environment" means vastly different things to different people. For sociologists and psychologists, it conjures up visions of social group interactions, family dynamics and maternal nurturing. Nutritionists might envision food pyramids and dietary supplements, whereas toxicologists think of water, soil and air pollutants ... [but scientists now have] evidence that these vastly different environments are all able to alter gene expression and change phenotype, in part by impinging on and modifying the epigenome.[23]

The take-home message is clear: Experiential factors can affect our epigenetic states, the structure of our chromatin can respond dynamically to our experiences, and each of us has a genome that effectively changes—develops—over time.

Lesson 4: Many Popular Metaphors About Genes Are Misleading.

A fourth lesson we can extract from epigenetics research is that some of the metaphors we use to think about the genome leave us with a distorted view of what causes our traits. A number of theorists expressed alarm about these metaphors long before the modern era of epigenetics research, but the epigenetics data have served to reinforce their conclusions. In discussing such concerns more than 25 years ago, Timothy D. Johnston, a psychologist at the University of North Carolina at Greensboro, wrote, "The road to confusion is paved with compelling but inaccurate metaphors."[24]

The specific metaphor Johnston was concerned with was the one proffered by the Nobel laureate Konrad Lorenz, who imagined that "information . . . provided by natural selection [is] . . . encoded in the genome as a genetic blueprint."[25] In his critique, Johnston makes a strong case that this metaphor "seriously [misrepresents] the nature of genetic involvement in development."[26] Nonetheless, the blueprint metaphor continues to be popular,[27] and its continuing popularity has led other critics to join the fray;[28a-28c] for instance, Massimo Pigliucci, a philosopher of science at the City College of New York, wrote in 2010 that the blueprint metaphor is "woefully inadequate [and] positively misleading."[29]

Of course, by 2010, several other theorists had adopted the critics' point of view and had started exploring the value of other metaphors. For example, one scientist opined in 2006, "Genomes are much more like knitting patterns or recipes than blueprints."[30] Unfortunately, the "recipe" metaphor is not much better than the blueprint metaphor, because it still suggests—incorrectly[31a-31b]—that natural selection has stored in our genomes encoded information that can be used in a context-independent way. The discovery that epigenetic marks can be influenced by experience has made such metaphors even less serviceable.

Yet another "information metaphor" suggests that genomes are computer programs that control the order in which developmental events occur. This metaphor is an improvement over the blueprint and recipe metaphors, because it can at least tolerate the fact that genomes are responsive to inputs from beyond the genome. But in other ways, it too has been found deficient.[32a-32c] One of the latest versions of this metaphor suggests that we should think of genes as being like "subroutines in a huge operating system."[33] However, according to the scientists involved in the ENCODE project, the ENCODE data do not "fit with the metaphor of the gene as a simple callable routine in a huge operating system,"[34] so this metaphor must be rejected as well. Given what we now know about epigenetics, are there any emerging analogies that might be able to fill our metaphor void?

In Nessa Carey's very good book on epigenetics,[35] she argued that the newest data on epigenetics suggest that DNA should be thought of as something like a script. She wrote:

> Think of *Romeo and Juliet*, for example. In 1936 George Cukor directed Leslie Howard and Norma Shearer in a film version. Sixty years later Baz Luhrmann directed Leonardo DiCaprio and Claire Danes in another movie version . . . Both productions used Shakespeare's script, yet the

two movies are entirely different. Identical starting points, different outcomes.[36]

Carey can be commended for trying to help readers understand that DNA is capable of being used by our bodies in a flexible way. But in the end, hers is an inadequate simile as well, because a script is typically written before a performance begins, and no director would dream of moving one of Shakespeare's lines from the middle of *Romeo and Juliet* to the end of the play while the performance is underway. Biological development, in contrast, is quite a bit less constrained than that; development occurs in real time—it is not preprogrammed—and genetic "information" really can be moved around to serve different functions in different contexts and at different times (alternative splicing, which I discussed in "Zooming in on DNA," is an excellent example of how this can happen). Ultimately, the script metaphor fails for the same reasons other information metaphors have failed.[37a-37c] DNA is only slightly more like a script than it is like a blueprint, and research on epigenetics has made the weaknesses of such information metaphors even more apparent than they already were to 20th-century developmental scientists.

The good news is that there are some newer metaphors that might be helpful in explaining how our bodies and minds come to have the characteristics they do. Van IJzendoorn and colleagues have suggested, "Child development might be conceptualized as experiences becoming sculpted in the organism's DNA through methylation";[38] importantly, this statement designates an essential role for experiences in the developmental process. Alternatively, a cancer genomics researcher has likened the ENCODE data set to Google Maps, saying "Now you can follow the roads and see the traffic circulation";[39] this metaphor, too, has some value, in that it captures the complexity of a system influenced by huge numbers of interacting elements, and thereby suggests that there are always multiple ways to produce a particular outcome.

Here is another metaphor that I think captures the in-the-moment, probabilistic way in which DNA actually functions: "Development is a spontaneous block party." At a spontaneous block party, there are people present with distinctive characteristics, and these characteristics affect how the interactions between the people unfold, and therefore influence the overall "flavor" of the event. (DNA segments, likewise, have distinctive characteristics that affect their interactions with the other molecules in their local environments.) It is difficult to predict exactly what the nature of the party will have been when all is said and done, because such parties can unfold in a variety of unforeseen ways. (And the same is true of development.) Of course, if your neighbors are all middle-aged professors, the party is unlikely to develop into a raging kegger (but it could!). So it is possible to make *reasonably* good predictions, and we can be confident that things will unfold in accord with the "laws of nature." (The same statements could be made of development.) But there is no overseer capable of controlling everything that happens at this sort of party, any more than there are "master molecules" capable of controlling everything that happens in a body. Likewise, the events that will occur at the party have not been "scripted," even if historical factors such as cultural norms do provide some constraints on what will transpire. (And analogous claims could be made about how genomes influence development.) Finally, there are external factors that can affect how the party will unfold (e.g., weather, the receipt of significant political news, the arrival of the police, etc.), which helps this metaphor fit the data on behavioral epigenetics. To the extent that this metaphor works, we can see why a genome is best *not* thought of as being like a script, blueprint, recipe, or computer program. Of course, there are other ways in which this metaphor does *not* work particularly well, but at least it captures some important aspects of the emergent quality of development.

In his book *The Music of Life*,[40] Denis Noble, a biologist, philosopher, and emeritus professor of computational physiology at the University of Oxford in England, provided some wonderful metaphors to help readers think about life processes. To his credit, he explicitly acknowledged,

> Each metaphor has its advantages and disadvantages . . . No metaphors map perfectly to the situation they are describing. They highlight certain aspects at the price of playing down others. The harm is done when we take the metaphors too literally, extend them beyond their range of application, and interpret them as uniquely correct scientifically.[41]

In a suggestion that makes it clear that Noble understands both the value and the danger of metaphors, his final chapter "recommends throwing all the metaphors away once we have used them to gain insight."[42] Thus, it is perhaps best for me to now leave the metaphors behind.

The Takeaway Messages of Behavioral Epigenetics

In thinking about the implications of behavioral epigenetics, different sets of conclusions are available for different readers; specifically, scientists and nonscientists can each be guided by this work in distinctive ways. For scientists, I think the most important advice to take from this work is "explore development." In comparison to a more deterministic worldview, the developmental worldview that is consistent with behavioral epigenetics can guide scientists down a very different—and more productive—path.

A deterministic worldview that sees some phenotypes as being caused primarily by genes can encourage a scientist to conduct twin studies like those traditionally conducted by behavioral geneticists, investigations that may be incorrectly thought to reveal which phenotypes can be influenced by environmental manipulations and which cannot. This scientist might believe that this approach will allow him or her to identify phenotypes that are "genetic" or that are "strongly influenced" by genes. Once these phenotypes are identified in this way, some people would disregard them, because of the mistaken belief that there is not much that can be done to influence them. If such a phenotype is typical of most of us, we would likely attribute it to "human nature," and if it is not, we would likely label it a "genetic abnormality." And either way, that would be the end of the investigation.

In contrast, a developmental worldview is likely to encourage a scientist to study how phenotypes *emerge* during development. According to this perspective, all of our characteristics develop as a result of mechanistic interactions between "inherited" factors, including our DNA *and* aspects of our environments (i.e., the environments outside of our developing bodies as well as the local environments surrounding our DNA). These factors are understood to interact in ways that produce changes that follow one after another in a long cascade of events that leads to the emergence of a phenotype, one that might be stable for a period of time or that might be a transitional state on the pathway to a different phenotype. For a scientist focused on development, this is the *beginning* of the investigation: The goal is to study how the phenotype comes into being through the interactions of previously existing factors.

Importantly, a developmental perspective provides mechanistic knowledge that can yield practical treatments for pathologies. In contrast, information about the "heritability" of a phenotype—the kind of information generated by twin studies—can never be as useful as information about the *development* of a phenotype, because only developmental information produces the kind of thorough understanding of a trait's emergence that can allow for successful interventions.[43] The discovery that our experiences can influence gene *expression* reinforces the role of development in the disposition of our characteristics. Research on epigenetics thus has the potentially far-reaching consequence of discouraging scientists from focusing exclusively on *correlations* between genes and phenotypes, and instead drawing their attention to how developmental processes actually *cause* phenotypes.

The practical conclusions that *non*scientists can harvest from epigenetics research are somewhat less clear, in part because the science of behavioral epigenetics is just getting underway. As one writer has characterized the state of our knowledge, "if research on epigenetics is in its infancy, research on *behavioral* epigenetics is in embryo."[44] Using currently available data, the advice that can be gleaned is no different from the advice attentive people would have given before learning about epigenetics at all: Eat a healthy diet with plenty of vegetables, stay calm, nurture friendships, avoid toxins. What we now understand is *how* these kinds of factors produce the effects they do, and this information will likely be useful to future healthcare professionals and, ultimately, to the people they are trying to help. But for now, this information will not change how most of us go about living our lives. If a person is gluttonous, will knowledge that they might be epigenetically harming their descendants change their behavior, if the knowledge that they are harming *themselves* has not changed their behavior? I doubt it. Should the expectation that memory-enhancing epigenetic drugs will be available in the future change how we currently feel about memory-impairing treatments like electroconvulsive therapy or medical marijuana? Probably not. Should the epigenetic work from the Meaney lab encourage mothers to engage in plenty of physical contact with their babies? Probably, but I would argue that we have already known for some time that this sort of contact is invaluable.

Understanding *how* biological processes work can change how we perceive each other, so even if we do not yet know how to productively change (or protect) our epigenetic states, being cognizant of the fact that these states influence behavior will likely have consequences. For instance, recent research has shown that US state trial judges hand down significantly different sentences for psychopaths depending on whether or not the judges are given information about the *biomechanism* responsible for the psychopath's behavior.[45] Thus, simply knowing that experiences affect gene expression—and therefore, brain chemistry, brain structure, and behavior—could influence how we view the people around us. But beyond these sorts of nonspecific effects of our emerging understanding of epigenetics, there is not yet much that can be said with certainty.

Even so, it has been clear for some time that the demise of genetic determinism should change how we think about human nature, and discoveries about epigenetics support this view. We are all profoundly influenced by the contexts in which we develop, and we have some control over those contexts; therefore, it is our responsibility to do what we can to help ourselves and others grow into compassionate, enlightened, and fulfilled individuals. The rise of epigenetics should help everyone hear these messages: Do not assume you are trapped by your biology. Strive. Nurture your children with care. Choose and construct your environments thoughtfully, and live your life in a way that fosters ongoing health and development, because what you do matters. These are beliefs sensible people have held for millennia, and there is little reason that a new understanding of *how* our experiences affect us should change the way we think about that wisdom. But even if the world's epigenetics laboratories have not yet produced any radical new insights about how we should live our lives, they are producing fascinating data at the dawn of the 21st century, and this new information is bound to touch all of us at some point in the not-too-distant future.

NOTES

1. Context

1. Kupperman, K. O. (1984). *Roanoke: The abandoned colony.* Lanham, MD: Rowman & Littlefield.

2. Stahle, D. W., Cleaveland, M. K., Blanton, D. B., Therrell, M. D., & Gay, D. A. (1998). The Lost Colony and Jamestown droughts. *Science, 280,* 564–567.

3. Stahle et al., 1998, p. 566.

4. Jones, E. E., & Harris, V. A. (1967). The attribution of attitudes. *Journal of Experimental Social Psychology, 3,* 1–24.

5. Stahle et al., 1998.

6. West, M. J., & King, A. P. (1987). Settling nature and nurture into an ontogenetic niche. *Developmental Psychobiology, 20,* 549–562.

7. Schneider, S. M. (2012). *The science of consequences: How they affect genes, change the brain, and impact our world.* Amherst, NY: Prometheus Books.

8. Needham, B. L., Epel, E. S., Adler, N. E., & Kiefe, C. (2010). Trajectories of change in obesity and symptoms of depression: The CARDIA study. *American Journal of Public Health, 100,* 1040–1046.

9. Dimsdale, J. E. (2008). Psychological stress and cardiovascular disease. *Journal of the American College of Cardiology, 51,* 1237–1246.

10. Dewsbury, D. A. (1991). Psychobiology. *American Psychologist, 46,* 198–205.

11. For more information, see Rice, W. R., Friberg, U., & Gavrilets, S. (2012). Homosexuality as a consequence of epigenetically canalized sexual development. *Quarterly Review of Biology, 87,* 343–368. I am citing this paper now because unlike the other topics listed here, I will not address homosexuality later in this book; I am not aware of any other scientific papers that have further addressed the relationship between epigenetics and sexual orientation.

12. Lester, B. M., Tronick, E., Nestler, E., Abel, T., Kosofsky, B., Kuzawa, C. W., . . . Wood, M. A. (2011). Behavioral epigenetics. *Annals of the New York Academy of Sciences, 1226,* 14–33.

13. See, for example, Maderspacher, F. (2010). Lysenko rising. *Current Biology, 20,* R835–R837.

14. Miller, G. (2010). The seductive allure of behavioral epigenetics. *Science, 329,* p. 24.

15a. Albert, P. R. (2010). Epigenetics in mental illness: Hope or hype? *Journal of Psychiatry and Neuroscience, 35,* 366–368.

15b. Buchen, L. (2010). In their nurture. *Nature, 467,* 146–148.

16. Ptashne, M. (2010). Questions over the scientific basis of epigenome project. *Nature, 464,* p. 487.

2. Phenotypes

1. Jolie, A. (2013, May 14). My medical choice. *New York Times*.
2. Dowd, M. (2013, May 14). Cascading confessions. *New York Times*.
3. National Cancer Institute. (2009, May 29). BRCA1 and BRCA2: Cancer risk and genetic testing. *National Cancer Institute Fact Sheet*. Retrieved July 13, 2013, from http://www.cancer.gov/cancertopics/factsheet/Risk/BRCA
4. Grady, D., Parker-Pope, T., & Belluck, P. (2013, May 14). Jolie's disclosure of preventive mastectomy highlights dilemma. *New York Times*.
5. Grady et al., 2013.
6a. Castéra, J., Abrougui, M., Nisiforou, O., Turcinaviciene, J., Sarapuu, T., Agorram, B., . . . Carvalho, G. (2008). Genetic determinism in school textbooks: A comparative study conducted among sixteen countries. *Science Education International, 19*, 163–184.
6b. dos Santos, V. C., Joaquim, L. M., & El-Hani, C. N. (2012). Hybrid deterministic views about genes in biology textbooks: A key problem in genetics teaching. *Science and Education, 21*, 543–578. doi:10.1007/s11191-011-9348-1
6c. Gericke, N. M., & Hagberg, M. (2010). Conceptual variation in the depiction of gene function in upper secondary school textbooks. *Science and Education, 19*, 963–994.
7. Kolata, G. (2013, July 18, 2:02 p.m. ET). Overweight? Maybe your genes really are at fault. *New York Times*.
8a. For information on the complex interactions that produce our **iris colors**, see Sturm, R. A., & Frudakis, T. N. (2004). Eye colour: Portals into pigmentation genes and ancestry. *Trends in Genetics, 20*, 327–332.
8b. For information on the complex interactions that produce our **bones**, see either Hall, B. K. (1988). The embryonic development of bone. *American Scientist, 76*(2), 174–181, or Gilbert, S. F. (2001). Ecological developmental biology: Developmental biology meets the real world. *Developmental Biology, 233*, 1–12.
8c. For information on the complex interactions that produce our **brains**, see Johnson, M. H. (2010). *Developmental Cognitive Neuroscience* (3rd ed.). Malden, MA: Wiley-Blackwell.
9a. Bateson, P., & Gluckman, P. (2011). *Plasticity, robustness, development and evolution*. Cambridge, England: Cambridge University Press.
9b. Blumberg, M. S. (2005). *Basic instinct: The genesis of behavior*. New York: Thunder's Mouth Press.
9c. Gottlieb, G. (2007). Probabilistic epigenesis. *Developmental Science, 10*, 1–11.
9d. Jablonka, E., & Lamb, M. J. (2005). *Evolution in four dimensions: Genetic, epigenetic, behavioral, and symbolic variation in the history of life*. Cambridge, MA: The MIT Press.
9e. Lewkowicz, D. J. (2011). The biological implausibility of the nature–nurture dichotomy and what it means for the study of infancy. *Infancy, 16*, 331–367.
9f. Lewontin, R. C. (2000). *The triple helix: Gene, organism, and environment*. Cambridge, MA: Harvard University Press.
9g. Lickliter, R. (2008). The growth of developmental thought: Implications for a new evolutionary psychology. *New Ideas in Psychology, 26*, 353–369.
9h. Lickliter, R. (2009). The fallacy of partitioning: Epigenetics' validation of the organism-environment system. *Ecological Psychology, 21*, 138–146.
9i. Meaney, M. J. (2010). Epigenetics and the biological definition of gene × environment interactions. *Child Development, 81*, 41–79.
9j. Moore, D. S. (2008a). Espousing interactions and fielding reactions: Addressing laypeople's beliefs about genetic determinism. *Philosophical Psychology, 21*, 331–348.
9k. Noble, D. (2006). *The music of life: Biology beyond genes*. New York: Oxford University Press.
9l. Oyama, S. (2000). *The ontogeny of information*. Durham, NC: Duke University Press.
9m. Robert, J. S. (2004). *Embryology, epigenesis, and evolution: Taking development seriously*. New York: Cambridge University Press.

9n. Spencer, J. P., Blumberg, M. S., McMurray, B., Robinson, S. R., Samuelson, L. K., & Tomblin, J. B. (2009). Short arms and talking eggs: Why we should no longer abide the nativist–empiricist debate. *Child Development Perspectives, 3*, 79–87.

10a-10e. To trace the origins of this idea from its earliest instantiation in the 20th century into the present, see the following five works:

10a. Driesch, H. A. E. (1910). Physiology of development. In *The Encyclopaedia Britannica* (11th ed., Vol. 9, pp. 329–331). London, England: Cambridge University Press.

10b. Beach, F. A. (1955). The descent of instinct. *Psychological Review, 62*, 401–410.

10c. Lehrman, D. S. (1953). A critique of Konrad Lorenz's theory of instinctive behavior. *Quarterly Review of Biology, 28*, 337–363.

10d. Gottlieb, G. (1991). Experiential canalization of behavioral development: Theory. *Developmental Psychology, 27*, 4–13.

10e. Lickliter, R., & Honeycutt, H. (2010). Rethinking epigenesis and evolution in light of developmental science. In M. S. Blumberg, J. H. Freeman, & S. R. Robinson (Eds.), *Oxford handbook of developmental behavioral neuroscience* (pp. 30–47). New York: Oxford University Press.

11. National Cancer Institute, 2009.

12. Lichtenstein, P., Holm, N. V., Verkasalo, P. K., Iliadou, A., Kaprio, J., Koskenvuo, M., . . . Hemminki, K. (2000). Environmental and heritable factors in the causation of cancer— Analyses of cohorts of twins from Sweden, Denmark, and Finland. *New England Journal of Medicine, 343*, 78–85.

13. Anand, P., Kunnumakara, A. B., Sundaram, C., Harikumar, K. B., Tharakan, S. T., Lai, O. S., . . . Aggarwal, B. B. (2008). Cancer is a preventable disease that requires major lifestyle changes. *Pharmaceutical Research, 25*, 2097–2116.

14. Feinberg, A. P., Ohlsson, R., & Henikoff, S. (2006). The epigenetic progenitor origin of human cancer. *Nature Reviews: Genetics, 7*, p. 24.

15. Mack, G. S. (2010). To selectivity and beyond. *Nature Biotechnology, 28*, p. 1262.

16a-16c. For more information on the history of the word "epigenesis"—from which the word "epigenetics" was derived—see the following three works:

16a. Gottlieb, G. (1992). *Individual development and evolution: The genesis of novel behavior.* New York: Oxford University Press.

16b. Gould, S. J. (1977). *Ontogeny and phylogeny.* Cambridge, MA: The Belknap Press of Harvard University Press.

16c. Robert, 2004.

17. Meaney, 2010.

18. Anand et al., 2008.

19. Waddington, C. H. (1968). The basic ideas of biology. In C. H. Waddington (Ed.), *Towards a Theoretical Biology* (Vol. 1: Prolegomena, pp. 1–32). Edinburgh: Edinburgh University Press.

20. Sweatt, J. D. (2009). Experience-dependent epigenetic modifications in the central nervous system. *Biological Psychiatry, 65*, p. 192.

21. Dawkins, R. (1987). *The Blind Watchmaker.* New York: Norton.

22. Keller, E. F. (2014). From gene action to reactive genomes. *Journal of Physiology, 592*, p. 2423.

3. Development

1. van Gorp, S., Leerink, M., Kakinohana, O., Platoshyn, O., Santucci, C., Galik, J., . . . Marsala, M. (2013). Amelioration of motor/sensory dysfunction and spasticity in a rat model of acute lumbar spinal cord injury by human neural stem cell transplantation. *Stem Cell Research and Therapy, 4*(3), 57.

2. Wilmut, I., Schnieke, A. E., McWhir, J., Kind, A. J., & Campbell, K. H. S. (1997). Viable offspring derived from fetal and adult mammalian cells. *Nature, 385*, 810–813.

3. Levenberg, S., Golub, J. S., Amit, M., Itskovitz-Eldor, J., & Langer, R. (2002). Endothelial cells derived from human embryonic stem cells. *Proceedings of the National Academy of Sciences USA, 99*, 4391–4396.

4. Gilbert, S. F. (2000). *Developmental Biology* (6th ed.). Sunderland, MA: Sinauer Associates.

5. Nüsslein-Volhard, C. (2006). *Coming to life: How genes drive development.* Carlsbad, CA: Kales Press, p. 21.

6a. Jablonka, E., & Lamb, M. J. (2002). The changing concept of epigenetics. *Annals of the New York Academy of Science, 981*, 82–96.

6b. Richards, E. J. (2006). Inherited epigenetic variation—Revisiting soft inheritance. *Nature Reviews: Genetics, 7*, 395–401.

6c. Van Speybroeck, L. (2002). From epigenesis to epigenetics: The case of C. H. Waddington. *Annals of the New York Academy of Science, 981*, 61–81.

7. Waddington, C. H. (1968). The basic ideas of biology. In C. H. Waddington (Ed.), *Towards a Theoretical Biology* (Vol. 1: Prolegomena, pp. 1–32). Edinburgh: Edinburgh University Press, pp. 9–10.

8. Waddington, 1968, p. 11.

9. Dawkins, R. (1999). *The extended phenotype: The long reach of the gene* (rev. ed.). Oxford, England: Oxford University Press.

10a. Gottlieb, G. (1991). Experiential canalization of behavioral development: Theory. *Developmental Psychology, 27*, 4–13.

10b. Gottlieb, G. (1992). *Individual development and evolution: The genesis of novel behavior.* New York: Oxford University Press.

10c. Gottlieb, G. (1997). *Synthesizing nature-nurture: Prenatal roots of instinctive behavior.* Mahwah, NJ: Erlbaum.

10d. Gottlieb, G. (1998). Normally occurring environmental and behavioral influences on gene activity: From central dogma to probabilistic epigenesis. *Psychological Review, 105*, 792–802.

11. Robert, J. S. (2008). Taking old ideas seriously: Evolution, development and human behavior. *New Ideas in Psychology, 26*, 387–404.

12a. Jablonka & Lamb, 2002.

12b. Jablonka, E., & Lamb, M. J. (2005). *Evolution in four dimensions: Genetic, epigenetic, behavioral, and symbolic variation in the history of life.* Cambridge, MA: MIT Press.

12c. Jablonka, E., & Lamb, M. J. (2007). Précis of evolution in four dimensions. *Behavioral and Brain Sciences, 30*, 353–392.

13. Canli, T., Qiu, M., Omura, K., Congdon, E., Haas, B. W., Amin, Z., . . . Lesch, K. P. (2006). Neural correlates of epigenesis. *Proceedings of the National Academy of Sciences USA, 103*, 16033–16038.

14a. Lickliter, R. (2008). The growth of developmental thought: Implications for a new evolutionary psychology. *New Ideas in Psychology, 26*, 353–369.

14b. Lickliter, R., & Honeycutt, H. (2013). A developmental evolutionary framework for psychology. *Review of General Psychology, 17*, 184–189.

15. Wu, C.-T., & Morris, J. R. (2001). Genes, genetics, and epigenetics: A correspondence. *Science, 293*, p. 1104.

16. Day, J. J., & Sweatt, J. D. (2010). DNA methylation and memory formation. *Nature Neuroscience, 13*, p. 1321.

17. Jablonka & Lamb, 2002, pp. 88–89.

18. Richards, 2006.

19. Carey, N. (2011). *The epigenetics revolution.* London, England: Icon Books, p. 42.

20. Lehrman, D. S. (1953). A critique of Konrad Lorenz's theory of instinctive behavior. *Quarterly Review of Biology, 28*, p. 359.

21. Moore, D. S. (2013c). Importing the homology concept from biology into developmental psychology. *Developmental Psychobiology, 55*, 13–21.

4. DNA

1a. Gericke, N. M., & Hagberg, M. (2010). Conceptual variation in the depiction of gene function in upper secondary school textbooks. *Science and Education, 19*, 963–994.

1b. Griffiths, P. E., & Neumann-Held, E. M. (1999). The many faces of the gene. *BioScience, 49*, 656–662.

1c. Keller, E. F. (2000). *The century of the gene.* Cambridge: Harvard University Press.

1d. Keller, E. F. (2014). From gene action to reactive genomes. *Journal of Physiology, 592*, 2423–2429.

2. Griffiths & Neumann-Held, 1999.

3. Watson, J. D., & Crick, F. H. C. (1953). Molecular structure of nucleic acids: A structure for deoxyribose nucleic acid. *Nature, 171*, 737–738.

4. Noble, D. (2008). Genes and causation. *Philosophical Transactions of the Royal Society A, 366*, 3001–3015.

5. Griffiths & Neumann-Held, 1999.

6. Oyama, S. (1992). Transmission and construction: Levels and the problem of heredity. In E. Tobach & G. Greenberg (Eds.), *Levels of social behavior: Evolutionary and genetic aspects: Award winning papers from the Third T. C. Schneirla Conference: Evolution of social behavior and integrative levels.* Wichita, KS: T.C. Schneirla Research Fund, p. 57.

7. A similar statement could be made about all of the other gene concepts developed by theorists in the life sciences, including those gene concepts that were developed before the classical molecular concept and those that have been developed more recently.

8. ENCODE is an acronym for the ENCyclopedia Of DNA Elements.

9. Gerstein, M. B., Bruce, C., Rozowsky, J. S., Zheng, D., Du, J., Korbel, J. O., . . . Snyder, M. (2007). What is a gene, post-ENCODE? History and updated definition. *Genome Research, 17*, 669–681.

10. Griffiths & Neumann-Held, 1999.

11. Gerstein et al., 2007, p. 669.

12. Keller, 2000, p. 69.

13. Quoted in Pennisi, E. (2007). DNA study forces rethink of what it means to be a gene. *Science, 316*, p. 1557.

14a. Jablonka, E., & Lamb, M. J. (2005). *Evolution in four dimensions: Genetic, epigenetic, behavioral, and symbolic variation in the history of life.* Cambridge, MA: MIT Press.

14b. Nijhout, H. F. (1990). Metaphors and the role of genes in development. *BioEssays, 12*, 441–446.

14c. Noble, D. (2006). *The music of life: Biology beyond genes.* New York: Oxford University Press.

14d. Pigliucci, M. (2010). Genotype–phenotype mapping and the end of the "genes as blueprint" metaphor. *Philosophical Transactions of the Royal Society B, 365*, 557–566.

15. For instance, in some cases a gene can be used to produce one kind of molecule after certain kinds of experiences, but that *same DNA segment* can be used to produce *a different form of the molecule* after other kinds of experiences (Lubin, Roth, & Sweatt, 2008). Clearly, the information in this gene does not "mean" only one thing.

5. Zooming in on DNA

1. Watson, J. D., & Crick, F. H. C. (1953). Molecular structure of nucleic acids: A structure for deoxyribose nucleic acid. *Nature, 171*, p. 737.

2. Gerstein, M. B., Bruce, C., Rozowsky, J. S., Zheng, D., Du, J., Korbel, J. O., . . . Snyder, M. (2007). What is a gene, post-ENCODE? History and updated definition. *Genome Research, 17*, 669–681.

3. Mattick, J. S., & Makunin, I. V. (2006). Non-coding RNA. *Human Molecular Genetics, 15*, R17–R29.

4. Ohno, S. (1972). So much "junk" DNA in our genome. In H. H. Smith (Ed.), *Evolution of genetic systems: Vol. 23. Brookhaven Symposia in Biology* (pp. 366–370). New York: Gordon & Breach.

5. Maher, B. (2012). The human encyclopaedia. *Nature, 489*, p. 46.

6a. Jacob, F., & Monod, J. (1961). Genetic regulatory mechanisms in the synthesis of proteins. *Journal of Molecular Biology, 3*, 318–356.

6b. Jacob, F., Perrin, D., Sanchez, C., & Monod, J. (1960). [Operon: A group of genes with the expression coordinated by an operator]. *Comptes Rendus Hebdomadaires des Séances de l'Académie des Sciences, 250*, 1727–1729.

7. Mattick & Makunin, 2006.

8. Mattick, J. S. (2005). The functional genomics of noncoding RNA. *Science, 309*, p. 1527.

9. Dinger, M. E., Pang, K. C., Mercer, T. R., & Mattick, J. S. (2008). Differentiating protein-coding and noncoding RNA: Challenges and ambiguities. *PLoS Computational Biology, 4, 1–5* (e1000176).

10. Mattick & Makunin, 2006.

11. Faghihi, M. A., Modarresi, F., Khalil, A. M., Wood, D. E., Sahagan, B. G., Morgan, T., . . . Wahlestedt, C. (2008). Expression of a noncoding RNA is elevated in Alzheimer's disease and drives rapid feed-forward regulation of β-secretase. *Nature Medicine, 14*, 723–730.

12. Sahoo, T., del Gaudio, D., German, J. R., Shinawi, M., Peters, S. U., Person, R. E., . . . Beaudet, A. L. (2008). Prader-Willi phenotype caused by paternal deficiency for the HBII-85 C/D/box small nucleolar RNA cluster. *Nature Genetics, 40*, 719–721.

13. Mattick & Makunin, 2006.

14a. Berget, S. M., Moore, C., & Sharp, P. A. (1977). Spliced segments at the 5' terminus of adenovirus 2 late mRNA. *Proceedings of the National Academy of Sciences USA, 74*, 3171–3175.

14b. Chow, L. T., Gelinas, R. E., Broker, T. R., & Roberts, R. J. (1977). An amazing sequence arrangement at the 5' ends of adenovirus 2 messenger RNA. *Cell, 12*, 1–8.

15. Gilbert, W. (1978). Why genes in pieces? *Nature, 271*, 501.

16. Noble, D. (2006). *The music of life: Biology beyond genes.* New York: Oxford University Press.

17. Wang, E. T., Sandberg, R., Luo, S., Khrebtukova, I., Zhang, L., Mayr, C., . . . Burge, C. B. (2008). Alternative isoform regulation in human tissue transcriptomes. *Nature, 456*, p. 470.

18. Amara, S. G., Jonas, V., Rosenfeld, M. B., Ong, E. S., & Evans, R. M. (1982). Alternative RNA processing in calcitonin gene expression generates mRNAs encoding different polypeptide products. *Nature, 298*, 240–244.

19. E. T. Wang et al., 2008.

20. Lubin, F. D., Roth, T. L., & Sweatt, J. D. (2008). Epigenetic regulation of *bdnf* gene transcription in the consolidation of fear memory. *Journal of Neuroscience, 28*, 10576–10586.

21. Johnson, J. M., Castle, J., Garrett-Engele, P., Kan, Z., Loerch, P. M., Armour, C. D., . . . Shoemaker, D. D. (2003). Genome-wide survey of human alternative pre-mRNA splicing with exon junction microarrays. *Science, 302*, p. 2141.

22. Christopher Burge, quoted in Trafton, A. (2008). Human genes sing different tunes in different tissues. *MIT TechTalk, 53*(8), p. 6.

23. E. T. Wang et al., 2008.

24. Pan, Q., Shai, O., Lee, L. J., Frey, B. J., & Blencowe, B. J. (2008). Deep surveying of alternative splicing complexity in the human transcriptome by high-throughput sequencing. *Nature Genetics, 40*, 1413–1415.

25. Gerstein et al., 2007, p. 671.

26. Noble, 2006.
27. Jablonka, E., & Lamb, M. J. (2007). Précis of evolution in four dimensions. *Behavioral and Brain Sciences, 30,* 353–392.
28. Gerstein et al., 2007, p. 671.
29. Gerstein et al., 2007, p. 677.

6. Regulation

1. Francis, R. C. (2011). *Epigenetics: The ultimate mystery of inheritance.* New York: Norton.
2. Karp, G. (2008). *Cell and molecular biology: Concepts and experiments* (5th ed.). New York: Wiley.
3. Beutler, E., Yeh, M., & Fairbanks, V. F. (1962). The normal human female as a mosaic of X-chromosome activity: Studies using the gene for G-6-PD deficiency as a marker. *Proceedings of the National Academy of Sciences of the USA, 48,* 9–16.
4. Lyon, M. F. (1961). Gene action in the X-chromosome of the mouse (*Mus musculus* L.). *Nature, 190,* 372–373.
5. van den Berg, I. M., Laven, J. S. E., Stevens, M., Jonkers, I., Galjaard, R., Gribnau, J., & van Doorninck, J. H. (2009). X chromosome inactivation is initiated in human preimplantation embryos. *American Journal of Human Genetics, 84,* 771–779.
6. Waddington, C. H. (1968). The basic ideas of biology. In C. H. Waddington (Ed.), *Towards a theoretical biology* (Vol. 1: Prolegomena, pp. 1–32). Edinburgh: Edinburgh University Press.
7. Karp, 2008.
8. Redon, C., Pilch, D., Rogakou, E., Sedelnikova, O., Newrock, K., & Bonner, W. (2002). Histone H2A variants H2AX and H2AZ. *Current Opinion in Genetics and Development, 12,* 162–169.
9. Gibbs, W. W. (2003). The unseen genome: Beyond DNA. *Scientific American, 289*(6), 106–113.
10. The epigenetic system we evolved to solve *both* our pluripotency-differentiation problem *and* our how-do-we-fit-this-super-long-molecule-into-this-tiny-cell problem has another feature that is useful for multicellular organisms: Cells inherit epigenetic information from the "parent" cell that divided to produce them. To illustrate this feature, consider a liver, which develops prenatally when immature stem cells differentiate and take on the distinctive characteristics of liver cells; this process begins with the epigenetic activation or repression of the specific DNA segments that must be activated or repressed for a cell to develop into a liver cell. The question is, when an *adult* needs to replace a liver cell that has been damaged, must she first produce an immature cell that then needs to go through this same process of differentiation? Or is there some way a liver cell can give rise directly to new liver cells? In fact, liver cells *can* give rise to new liver cells directly (Otu et al., 2007), because the epigenetic state of a differentiated cell is passed on to the "daughter" cells that arise when a parent cell divides. That is, a cell typically divides into daughter cells that are epigenetically like their parent, because the daughter cells *inherit* their parent's epigenetic state (Reik, Dean, & Walter, 2001). It is this type of epigenetic inheritance that allows epigenetic states established early in development to remain stable thereafter; this is why skin cells, for instance, always remain skin cells and never spontaneously turn into neurons. (Epigenetic inheritance in which a daughter *cell* inherits characteristics of a parent *cell* is different from the sort of epigenetic inheritance in which offspring inherit epigenetic states from their parents, a kind of inheritance that will be the focus of part III of this book.)
11. Martin, C., & Zhang, Y. (2007). Mechanisms of epigenetic inheritance. *Current Opinion in Cell Biology, 19,* 266–272.
12. Razin, A. (1998). CpG methylation, chromatin structure, and gene silencing—a three-way connection. *EMBO Journal, 17,* 4905–4908.

13. Daxinger, L., & Whitelaw, E. (2012). Understanding transgenerational epigenetic inheritance via the gametes in mammals. *Nature Reviews: Genetics, 13,* 153–162.

14a. Borrelli, E., Nestler, E. J., Allis, C. D., & Sassone-Corsi, P. (2008). Decoding the epigenetic language of neuronal plasticity. *Neuron, 60,* 961–974.

14b. Day, J. J., & Sweatt, J. D. (2011). Epigenetic mechanisms in cognition. *Neuron, 70,* 813–829.

15. Martin & Zhang, 2007.

16. Myzak, M. C., & Dashwood, R. H. (2006). Histone deacetylases as targets for dietary cancer preventive agents: Lessons learned with butyrate, diallyl disulfide, and sulforaphane. *Current Drug Targets, 7,* 443–452.

17. Gibbs, 2003.

18. Day, J. J., & Sweatt, J. D. (2010). DNA methylation and memory formation. *Nature Neuroscience, 13,* 1319–1323.

19. Santos, K. F., Mazzola, T. N., & Carvalho, H. F. (2005). The prima donna of epigenetics: The regulation of gene expression by DNA methylation. *Brazilian Journal of Medical and Biological Research, 38,* 1531–1541.

20a. Daxinger & Whitelaw, 2012.

20b. González-Pardo, H., & Álvarez, M. P. (2013). Epigenetics and its implications for psychology. *Psicothema, 25,* 3–12.

21. McDaniel, I. E., Lee, J. M., Berger, M. S., Hanagami, C. K., & Armstrong, J. A. (2008). Investigations of CHD1 function in transcription and development of *Drosophila melanogaster. Genetics, 178,* 583–587.

22. Borrelli et al., 2008, p. 964.

23. Berger, S. L. (2007). The complex language of chromatin regulation during transcription. *Nature, 447,* 407–412.

24. Fiering, S., Whitelaw, E., & Martin, D. I. K. (2000). To be or not to be active: The stochastic nature of enhancer action. *BioEssays, 22,* 381–387.

25a. Pandya, K., Cowhig, J., Brackhan, J., Kim, H. S., Hagaman, J., Rojas, M., . . . Smithies, O. (2008). Discordant on/off switching of gene expression in myocytes during cardiac hypertrophy in vivo. *Proceedings of the National Academy of Sciences USA, 105,* 13063–13068.

25b. Zhang, Q., Andersen, M. E., & Conolly, R. B. (2006). Binary gene induction and protein expression in individual cells. *Theoretical Biology and Medical Modelling, 3*(18). doi:10.1186/1742-4682-3-18

26. Pirone, J. R., & Elston, T. C. (2004). Fluctuations in transcription factor binding can explain the graded and binary responses observed in inducible gene expression. *Journal of Theoretical Biology, 226,* 111–121.

27. Remarkably, even this more finely rendered portrait is not as nuanced as it could be, because in some cases, the active and inactive states of chromatin are not clearly defined. Instead, epigenetic modifications sometimes have complex effects on chromatin, leading some theorists to believe "that the presence of certain modifications may not indicate a unique regulatory status (that is, 'on' or 'off')" (Berger, 2007, p. 407). Said another way, some epigenetic marks are associated with *both* increased genetic expression and decreased genetic expression. This is a very complex system indeed.

28. Pirone & Elston, 2004.

29. Lickliter, R. (2009). The fallacy of partitioning: Epigenetics' validation of the organism-environment system. *Ecological Psychology, 21,* p. 140, emphasis added.

7. Zooming in on Regulation

1. Gurdon, J. B., Laskey, R. A., & Reeves, O. R. (1975). The developmental capacity of nuclei transplanted from keratinized skin cells of adult frogs. *Journal of Embryology and Experimental Morphology, 34,* p. 93.

2. Wilmut, I., Schnieke, A. E., McWhir, J., Kind, A. J., & Campbell, K. H. S. (1997). Viable offspring derived from fetal and adult mammalian cells. *Nature, 385,* 810–813.

3. Wilmut et al., 1997.

4. Wilmut et al., 1997, p. 812.

5. Baron, D. (2000, February 11). *Clones may not be identical* [Audio podcast]. Retrieved from http://www.npr.org/templates/story/story.php?storyId=1070242

6. Holden, C. (2002). Carbon-Copy clone is the real thing. *Science, 295,* 1443–1444.

7. Takahashi, K., & Yamanaka, S. (2006). Induction of pluripotent stem cells from mouse embryonic and adult fibroblast cultures by defined factors. *Cell, 126,* 663–676.

8. Takahashi and Yamanaka's method required four gene products, but Kim and colleagues succeeded in 2008 with only two gene products, because they started with a different kind of adult cell; see Kim, J. B., Zaehres, H., Wu, G., Gentile, L., Ko, K., Sebastiano, V., . . . Schöler, H. R. (2008). Pluripotent stem cells induced from adult neural stem cells by reprogramming with two factors. *Nature, 454,* 646–650.

9. Gallagher, J. (2013, July 19). Pioneering adult stem cell trial approved by Japan. *BBC News.* Retrieved from http://www.bbc.co.uk/news/health-23374622

10. Carey, N. (2011). *The epigenetics revolution.* London, England: Icon Books.

11. Cassidy, S. B. (1997). Prader-Willi syndrome. *Journal of Medical Genetics, 34,* 917–923.

12a. Holm, V. A., Cassidy, S. B., Butler, M. G., Hanchett, J. M., Greenswag, L. R., Whitman, B. Y., & Greenberg, F. (1993). Prader-Willi syndrome: Consensus diagnostic criteria. *Pediatrics, 91,* 398–402.

12b. Wadsworth, J. S., McBrien, D. M., & Harper, D. C. (2003). Vocational guidance and employment of persons with a diagnosis of Prader-Willi syndrome. *Journal of Rehabilitation, 69,* 15–21.

13a. Nicholls, R. D., Knoll, J. H. M., Butler, M. G., Karam, S., & Lalande, M. (1989). Genetic imprinting suggested by maternal heterodisomy in non-deletion Prader-Willi syndrome. *Nature, 342,* 281–285.

13b. Sahoo, T., del Gaudio, D., German, J. R., Shinawi, M., Peters, S. U., Person, R. E., . . . Beaudet, A. L. (2008). Prader-Willi phenotype caused by paternal deficiency for the HBII-85 C/D/box small nucleolar RNA cluster. *Nature Genetics, 40,* 719–721.

14. Knoll, J. H. M., Nicholls, R. D., Magenis, R. E., Graham, J. M., Lalande, M., Latt, S. A., . . . Reynolds, J. F. (1989). Angelman and Prader-Willi syndromes share a common chromosome 15 deletion but differ in parental origin of the deletion. *American Journal of Medical Genetics, 32,* 285–290.

15. Francis, R. C. (2011). *Epigenetics: The ultimate mystery of inheritance.* New York: Norton.

16a. Li, E., Beard, C., & Jaenisch, R. (1993). Role for DNA methylation in genomic imprinting. *Nature, 366,* 362–365.

16b. Sapienza, C., Peterson, A. C., Rossant, J., & Balling, R. (1987). Degree of methylation of transgenes is dependent on gamete of origin. *Nature, 328,* 251–254.

17. Surani, M. A. H., Barton, S. C., & Norris, M. L. (1987). Influence of parental chromosomes on spatial specificity in androgenetic ↔parthenogenetic chimaeras in the mouse. *Nature, 326,* 395–397.

18. Cassidy, 1997.

19. Cassidy, 1997.

20. Nicholls et al., 1989.

21. Holm et al., 1993.

22. Williams, C. A., Beaudet, A. L., Clayton-Smith, J., Knoll, J. H., Kyllerman, M., Laan, L. A., . . . Wagstaff, J. (2006). Angelman syndrome 2005: Updated consensus for diagnostic criteria. *American Journal of Medical Genetics, 140A,* 413–418.

23. Feinberg, A. P. (2007). Phenotypic plasticity and the epigenetics of human disease. *Nature, 447,* 433–440.

24. van den Berg, I. M., Laven, J. S. E., Stevens, M., Jonkers, I., Galjaard, R., Gribnau, J., & van Doorninck, J. H. (2009). X chromosome inactivation is initiated in human preimplantation embryos. *American Journal of Human Genetics, 84*, 771–779.

25. Reik, W., Dean, W., & Walter, J. (2001). Epigenetic reprogramming in mammalian development. *Science, 293*, 1089–1093.

26. Francis, 2011.

27. Carey, 2011.

28. Early studies led researchers to estimate that between approximately 130 (Wilkinson, 2010) and 230 (Carey, 2011; Francis, 2011) of our genes are imprinted. However, recent research on genetic expression in mammalian brain cells uncovered more than 1,300 genes that behave as if they are imprinted (Gregg et al., 2010), so our understanding of the frequency of imprinting in the human genome is currently in flux.

29. Interestingly enough, it is only the cells of a female embryo itself that ignore the X chromosome's parental origin. In the cells of the *placenta* belonging to a female embryo, it is always the paternally provided X chromosome that is inactivated (Cheng & Disteche, 2004; van den Berg, et al., 2009).

30. Lyon, M. F. (1962). Sex chromatin and gene action in the mammalian X-chromosome. *American Journal of Human Genetics, 14*, 135–148.

31. Travis, J. (2000). Silence of the Xs: Does junk DNA help women muffle one X chromosome? *Science News, 158*, 92–94.

32. Carey, 2011.

33. Karp, G. (2008). *Cell and molecular biology: Concepts and experiments* (5th ed.). New York: Wiley.

34. Holden, 2002.

35a. Cattanach, B. M., & Isaacson, J. H. (1967). Controlling elements in the mouse X chromosome. *Genetics, 57*, 331–346.

35b. Russell, L. B. (1963). Mammalian X-chromosome action: Inactivation limited in spread and in region of origin. *Science, 140*, 976–978.

36. Rastan, S., & Robertson, E. J. (1985). X-chromosome deletions in embryo-derived (EK) cell lines associated with lack of X-chromosome inactivation. *Journal of Embryology and Experimental Morphology, 90*, 379–388.

37. Brown, C. J., Ballabio, A., Rupert, J. L., Lafreniere, R. G., Grompe, M., Tonlorenzi, R., & Willard, H. F. (1991). A gene from the region of the human X inactivation centre is expressed exclusively from the inactive X chromosome. *Nature, 349*, 38–44.

38a. Carey, 2011.

38b. Francis, 2011.

39. Popova, B. C., Tada, T., Takagi, N., Brockdorff, N., & Nesterova, T. B. (2006). Attenuated spread of X-inactivation in an X;autosome translocation. *Proceedings of the National Academy of Sciences USA, 103*, 7706–7711.

40. Popova et al., 2006, p. 7706.

41. Zhang, T.-Y., & Meaney, M. J. (2010). Epigenetics and the environmental regulation of the genome and its function. *Annual Review of Psychology, 61*, 439–466.

42. Karp, 2008.

43. Cropley, J. E., Suter, C. M., Beckman, K. B., & Martin, D. I. I. (2006). Germ-line epigenetic modification of the murine Avy allele by nutritional supplementation. *Proceedings of the National Academy of Sciences of the USA, 103*, 17308–17312.

44. McCarthy, M. M., Auger, A. P., Bale, T. L., De Vries, G. J., Dunn, G. A., Forger, N. G., . . . Wilson, M. E. (2009). The epigenetics of sex differences in the brain. *Journal of Neuroscience, 29*, 12815–12823.

8. *Epigenetics*

1. Fraga, M. F., Ballestar, E., Paz, M. F., Ropero, S., Setien, F., Ballestar, M. L., . . . Esteller, M. (2005). Epigenetic differences arise during the lifetime of monozygotic twins. *Proceedings of the National Academy of Sciences of the USA, 102*, 10604–10609.

2. Fraga et al., 2005, p. 10608.

3a. Masterpasqua, F. (2009). Psychology and epigenetics. *Review of General Psychology, 13,* 194–201.

3b. Roth, T. L. (2012). Epigenetics of neurobiology and behavior during development and adulthood. *Developmental Psychobiology, 54,* 590–597.

3c. Szyf, M., McGowan, P., & Meaney, M. J. (2008). The social environment and the epigenome. *Environmental and Molecular Mutagenesis, 49,* 46–60.

4a. Gordon, L., Joo, J. E., Powell, J. E., Ollikainen, M., Novakovic, B., Li, X., . . . Saffery, R. (2012). Neonatal DNA methylation profile in human twins is specified by a complex interplay between intrauterine environmental and genetic factors, subject to tissue-specific influence. *Genome Research, 22,* 1395–1406.

4b. Ollikainen, M., Smith, K. R., Joo, E. J., Ng, H. K., Andronikos, R., Novakovic, B., . . . Craig, J. M. (2010). DNA methylation analysis of multiple tissues from newborn twins reveals both genetic and intrauterine components to variation in the human neonatal epigenome. *Human Molecular Genetics, 19,* 4176–4188.

5a. Bjornsson, H. T., Sigurdsson, M. I., Fallin, M. D., Irizarry, R. A., Aspelund, T., Cui, H., . . . Feinberg, A. P. (2008). Intra-individual change over time in DNA methylation with familial clustering. *Journal of the American Medical Association, 299,* 2877–2883.

5b. Boks, M. P., Derks, E. M., Weisenberger, D. J., Strengman, E., Janson, E., Sommer, I. E., . . . Ophoff, R. A. (2009). The relationship of DNA methylation with age, gender and genotype in twins and healthy controls. *PLoS ONE, 4*(8), e6767. doi:10.1371/journal.pone.0006767

5c. Christensen, B. C., Houseman, E. A., Marsit, C. J., Zheng, S., Wrensch, M. R., Wiemels, J. L., . . . Kelsey, K. T. (2009). Aging and environmental exposures alter tissue-specific DNA methylation dependent upon CpG island context. *PLoS Genetics, 5*(8), e1000602. doi:10.1371/journal.pgen.1000602

5d. Rakyan, V. K., Down, T. A., Maslau, S., Andrew, T., Yang, T.-P., Beyan, H., . . . Spector, T. D. (2010). Human aging-associated DNA hypermethylation occurs preferentially at bivalent chromatin domains. *Genome Research, 20,* 434–439.

5e. Wong, C. C. Y., Caspi, A., Williams, B., Craig, I. W., Houts, R., Ambler, A., . . . Mill, J. (2010). A longitudinal study of epigenetic variation in twins. *Epigenetics, 5,* 516–526.

6. Petronis, A., Gottesman, I. I., Kan, P., Kennedy, J. L., Basile, V. S., Paterson, A. D., & Popendikyte, V. (2003). Monozygotic twins exhibit numerous epigenetic differences: Clues to twin discordance? *Schizophrenia Bulletin, 29,* 169–178.

7. Although epigenetic differences appear to explain some instances of discordance, do note that studies of other pathological conditions—for example, multiple sclerosis—indicate that epigenetic differences are not always the culprit; see Baranzini, S. E., Mudge, J., van Velkinburgh, J. C., Khankhanian, P., Khrebtukova, I., Miller, N. A., . . . Kingsmore, S. F. (2010). Genome, epigenome and RNA sequences of monozygotic twins discordant for multiple sclerosis. *Nature, 464,* 1351–1356.

8. Cubas, P., Vincent, C., & Coen, E. (1999). An epigenetic mutation responsible for natural variation in floral symmetry. *Nature, 401,* 157–161.

9. Gokhman, D., Lavi, E., Prüfer, K., Fraga, M. F., Riancho, J. A., Kelso, J., . . . Carmel, L. (2014). Reconstructing the DNA methylation maps of the Neandertal and the Denisovan. *Science, 344,* 523–527.

10. Carey, N. (2011). *The epigenetics revolution.* London, England: Icon Books.

11. Shuel, R. W., & Dixon, S. E. (1960). The early establishment of dimorphism in the female honeybee, *Apis mellifera,* L. *Insectes Sociaux, 7,* 265–282.

12. Carey, 2011.

13. Kamakura, M. (2011). Royalactin induces queen differentiation in honeybees. *Nature, 473,* 478–483.

14. Evans, J. D., & Wheeler, D. E. (2001). Gene expression and the evolution of insect polyphenisms. *BioEssays, 23,* 62–68.

15. Kucharski, R., Maleszka, J., Foret, S., & Maleszka, R. (2008). Nutritional control of reproductive status in honeybees via DNA methylation. *Science, 319,* 1827–1830.

16. Carey, 2011.

17a. Duhl, D. M. J., Vrieling, H., Miller, K. A., Wolff, G. L., & Barsh, G. S. (1994). Neomorphic *agouti* mutations in obese yellow mice. *Nature Genetics, 8,* 59–65.

17b. Waterland, R. A., & Jirtle, R. L. (2003). Transposable elements: Targets for early nutritional effects on epigenetic gene regulation. *Molecular and Cellular Biology, 23,* 5293–5300.

18a. Crews, D. (2010). Epigenetics, brain, behavior, and the environment. *Hormones, 9,* 41–50.

18b. Yokota, S., Hori, H., Umezawa, M., Kubota, N., Niki, R., Yanagita, S., & Takeda, K. (2013). Gene expression changes in the olfactory bulb of mice induced by exposure to diesel exhaust are dependent on animal rearing environment. *PLoS ONE, 8*(8), e70145. doi:10.1371/journal.pone.0070145

19. Maze, I., & Nestler, E. J. (2011). The epigenetic landscape of addiction. *Annals of the New York Academy of Sciences, 1216,* 99–113.

20a. Abel, J. L., & Rissman, E. F. (2013). Running-induced epigenetic and gene expression changes in the adolescent brain. *International Journal of Developmental Neuroscience, 31,* 382–390.

20b. Gomez-Pinilla, F., Zhuang, Y., Feng, J., Ying, Z., & Fan, G. (2011). Exercise impacts brain-derived neurotrophic factor plasticity by engaging mechanisms of epigenetic regulation. *European Journal of Neuroscience, 33,* 383–390.

20c. Lovatel, G. A., Elsner, V. R., Bertoldi, K., Vanzella, C., Moysés, F. D. S., Vizuete, A., . . . Siqueira, I. R. (2013). Treadmill exercise induces age-related changes in aversive memory, neuroinflammatory and epigenetic processes in the rat hippocampus. *Neurobiology of Learning and Memory, 101,* 94–102.

20d. McGee, S. L., Fairlie, E., Garnham, A. P., & Hargreaves, M. (2009). Exercise-induced histone modifications in human skeletal muscle. *Journal of Physiology, 587,* 5951–5958.

21. Meaney, M. J. (2010). Epigenetics and the biological definition of gene × environment interactions. *Child Development, 81,* 41–79.

22. Jaenisch, R., & Bird, A. (2003). Epigenetic regulation of gene expression: How the genome integrates intrinsic and environmental signals. *Nature Genetics Supplement, 33,* p. 245.

23. Jaenisch & Bird, 2003, p. 251.

24. Katada, S., & Sassone-Corsi, P. (2010). The histone methyltransferase MLL1 permits the oscillation of circadian gene expression. *Nature Structural and Molecular Biology, 17,* p. 1414–1421.

25. Katada & Sassone-Corsi, 2010.

26. Konopka, R. J., & Benzer, S. (1971). Clock mutants of *Drosophila melanogaster. Proceedings of the National Academy of Sciences USA, 68,* 2112–2116.

27. Nakahata, Y., Kaluzova, M., Grimaldi, B., Sahar, S., Hirayama, J., Chen, D., ... Sassone-Corsi, P. (2008). The NAD+-dependent deacetylase SIRT1 modulates CLOCK-mediated chromatin remodeling and circadian control. *Cell, 134,* 329–340.

28. Nagoshi, E., Saini, C., Bauer, C., Laroche, T., Naef, F., & Schibler, U. (2004). Circadian gene expression in individual fibroblasts: Cell-autonomous and self-sustained oscillators pass time to daughter cells. *Cell, 119,* 693–705.

29. Because cells depend on RNA to convey sequence information needed for protein construction, the amount of relevant RNA in these neurons also varies across a 24-hour cycle, peaking regularly several hours before the peaks in protein concentrations; see Hardin, P. E., Hall, J. C., & Rosbash, M. (1990). Feedback of the *Drosophila* period gene product on circadian cycling of its messenger RNA levels. *Nature, 343,* 536–540.

30. Reppert, S. M., & Weaver, D. R. (2002). Coordination of circadian timing in mammals. *Nature, 418,* 935–941.

31. Rusak, B., Robertson, H. A., Wisden, W., & Hunt, S. P. (1990). Light pulses that shift rhythms induce gene expression in the suprachiasmatic nucleus. *Science, 248,* 1237–1240.

32. Naruse, Y., Oh-hashi, K., Iijima, N., Naruse, M., Yoshioka, H., & Tanaka, M. (2004). Circadian and light-induced transcription of clock gene Per1 depends on histone acetylation and deacetylation. *Molecular and Cellular Biology, 24*, 6278–6287.

33. Naruse et al., 2004, p. 6278.

34. Katada & Sassone-Corsi, 2010.

35. Orozco-Solis, R., & Sassone-Corsi, P. (2014). Epigenetic control and the circadian clock: Linking metabolism to neuronal responses. *Neuroscience, 264*, 76–87.

36. Day, J. J., & Sweatt, J. D. (2010). DNA methylation and memory formation. *Nature Neuroscience, 13*, 1319–1323.

37a. Roth, 2012.

37b. Zhang, T.-Y., & Meaney, M. J. (2010). Epigenetics and the environmental regulation of the genome and its function. *Annual Review of Psychology, 61*, 439–466.

38. Cloud, J. (2010, January 6). Why your DNA isn't your destiny. *Time Magazine*. Retrieved from www.time.com/time/magazine/

39. Begley, S. (2010, October 30). Sins of the grandfathers. *Newsweek Magazine*. Retrieved from http://www.thedailybeast.com/newsweek/2010/10/30/how-your-experiences-change-y our-sperm-and-eggs.html

40. Buchen, L. (2010). In their nurture. *Nature, 467*, p. 146.

41. Albert, P. R. (2010). Epigenetics in mental illness: Hope or hype? *Journal of Psychiatry and Neuroscience, 35*, p. 366.

42. Miller, G. (2010). The seductive allure of behavioral epigenetics. *Science, 329*, p. 24.

43. Day & Sweatt, 2010.

9. Zooming in on Epigenetics

1a. Lum, T. E., & Merritt, T. J. S. (2011). Nonclassical regulation of transcription: Interchromosomal interactions at the *Malic enzyme* locus of *Drosophila melanogaster*. *Genetics, 189*, 837–849.

1b. Spilianakis, C. G., Lalioti, M. D., Town, T., Lee, G. R., & Flavell, R. A. (2005). Interchromosomal associations between alternatively expressed loci. *Nature, 435*, 637–645.

2. Karp, G. (2008). *Cell and molecular biology: Concepts and experiments* (5th ed.). New York: Wiley, p. 518.

3. Karp, 2008, p. 518, emphasis in original.

4. See also Clayton, D. F. (2000). The genomic action potential. *Neurobiology of Learning and Memory, 74*, 185–216.

5. Myzak, M. C., & Dashwood, R. H. (2006). Histone deacetylases as targets for dietary cancer preventive agents: Lessons learned with butyrate, diallyl disulfide, and sulforaphane. *Current Drug Targets, 7*, 443–452.

6. Zhang, T.-Y., & Meaney, M. J. (2010). Epigenetics and the environmental regulation of the genome and its function. *Annual Review of Psychology, 61*, 439–466.

7a. Gibbs, W. W. (2003). The unseen genome: Beyond DNA. *Scientific American, 289*(6), 106–113.

7b. Weaver, I. C. G. (2007). Epigenetic programming by maternal behavior and pharmacological intervention: Nature versus nurture: Let's call the whole thing off. *Epigenetics, 2*, 22–28.

8. Zhang & Meaney, 2010.

9. Karp, 2008.

10a. Borrelli, E., Nestler, E. J., Allis, C. D., & Sassone-Corsi, P. (2008). Decoding the epigenetic language of neuronal plasticity. *Neuron, 60*, 961–974.

10b. Carey, N. (2011). *The epigenetics revolution*. London, England: Icon Books.

11. Berger, S. L. (2007). The complex language of chromatin regulation during transcription. *Nature, 447,* 407–412.

12. Lee, K. K., & Workman, J. L. (2007). Histone acetyltransferase complexes: One size doesn't fit all. *Nature Reviews: Molecular Cell Biology, 8,* 284–295.

13. Carey, 2011.

14. Zhang & Meaney, 2010.

15. Borrelli et al., 2008.

16. Day, J. J., & Sweatt, J. D. (2011). Epigenetic mechanisms in cognition. *Neuron, 70,* 813–829.

17. For example, di- or trimethylation of the lysine in the fourth position in the tail of H3 activates gene expression, but di- or trimethylation of the lysine in the *ninth* position on that same tail is repressive; see Sun, J.-M., Chen, H. Y., Espino, P. S., & Davie, J. R. (2007). Phosphorylated serine 28 of histone H3 is associated with destabilized nucleosomes in transcribed chromatin. *Nucleic Acids Research, 35,* 6640–6647; or Mack, G. S. (2010). To selectivity and beyond. *Nature Biotechnology, 28,* 1259–1266.

18. Borrelli et al., 2008.

19. Choi, S.-W., & Friso, S. (2010). Epigenetics: A new bridge between nutrition and health. *Advances in Nutrition, 1,* 8–16.

20. Martin, C., & Zhang, Y. (2007). Mechanisms of epigenetic inheritance. *Current Opinion in Cell Biology, 19,* 266–272.

21. Carey, 2011, p. 68.

22. Wang, Z., Zang, C., Rosenfeld, J. A., Schones, D. E., Barski, A., Cuddapah, S., . . . Zhao, K. (2008). Combinatorial patterns of histone acetylations and methylations in the human genome. *Nature Genetics, 40,* 897–903.

23. Carey, 2011, pp. 68–69.

24a. Strahl, B. D., & Allis, D. (2000). The language of covalent histone modifications. *Nature, 403,* 41–45.

24b. Taverna, S. D., Li, H., Ruthenburg, A. J., Allis, C. D., & Patel, D. J. (2007). How chromatin-binding modules interpret histone modifications: Lessons from professional pocket pickers. *Nature Structural and Molecular Biology, 14,* 1025–1040.

25. Dulac, C. (2010). Brain function and chromatin plasticity. *Nature, 465,* p. 732.

26. Globisch, D., Münzel, M., Müller, M., Michalakis, S., Wagner, M., Koch, S., . . . Carell, T. (2010). Tissue distribution of 5-hydroxymethylcytosine and search for active demethylation intermediates. *PLoS ONE, 5*(12), e15367. doi:10.1371/journal.pone.0015367

27. Eckhardt, F., Lewin, J., Cortese, R., Rakyan, V. K., Attwood, J., Burger, M., . . . Beck, S. (2006). DNA methylation profiling of human chromosomes 6, 20 and 22. *Nature Genetics, 38,* 1378–1385.

28a. McGowan, P. O., Sasaki, A., D'Alessio, A. C., Dymov, S., Labonté, B., Szyf, M., . . . Meaney, M. J. (2009). Epigenetic regulation of the glucocorticoid receptor in human brain associates with childhood abuse. *Nature Neuroscience, 12,* 342–348.

28b. Provençal, N., Suderman, M. J., Guillemin, C., Massart, R., Ruggiero, A., Wang, D., . . . Szyf, M. (2012). The signature of maternal rearing in the methylome in rhesus macaque prefrontal cortex and T cells. *Journal of Neuroscience, 32,* 15626–15642.

29. Richards, E. J. (2006). Inherited epigenetic variation—Revisiting soft inheritance. *Nature Reviews: Genetics, 7,* 395–401.

30. Choi, J. D., & Lee, J.-S. (2013). Interplay between epigenetics and genetics in cancer. *Genomics and Informatics, 11,* 164–173.

31a. Kerkel, K., Spadola, A., Yuan, E., Kosek, J., Jiang, L., Hod, E., . . . Tycko, B. (2008). Genomic surveys by methylation-sensitive SNP analysis identify sequence-dependent allele-specific DNA methylation. *Nature Genetics, 40,* 904–908.

31b. Klengel, T., Pape, J., Binder, E. B., & Mehta, D. (2014). The role of DNA methylation in stress-related psychiatric disorders. *Neuropharmacology, 80,* 115–132.

32a. Choi & Lee, 2013.

32b. Klengel et al., 2014.

33. Karp, 2008.

34. Heard, E. (2004). Recent advances in X-chromosome inactivation. *Current Opinion in Cell Biology, 16,* 247–255.

35. Carey, 2011.

36. Popova, B. C., Tada, T., Takagi, N., Brockdorff, N., & Nesterova, T. B. (2006). Attenuated spread of X-inactivation in an X;autosome translocation. *Proceedings of the National Academy of Sciences USA, 103,* 7706–7711.

37. This sequence of events has led some researchers to conclude that one of the major functions of DNA methylation is to orchestrate additional epigenetic activity on the histones, that is, to effectively guide this other activity to an appropriate place in the genome; see Karp (2008) and Richards (2006). In addition, see Carey (2011) and Mattick (2010).

38. Zhang & Meaney, 2010.

39. Carey, 2011, p. 253.

40. Zhang & Meaney, 2010.

41. Zhang & Meaney, 2010.

42. See, for example, Buchen, L. (2010). In their nurture. *Nature, 467,* 146–148.

43. Mayer, W., Niveleau, A., Walter, J., Fundele, R., & Haaf, T. (2000). Demethylation of the zygotic paternal genome. *Nature, 403,* 501–502.

44. Ooi, S. K. T., & Bestor, T. H. (2008). The colorful history of active DNA demethylation. *Cell, 133,* 1145–1148.

45. Day, J. J., & Sweatt, J. D. (2010). DNA methylation and memory formation. *Nature Neuroscience, 13,* p. 1321.

46. Sweatt, J. D. (2009). Experience-dependent epigenetic modifications in the central nervous system. *Biological Psychiatry, 65,* 191–197.

47. Anway, M. D., Cupp, A. S., Uzumcu, M., & Skinner, M. K. (2005). Epigenetic transgenerational actions of endocrine disruptors and male fertility. *Science, 308,* 1466–1469.

48. Weaver, 2007.

49. Several laboratories have reported active DNA demethylation in nondividing vertebrate cells; see Carey (2011) and Ooi & Bestor (2008). These demonstrations have not yielded subsequent characterization of the putative demethylating enzymes; see Ooi & Bestor (2008).

50a. Kriaucionis, S., & Heintz, N. (2009). The nuclear DNA base 5-hydroxymethylcytosine is present in Purkinje neurons and the brain. *Science, 324,* 929–930.

50b. Lister, R., Mukamel, E. A., Nery, J. R., Urich, M., Puddifoot, C. A., Johnson, N. D., . . . Ecker, J. R. (2013). Global epigenomic reconfiguration during mammalian brain development. *Science, 341,* 1237905. doi:10.1126/science.1237905

50c. Klengel et al., 2014.

51. Szyf, M., & Bick, J. (2013). DNA methylation: A mechanism for embedding early life experiences in the genome. *Child Development, 84,* 49–57.

52a. Li, W., & Liu, M. (2011). Distribution of 5-hydroxymethylcytosine in different human tissues. *Journal of Nucleic Acids, 2011,* 870726. doi:10.4061/2011/870726

52b. Globisch et al., 2010.

53. Klengel et al., 2014.

54. Skinner, M. K. (2011). Role of epigenetics in developmental biology and transgenerational inheritance. *Birth Defects Research (Part C), 93,* 51–55.

55a. Kriaucionis & Heintz, 2009.

55b. Day & Sweatt, 2011.

55c. Shen, L., & Zhang, Y. (2012). Enzymatic analysis of Tet proteins: Key enzymes in the metabolism of DNA methylation. *Methods in Enzymology, 512,* 93–105.

55d. Alvarado, S., Fernald, R. D., Storey, K. B., & Szyf, M. (2014). The dynamic nature of DNA methylation: A role in response to social and seasonal variation. *Integrative and Comparative Biology, 54,* 68–76.

55e. Guo, J. U., Su, Y., Zhong, C., Ming, G.-L., & Song, H. (2011). Emerging roles of TET proteins and 5-Hydroxymethylcytosines in active DNA demethylation and beyond. *Cell Cycle*,
10, 2662–2668.

56. Guo, J. U., Su, Y., Zhong, C., Ming, G.-L., & Song, H. (2011). Hydroxylation of 5-methylcytosine
by Tet1 promotes active DNA demethylation in the adult brain. *Cell*, *145*, 423–434.

57. Lister et al., 2013.

58. Massart, R., Suderman, M., Provençal, N., Yi, C., Bennett, A. J., Suomi, S., & Szyf, M.
(2014). Hydroxymethylation and DNA methylation profiles in the prefrontal cortex of the
non-human primate rhesus macaque and the impact of maternal deprivation on hydroxy-
methylation. *Neuroscience*, *268*, 139–148.

59. Quoted in Buchen, 2010, p. 148.

10. Experience

1. Masten, A. S. (2001). Ordinary magic: Resilience processes in development. *American
Psychologist*, *56*, 227–238.

2a. Neigh, G. N., Gillespie, C. F., & Nemeroff, C. B. (2009). The neurobiological toll of child
abuse and neglect. *Trauma, Violence, and Abuse*, *10*, 389–410.

2b. Lutz, P.-E., & Turecki, G. (2014). DNA methylation and childhood maltreatment: From
animal models to human studies. *Neuroscience*, *264*, 142–156.

3. Harlow, H. F., Dodsworth, R. O., & Harlow, M. K. (1965). Total social isolation in monkeys. *Proceedings of the National Academy of Sciences USA*, *54*, p. 90.

4. Harlow, H. F. (1958). The nature of love. *American Psychologist*, *13*, p. 675.

5. Scafidi, F. A., Field, T. M., Schanberg, S. M., Bauer, C. R., Tucci, K., Roberts, J., ... & Kuhn,
C. M. (1990). Massage stimulates growth in preterm infants: A replication. *Infant Behavior
and Development*, *13*, 167–188.

6. Hernandez-Reif, M., Diego, M., & Field, T. (2007). Preterm infants show reduced stress
behaviors and activity after 5 days of massage therapy. *Infant Behavior and Development*, *30*,
557–561.

7. Diego, M. A., Field, T., & Hernandez-Reif, M. (2009). Procedural pain heart rate responses
in massaged preterm infants. *Infant Behavior and Development*, *32*, 226–229.

8. Borghol, N., Suderman, M., McArdle, W., Racine, A., Hallett, M., Pembrey, M., ... Szyf, M.
(2012). Associations with early-life socio-economic position in adult DNA methylation.
International Journal of Epidemiology, *41*, 62–74.

9. Hackman, D. A., Farah, M. J., & Meaney, M. J. (2010). Socioeconomic status and the
brain: Mechanistic insights from human and animal research. *Nature Reviews: Neuroscience*,
11, 651–659.

10. Smith, L. B. (1999). Do infants possess innate knowledge structures? The con side.
Developmental Science, *2*, p. 140.

11a. Meaney, M. J. (2010). Epigenetics and the biological definition of gene × environment
interactions. *Child Development*, *81*, 41–79.

11b. Meaney, M. J., & Szyf, M. (2005). Maternal care as a model for experience-dependent
chromatin plasticity? *Trends in Neurosciences*, *28*, 456–463.

12. Curley, J. P., Jensen, C. L., Mashoodh, R., & Champagne, F. A. (2011). Social influences on neurobiology and behavior: Epigenetic effects during development.
Psychoneuroendocrinology, *36*, 352–371.

13a. Coplan, J. D., Andrews, M. W., Rosenblum, L. A., Owens, M. J., Friedman, S., Gorman,
J. M., & Nemeroff, C. B. (1996). Persistent elevations of cerebrospinal fluid concentrations
of corticotropin-releasing factor in adult nonhuman primates exposed to early-life stressors: Implications for the pathophysiology of mood and anxiety disorders. *Proceedings of the
National Academy of Sciences of the USA*, *93*, 1619–1623.

13b. Francis, D. D., Caldji, C., Champagne, F., Plotsky, P. M., & Meaney, M. J. (1999a). The
role of corticotropin-releasing factor—norepinephrine systems in mediating the effects

of early experience on the development of behavioral and endocrine responses to stress. *Biological Psychiatry, 46*, 1153–1166.

13c. Lee, R., Geracioti, T. D., Kasckow, J. W., & Coccaro, E. F. (2005). Childhood trauma and personality disorder: Positive correlation with adult CSF corticotropin-releasing factor concentrations. *American Journal of Psychiatry, 162*, 995–997.

14. Francis et al., 1999a.

15. Francis et al., 1999a.

16a. Caldji, C., Tannenbaum, B., Sharma, S., Francis, D., Plotsky, P. M., & Meaney, M. J. (1998). Maternal care during infancy regulates the development of neural systems mediating the expression of fearfulness in the rat. *Proceedings of the National Academy of Sciences of the USA, 95*, 5335–5340.

16b. Francis et al., 1999a.

17. Francis, D., Diorio, J., Liu, D., & Meaney, M. J. (1999b). Nongenomic transmission across generations of maternal behavior and stress responses in the rat. *Science, 286*, 1155–1158.

18. For example, see Champagne, F. A., Weaver, I. C. G., Diorio, J., Dymov, S., Szyf, M., & Meaney, M. J. (2006). Maternal care associated with methylation of the estrogen receptor-α1b promoter and estrogen receptor-α expression in the medial preoptic area of female offspring. *Endocrinology, 147*, 2909–2915.

19. Meaney, 2010, p. 63.

20a. Ho, M. (1984). Environment and heredity in development and evolution. In M. Ho & P. T. Saunders (Eds.), *Beyond neo-Darwinism: An introduction to the new evolutionary paradigm* (pp. 267–289). London: Academic Press.

20b. Lickliter, R., & Honeycutt, H. (2003). Developmental dynamics: Toward a biologically plausible evolutionary psychology. *Psychological Bulletin, 129*, 819–835.

21. Several other nongenomic modes of intergenerational transmission have been detected as well. Part III of this book will consider issues of intergenerational transmission. An excellent source for anyone interested in these issues is Jablonka, E., & Lamb, M. J. (2005). *Evolution in four dimensions: Genetic, epigenetic, behavioral, and symbolic variation in the history of life.* Cambridge, MA: MIT Press.

22. Weaver, I. C. G., Cervoni, N., Champagne, F. A., D'Alessio, A. C., Sharma, S., Seckl, J. R., . . . Meaney, M. J. (2004a). Epigenetic programming by maternal behavior. *Nature Neuroscience, 7*, 847–854.

23. Curley et al., 2011.

24. Weaver et al., 2004a.

25. Zhang, T.-Y., Bagot, R., Parent, C., Nesbitt, C., Bredy, T. W., Caldji, C., . . . Meaney, M. J. (2006). Maternal programming of defensive responses through sustained effects on gene expression. *Biological Psychology, 73*, 72–89.

26. Liu, D., Diorio, J., Day, J. C., Francis, D. D., & Meaney, M. J. (2000). Maternal care, hippocampal synaptogenesis and cognitive development in rats. *Nature Neuroscience, 3*, 799–806.

27. Liu et al., 2000.

28. Day, J. J., & Sweatt, J. D. (2010). DNA methylation and memory formation. *Nature Neuroscience, 13*, p. 1321.

29. Szyf, M., & Bick, J. (2013). DNA methylation: A mechanism for embedding early life experiences in the genome. *Child Development, 84*, 49–57.

11. Zooming In On Experience

1. Olshansky, S. J. (2011). Aging of US presidents. *Journal of the American Medical Association, 306*, 2328–2329.

2a. Ballantyne, C. (2007, October 24). Fact or fiction? Stress causes gray hair. *Scientific American.* Retrieved from http://www.scientificamerican.com

2b. Parker-Pope, T. (2009, March 9). Unlocking the secrets of gray hair. *New York Times.*

3. McEwen, B. S. (2008). Central effects of stress hormones in health and disease: Understanding the protective and damaging effects of stress and stress mediators. *European Journal of Pharmacology, 583,* 174–185.

4. Chrousos, G. P. (2009). Stress and disorders of the stress system. *Nature Reviews: Endocrinology, 5,* 374–381.

5. McEwen, 2008.

6. Chrousos, 2009.

7. McEwen, 2008.

8. Chrousos, 2009.

9. McEwen, 2008.

10. Neigh, G. N., Gillespie, C. F., & Nemeroff, C. B. (2009). The neurobiological toll of child abuse and neglect. *Trauma, Violence, and Abuse 10,* 389–410.

11. Vale, W., Spiess, J., Rivier, C., & Rivier, J. (1981). Characterization of a 41-residue ovine hypothalamic peptide that stimulates secretion of corticotropin and β-endorphin. *Science, 213,* 1394–1397.

12. Chrousos, 2009.

13. Francis, D. D., Caldji, C., Champagne, F., Plotsky, P. M., & Meaney, M. J. (1999a). The role of corticotropin-releasing factor—norepinephrine systems in mediating the effects of early experience on the development of behavioral and endocrine responses to stress. *Biological Psychiatry, 46,* 1153–1155.

14. Liu, D., Diorio, J., Tannenbaum, B., Caldji, C., Francis, D., Freedman, A., . . . Meaney, M. J. (1997). Maternal care, hippocampal glucocorticoid receptors and hypothalamic-pituitary-adrenal responses to stress. *Science, 277,* 1659–1662.

15a. Francis et al., 1999a.

15b. Meaney, M. J. (2001). Maternal care, gene expression, and the transmission of individual differences in stress reactivity across generations. *Annual Review of Neuroscience, 24,* 1161–1192.

15c. Weaver, I. C. G., Cervoni, N., Champagne, F. A., D'Alessio, A. C., Sharma, S., Seckl, J. R., . . . Meaney, M. J. (2004a). Epigenetic programming by maternal behavior. *Nature Neuroscience, 7,* 847–854.

16. Liu et al., 1997, p. 1660.

17. Chrousos, 2009.

18. Buckingham, J. C. (2006). Glucocorticoids: Exemplars of multi-tasking. *British Journal of Pharmacology, 147,* S258–S268.

19. Karp, G. (2008). *Cell and molecular biology: Concepts and experiments* (5th ed.). New York: Wiley, p. 518.

20. Buckingham, 2006.

21. Reddy, T. E., Pauli, F., Sprouse, R. O., Neff, N. F., Newberry, K. M., Garabedian, M. J., & Myers, R. M. (2009). Genomic determination of the glucocorticoid response reveals unexpected mechanisms of gene regulation. *Genome Research, 19,* 2163–2171.

22. Buckingham, 2006.

23. Buckingham, 2006, p. S264.

24a. Weaver et al., 2004a.

24b. Weaver, I. C. G., Diorio, J., Seckl, J. R., Szyf, M., & Meaney, M. J. (2004b). Early environmental regulation of hippocampal glucocorticoid receptor gene expression: Characterization of intracellular mediators and potential genomic target sites. *Annals of the New York Academy of Science, 1024,* 182–212.

25. Weaver et al., 2004a.

26. Weaver et al., 2004a.

27. Weaver et al., 2004a.

28a. Radiolab (Producer). (2012a, November 19). *Leaving your Lamarck* [Audio podcast]. Retrieved from http://www.radiolab.org/2012/nov/19/leaving-lamarck/

28b. Weaver, I. C. G., D'Alessio, A. C., Brown, S. E., Hellstron, I. C., Dymov, S., Sharma, S., . . . Meaney, M. J. (2007). The transcription factor nerve growth factor-inducible protein A mediates epigenetic programming: Altering epigenetic marks by immediate-early genes. *Journal of Neuroscience, 27*, 1756–1768.

29a. Kandel, E. R. (2001). The molecular biology of memory storage: A dialogue between genes and synapses. *Science, 294*, 1030–1038.

29b. Zhang, T.-Y., & Meaney, M. J. (2010). Epigenetics and the environmental regulation of the genome and its function. *Annual Review of Psychology, 61*, 439–466.

30. Weaver et al., 2004a, p. 849.

31. Murgatroyd, C., Patchev, A. V., Wu, Y., Micale, V., Bockmühl, Y., Fischer, D., . . . Spengler, D. (2009). Dynamic DNA methylation programs persistent adverse effects of early-life stress. *Nature Neuroscience, 12*, 1559–1566.

32. Harlow, H. F., Dodsworth, R. O., & Harlow, M. K. (1965). Total social isolation in monkeys. *Proceedings of the National Academy of Sciences USA, 54*, 90–97.

33. Lee, R., Geracioti, T. D., Kasckow, J. W., & Coccaro, E. F. (2005). Childhood trauma and personality disorder: Positive correlation with adult CSF corticotropin-releasing factor concentrations. *American Journal of Psychiatry, 162*, 995–997.

34. Murgatroyd et al., 2009.

35. Murgatroyd et al., 2009, p. 1559.

36. Mueller, B. R., & Bale, T. L. (2008). Sex-specific programming of offspring emotionality after stress early in pregnancy. *Journal of Neuroscience, 28*, 9055–9065.

37. Carey, N. (2011). *The epigenetics revolution*. London, England: Icon Books.

38. Roth, T. L., Lubin, F. D., Funk, A. J., & Sweatt, J. D. (2009). Lasting epigenetic influence of early-life adversity on the BDNF gene. *Biological Psychiatry, 65*, 760–769.

39. Roth et al., 2009.

40. Heijmans, B. T., Tobi, E. W., Lumey, L. H., & Slagboom, P. E. (2009). The epigenome: Archive of the prenatal environment. *Epigenetics, 4*, 526–531.

12. Primates

1. Keeley, B. L. (2004). Anthropomorphism, primatomorphism, mammalomorphism: Understanding cross-species comparisons. *Biology and Philosophy, 19*, p. 523.

2. Gottlieb, G., & Lickliter, R. (2004). The various roles of animal models in understanding human development. *Social Development, 13*, p. 312, emphasis added.

3. Chrousos, G. P., Schuermeyer, T. H., Doppman, J., Oldfield, E. H., Schulte, H. M., Gold, P. W., & Loriaux, D. L. (1985). NIH conference: Clinical applications of corticotropin-releasing factor. *Annals of Internal Medicine, 102*, 344–358.

4. Dawkins, R. (2004). *The ancestor's tale: A pilgrimage to the dawn of evolution*. New York: Houghton Mifflin.

5. Gottlieb & Lickliter, 2004, p. 312.

6a. Keller, S., Sarchiapone, M., Zarrilli, F., Videtič, A., Ferraro, A., Carli, V., . . . Chiariotti, L. (2010). Increased *BDNF* promoter methylation in the Wernicke area of suicide subjects. *Archives of General Psychiatry, 67*, 258–267.

6b. Poulter, M. O., Du, L., Weaver, I. C. G., Palkovits, M., Faludi, G., Merali, Z., . . . Anisman, H. (2008). GABAA receptor promoter hypermethylation in suicide brain: Implications for the involvement of epigenetic processes. *Biological Psychiatry, 64*, 645–652.

7. Poulter et al., 2008, p. 651.

8. Keller et al., 2010, p. 266.

9. McGowan, P. O., Sasaki, A., D'Alessio, A. C., Dymov, S., Labonté, B., Szyf, M., . . . Meaney, M. J. (2009). Epigenetic regulation of the glucocorticoid receptor in human brain associates with childhood abuse. *Nature Neuroscience, 12*, p. 342.

10. McGowan et al., 2009.

11. Weaver, I. C. G., Cervoni, N., Champagne, F. A., D'Alessio, A. C., Sharma, S., Seckl, J. R., . . . Meaney, M. J. (2004a). Epigenetic programming by maternal behavior. *Nature Neuroscience, 7,* 847–854.

12. McGowan et al., 2009, p. 342.

13. McGowan et al., 2009, p. 346.

14. For example, see Kasl, S. V., Evans, A. S., & Niederman, J. C. (1979). Psychosocial risk factors in the development of infectious mononucleosis. *Psychosomatic Medicine, 41,* 445–466.

15. Glaser, R., Rice, J., Sheridan, J., Fertel, R., Stout, J., Speicher, C., . . . Kiecolt-Glaser, J. (1987). Stress-related immune suppression: Health implications. *Brain, Behavior, and Immunity, 1,* 7–20.

16. Glaser, R., Kennedy, S., Lafuse, W. P., Bonneau, R. H., Speicher, C., Hillhouse, J., & Kiecolt-Glaser, J. K. (1990). Psychological stress-induced modulation of interleukin 2 receptor gene expression and interleukin 2 production in peripheral blood leukocytes, *Archives of General Psychiatry, 47,* p. 707.

17a. Tylee, D. S., Kawaguchi, D. M., & Glatt, S. J. (2013). On the outside, looking in: A review and evaluation of the comparability of blood and brain "-omes." *American Journal of Medical Genetics Part B: Neuropsychiatric Genetics, 162B,* 595–603.

17b. Nikolova, Y. S., Koenen, K. C., Galea, S., Wang, C.-M., Seney, M. L., Sibille, E., . . . Hariri, A. R. (2014). Beyond genotype: Serotonin transporter epigenetic modification predicts human brain function. *Nature Neuroscience.* Advance online publication. doi:10.1038/nn.3778

18a. Van IJzendoorn, M. H., Bakermans-Kranenburg, M. J., & Ebstein, R. P. (2011). Methylation matters in child development: Toward developmental behavioral epigenetics. *Child Development Perspectives, 5,* 305–310.

18b. Provençal, N., Suderman, M. J., Guillemin, C., Massart, R., Ruggiero, A., Wang, D., . . . Szyf, M. (2012). The signature of maternal rearing in the methylome in rhesus macaque prefrontal cortex and T cells. *Journal of Neuroscience, 32,* 15626–15642.

19. Provençal et al., 2012.

20. Provençal et al., 2012, p. 15626.

21. Provençal et al., 2012.

22. Other investigations have explored the correspondence between methylation in brain cells and methylation in blood cells, and these studies—which used different approaches than Provençal et al. (2012)—have found that methylation levels in brain and blood are highly correlated; see Tylee et al., 2013.

23. Tung, J., Barreiro, L. B., Johnson, Z. P., Hansen, K. D., Michopoulos, V., Toufexis, D., . . . Gilad, Y. (2012). Social environment is associated with gene regulatory variation in the rhesus macaque immune system. *Proceedings of the National Academy of Sciences USA, 109,* 6490–6495.

24. Sapolsky, R. M. (2005). The influence of social hierarchy on primate health. *Science, 308,* 648–652.

25. Tung et al., 2012.

26. Tung et al., 2012, p. 6494.

27. Tung et al., 2012, p. 6494.

28. Fredrickson, B. L., Grewen, K. M., Coffey, K. A., Algoe, S. B., Firestine, A. M., Arevalo, J. M. G., . . . Cole, S. W. (2013). A functional genomic perspective on human well-being. *Proceedings of the National Academy of Sciences USA, 110,* 13684–13689.

29. Fraga, M. F., Ballestar, E., Paz, M. F., Ropero, S., Setien, F., Ballestar, M. L., . . . Esteller, M. (2005). Epigenetic differences arise during the lifetime of monozygotic twins. *Proceedings of the National Academy of Sciences of the USA, 102,* 10604–10609.

30a. Gordon, L., Joo, J. E., Powell, J. E., Ollikainen, M., Novakovic, B., Li, X., . . . Saffery, R. (2012). Neonatal DNA methylation profile in human twins is specified by a complex interplay between intrauterine environmental and genetic factors, subject to tissue-specific influence. *Genome Research, 22,* 1395–1406.

30b. Ollikainen, M., Smith, K. R., Joo, E. J., Ng, H. K., Andronikos, R., Novakovic, B., ... Craig, J. M. (2010). DNA methylation analysis of multiple tissues from newborn twins reveals both genetic and intrauterine components to variation in the human neonatal epigenome. *Human Molecular Genetics, 19,* 4176–4188.

30c. Wong, C. C. Y., Caspi, A., Williams, B., Craig, I. W., Houts, R., Ambler, A., ... Mill, J. (2010). A longitudinal study of epigenetic variation in twins. *Epigenetics, 5,* 516–526.

31. Ollikainen et al., 2010.

32. Newer research by Gordon and colleagues (2012) found similar effects in a genome-scale study of twins that examined approximately 20,000 different DNA segments.

33. Van IJzendoorn et al., 2011.

34. Oberlander, T. F., Weinberg, J., Papsdorf, M., Grunau, R., Misri, S., & Devlin, A. M. (2008). Prenatal exposure to maternal depression, neonatal methylation of human glucocorticoid receptor gene (*NR3C1*) and infant cortisol stress responses. *Epigenetics, 3,* 97–106.

35. For example, see Ansorge, M. S., Zhou, M., Lira, A., Hen, R., & Gingrich, J. A. (2004). Early-life blockade of the 5-HT transporter alters emotional behavior in adult mice. *Science, 306,* 879–881.

36. Devlin, A. M., Brain, U., Austin, J., & Oberlander, T. F. (2010). Prenatal exposure to maternal depressed mood and the *MTHFR* C677T variant affect *SLC6A4* methylation in infants at birth. *PLoS ONE, 5*(8), e12201. doi:10.1371/journal.pone.0012201

37. Devlin et al., 2010, p. 6.

38. Beach, S. R. H., Brody, G. H., Todorov, A. A., Gunter, T. D., & Philibert, R. A. (2010). Methylation at *SLC6A4* is linked to family history of child abuse: An examination of the Iowa adoptee sample. *American Journal of Medical Genetics Part B, 153B,* 710–713.

39. Perroud, N., Paoloni-Giacobino, A., Prada, P. Olié, E., Salzmann, A., Nicastro, R., ... Malafosse, A. (2011). Increased methylation of glucocorticoid receptor gene (*NR3C1*) in adults with a history of childhood maltreatment: A link with the severity and type of trauma. *Translational Psychiatry, 1,* e59. doi:10.1038/tp.2011.60

40a. Labonté, B., Suderman, M., Maussion, G., Navaro, L., Yerko, V., Mahar, I., ... Turecki, G. (2012). Genome-wide epigenetic regulation by early-life trauma. *Archives of General Psychiatry, 69,* 722–731.

40b. Suderman, M., Borghol, N., Pappas, J. J., Pereira, S. M. P., Pembrey, M., Hertzman, C., ... Szyf, M. (2014). Childhood abuse is associated with methylation of multiple loci in adult DNA. *BMC Medical Genomics, 7,* 13. doi:10.1186/1755-8794-7-13

41. Lutz, P.-E., & Turecki, G. (2014). DNA methylation and childhood maltreatment: From animal models to human studies. *Neuroscience, 264,* 142–156.

42. Nikolova et al., 2014.

43. Beach et al., 2010.

44. Radtke, K. M., Ruf, M., Gunter, H. M., Dohrmann, K., Schauer, M., Meyer, A., & Elbert, T. (2011). Transgenerational impact of intimate partner violence on methylation in the promoter of the glucocorticoid receptor. *Translational Psychiatry, 1,* e21. doi:10.1038/tp.2011.21

45. For the purposes of this study, violence was defined as "any behavior within an intimate relationship that causes physical, psychological or sexual harm to those in the relationship" (Radtke et al., 2011, p. 4).

46. Radtke et al., 2011, p. 4.

47. Alvarado, S., Fernald, R. D., Storey, K. B., & Szyf, M. (2014). The dynamic nature of DNA methylation: A role in response to social and seasonal variation. *Integrative and Comparative Biology, 54,* 68–76.

48. For example, see Essex, M. J., Boyce, W. T., Hertzman, C., Lam, L. L., Armstrong, J. M., Neumann, S. M. A., & Kobor, M. S. (2013). Epigenetic vestiges of early developmental adversity: Childhood stress exposure and DNA methylation in adolescence. *Child Development, 84,* 58–75.

49. House, J. S., Landis, K. R., & Umberson, D. (1988). Social relationships and health. *Science*, *241*, p. 541.

50. Cole, S. W., Hawkley, L. C., Arevalo, J. M., Sung. C. Y., Rose, R. M., & Cacioppo, J. T. (2007). Social regulation of gene expression in human leukocytes. *Genome Biology*, *8*, R189.

51. Miller, G. E., Chen, E., Fok, A. K., Walker, H., Lim, A., Nicholls, E. F., . . . Kobor, M. S. (2009). Low early-life social class leaves a biological residue manifested by decreased glucocorticoid and increased proinflammatory signaling. *Proceedings of the National Academy of Sciences USA*, *106*, 14716–14721.

52. I should point out here that the absence of evidence about epigenetics from the Miller lab does not mean his group is not looking for such evidence. They are, but have simply not found any yet. In an interview about this research, Miller provided some additional information about his team's efforts to trace the effects of early-life SES back to epigenetic alterations. He said, "We spent the last few years trying to see if we could find evidence of epigenetic alterations in the immune system that are related to early life experience. . . . This work is still ongoing, so I think it would be premature to conclude anything definitively, but we've had less success than we'd hoped and imagined" (Miller, 2010, p. 27). Clearly, there is still more work to be done, because *something* is responsible for the reduced GR activity observed!

53. Borghol, N., Suderman, M., McArdle, W., Racine, A., Hallett, M., Pembrey, M., . . . Szyf, M. (2012). Associations with early-life socio-economic position in adult DNA methylation. *International Journal of Epidemiology*, *41*, 62–74.

54. Borghol et al., 2012, p. 71.

55. Hackman, D. A., Farah, M. J., & Meaney, M. J. (2010). Socioeconomic status and the brain: Mechanistic insights from human and animal research. *Nature Reviews: Neuroscience*, *11*, 651–659.

56. Kuzawa, C. W., & Sweet, E. (2009). Epigenetics and the embodiment of race: Developmental origins of US racial disparities in cardiovascular health. *American Journal of Human Biology*, *21*, 2–15.

57. Terry, M. B., Ferris, J. S., Pilsner, R., Flom, J. D., Tehranifar, P., Santella, R. M., . . . Susser, E. (2008). Genomic DNA methylation among women in a multiethnic New York City birth cohort. *Cancer Epidemiology, Biomarkers and Prevention*, *17*, 2306–2310.

58. Kuzawa & Sweet, 2009.

59. Kuzawa & Sweet, 2009.

60. Kuzawa & Sweet, 2009, p. 3–4.

61. Curley, J. P., Jensen, C. L., Mashoodh, R., & Champagne, F. A. (2011). Social influences on neurobiology and behavior: Epigenetic effects during development. *Psychoneuroendocrinology*, *36*, 352–371.

62. Brena, R. M., Huang, T. H-M., & Plass, C. (2006). Toward a human epigenome. *Nature Genetics*, *38*, 1359–1360.

63. Human Epigenome Consortium (2013). *The human epigenome project*. Retrieved from http://www.epigenome.org/index.php?page=project

64. Gomase, V. S., & Tagore, S. (2008). Epigenomics. *Current Drug Metabolism*, *9*, 232–237.

65. Maher, B. (2012). The human encyclopaedia. *Nature*, *489*, p. 46.

13. Memory

1. Miller, C. A., & Sweatt, J. D. (2006). Amnesia or retrieval deficit? Implications of a molecular approach to the question of reconsolidation. *Learning and Memory*, *13*, 498–505.

2a. Dębiec, J., Doyère, V., Nader, K., & LeDoux, J. E. (2006). Directly reactivated, but not indirectly reactivated, memories undergo reconsolidation in the amygdala. *Proceedings of the National Academy of Sciences of the USA*, *102*, 3428–3433.

2b. Doyère, V., Dębiec, J., Monfils, M., Schafe, G. E., & LeDoux, J. E. (2007). Synapse-specific reconsolidation of distinct fear memories in the lateral amygdala. *Nature Neuroscience, 10,* 414–416.

3. Kandel, E. R. (2001). The molecular biology of memory storage: A dialogue between genes and synapses. *Science, 294,* p. 1030.

4. Kandel, 2001, pp. 1030–1031.

5. Kandel, 2001, p. 1038.

6. Kandel, 2001, p. 1030.

7. Kandel, 2001, p. 1030.

8. Pinsker, H. M., Hening, W. A., Carew, T. J., & Kandel, E. R. (1973). Long-term sensitization of a defensive withdrawal reflex in Aplysia. *Science, 182,* 1039–1042.

9. Castellucci, V. F., Blumenfeld, H., Goelet, P., & Kandel, E. R. (1989). Inhibitor of protein synthesis blocks longterm behavioral sensitization in the isolated gill-withdrawal reflex of *Aplysia. Journal of Neurobiology, 20,* 1–9.

10. Atkinson, R. C., & Shiffrin, R. M. (1968). Human memory: A proposed system and its control processes. In K. W. Spence, Ed.), *The psychology of learning and motivation: Advances in research and theory* (pp. 89–195). New York, NY: Academic Press.

11. Flexner, L. B., & Flexner, J. B. (1966). Effect of acetoxycycloheximide and of an acetoxycycloheximide-puromycin mixture on cerebral protein synthesis and memory in mice. *Proceedings of the National Academy of Sciences of the USA, 55,* 369–374.

12. Bailey, C. H., & Chen, M. (1988). Long-term memory in *Aplysia* modulates the total number of varicosities of single identified sensory neurons. *Proceedings of the National Academy of Sciences USA, 85,* 2373–2377.

13. Zhang, T.-Y., & Meaney, M. J. (2010). Epigenetics and the environmental regulation of the genome and its function. *Annual Review of Psychology, 61,* 439–466.

14. Kandel, E. R. (2001). The molecular biology of memory storage: A dialogue between genes and synapses. *Science, 294,* 1030–1038.

15. Mattick, J. S. (2010). RNA as the substrate for epigenome-environment interactions. *BioEssays, 32,* 548–552.

16. Jacob, F. (1977). Evolution and tinkering. *Science, 196,* 1163–1164.

17. Levenson, J. M., & Sweatt, J. D. (2005). Epigenetic mechanisms in memory formation. *Nature Reviews: Neuroscience, 6,* 108–118.

18. Feinberg, A. P. (2008). Epigenetics at the epicenter of modern medicine. *Journal of the American Medical Association, 299,* 1345–1350.

19. Gould, S. J., & Vrba, E. S. (1982). Exaptation—A missing term in the science of form. *Paleobiology, 8,* p. 4.

20. Day, J. J., & Sweatt, J. D. (2011). Epigenetic mechanisms in cognition. *Neuron, 70,* 813–829.

21. Levenson & Sweatt, 2005, p. 116.

22. Levenson & Sweatt, 2005, p. 109.

23. Guan, Z., Giustetto, M., Lomvardas, S., Kim, J.-H., Miniaci, M. C., Schwartz, J. H., . . . Kandel, E. R. (2002). Integration of long-term-memory-related synaptic plasticity involves bidirectional regulation of gene expression and chromatin structure. *Cell, 111,* 483–493.

24. Alarcón, J. M., Malleret, G., Touzani, K., Vronskaya, S., Ishii, S., Kandel, E. R., & Barco, A. (2004). Chromatin acetylation, memory, and LTP are impaired in CBP+/- mice: A model for the cognitive deficit in Rubinstein-Taybi syndrome and its amelioration. *Neuron, 42,* 947–959.

25. Levenson, J. M., O'Riordan, K. J., Brown, K. D., Trinh, M. A., Molfese, D. L., & Sweatt, J. D. (2004). Regulation of histone acetylation during memory formation in the hippocampus. *Journal of Biological Chemistry, 279,* 40545–40559.

26. Scoville, W. B., & Milner, B. (1957). Loss of recent memory after bilateral hippocampal lesions. *Journal of Neurology, Neurosurgery, and Psychiatry, 20,* 11–21.

27. Scoville & Milner, 1957.

28. Scoville & Milner, 1957, p. 14.

29. Scoville & Milner, 1957, p. 14

30. Miller, C. A., Gavin, C. F., White, J. A., Parrish, R. R., Honasoge, A., Yancey, C. R., . . . Sweatt, J. D. (2010). Cortical DNA methylation maintains remote memory. *Nature Neuroscience, 13*, 664–666.

31. Levenson et al., 2004.

32. Levenson et al., 2004.

33. Levenson & Sweatt, 2005, p. 113.

34. Gupta, S., Kim, S. Y., Artis, S., Molfese, D. L., Schumacher, A., Sweatt, J. D., . . . Lubin, F. D. (2010). Histone methylation regulates memory formation. *Journal of Neuroscience, 30*, 3589–3599.

35. Day & Sweatt, 2011, p. 815.

36. Sweatt, J. D. (2009). Experience-dependent epigenetic modifications in the central nervous system. *Biological Psychiatry, 65*, 191–197.

37a. Borrelli, E., Nestler, E. J., Allis, C. D., & Sassone-Corsi, P. (2008). Decoding the epigenetic language of neuronal plasticity. *Neuron, 60*, 961–974.

37b. Levenson, J. M., Roth, T. L., Lubin, F. D., Miller, C. A., Huang, I.-C., Desai, P., . . . Sweatt, J. D. (2006). Evidence that DNA (cytosine-5) methyltransferase regulates synaptic plasticity in the hippocampus. *Journal of Biological Chemistry, 281*, 15763–15773.

37c. Lubin, F. D., Roth, T. L., & Sweatt, J. D. (2008). Epigenetic regulation of bdnf gene transcription in the consolidation of fear memory. *Journal of Neuroscience, 28*, 10576–10586.

38. Miller et al., 2010.

39. Lubin et al., 2008.

40. Day, J. J., & Sweatt, J. D. (2010). DNA methylation and memory formation. *Nature Neuroscience, 13*, p. 1322, emphasis added.

41. Day & Sweatt, 2010, p. 1322.

42. Levenson et al., 2006.

43. Day & Sweatt, 2011, p. 816.

44. Day & Sweatt, 2011, p. 813.

45. Levenson & Sweatt, 2005, p. 114.

46. Levenson & Sweatt, 2005.

47. Rudenko, A., & Tsai, L.-H. (2014). Epigenetic regulation in memory and cognitive disorders. *Neuroscience, 264*, 51–63.

48. Levenson et al., 2004.

49. Gräff, J., Rei, D., Guan, J.-S., Wang, W.-Y., Seo, J., Hennig, K. M., . . . Tsai, L.-H. (2012). An epigenetic blockade of cognitive functions in the neurodegenerating brain. *Nature, 483*, 222–226.

50. Fischer, A., Sananbenesi, F., Wang, X., Dobbin, M., & Tsai, L.-H. (2007). Recovery of learning and memory is associated with chromatin remodeling. *Nature, 447*, 178–182.

14. Zooming in on Memory

1. Gräff, J., Rei, D., Guan, J.-S., Wang, W.-Y., Seo, J., Hennig, K. M., . . . Tsai, L.-H. (2012). An epigenetic blockade of cognitive functions in the neurodegenerating brain. *Nature, 483*, p. 222.

2. Kandel, E. R. (2001). The molecular biology of memory storage: A dialogue between genes and synapses. *Science, 294*, 1030–1038.

3. Dulac, C. (2010). Brain function and chromatin plasticity. *Nature, 465*, 728–735.

4. Alarcón, J. M., Malleret, G., Touzani, K., Vronskaya, S., Ishii, S., Kandel, E. R., & Barco, A. (2004). Chromatin acetylation, memory, and LTP are impaired in CBP+/- mice: A model for the cognitive deficit in Rubinstein-Taybi syndrome and its amelioration. *Neuron, 42*, 947–959.

5a. Borrelli, E., Nestler, E. J., Allis, C. D., & Sassone-Corsi, P. (2008). Decoding the epigenetic language of neuronal plasticity. *Neuron, 60,* 961–974.

5b. Dulac, 2010.

5c. Zhang, T.-Y., & Meaney, M. J. (2010). Epigenetics and the environmental regulation of the genome and its function. *Annual Review of Psychology, 61,* 439–466.

6. Alarcón et al., 2004.

7. Tanaka, Y., Naruse, I., Maekawa, T., Masuya, H., Shiroishi, T., & Ishii, S. (1997). Abnormal skeletal patterning in embryos lacking a single *Cbp* allele: A partial similarity with Rubinstein-Taybi syndrome. *Proceedings of the National Academy of Sciences USA, 94,* 10215–10220.

8. Tanaka et al., 1997.

9. Alarcón et al., 2004.

10. Alarcón et al., 2004.

11. Alarcón et al., 2004, p. 947.

12. Alvarez-Breckenridge, C. A., Yu, J., Price, R., Wei, M., Wang, Y., Nowicki, M. O., . . . Chiocca, E. A. (2012). The histone deacetylase inhibitor valproic acid lessens NK cell action against oncolytic virus-infected glioblastoma cells by inhibition of STAT5/T-BET signaling and generation of gamma interferon. *Journal of Virology, 86,* 4566–4577.

13. Alarcón et al., 2004.

14. Alarcón et al., 2004.

15a. Borrelli et al., 2008.

15b. Guan, J.-S., Haggarty, S. J., Giacometti, E., Dannenberg, J.-H., Joseph, N., Gao, J., . . . Tsai, L.-H. (2009). HDAC2 negatively regulates memory formation and synaptic plasticity. *Nature, 459,* 55–60.

15c. Levenson, J. M., O'Riordan, K. J., Brown, K. D., Trinh, M. A., Molfese, D. L., & Sweatt, J. D. (2004). Regulation of histone acetylation during memory formation in the hippocampus. *Journal of Biological Chemistry, 279,* 40545–40559.

15d. Levenson, J. M., & Sweatt, J. D. (2005). Epigenetic mechanisms in memory formation. *Nature Reviews: Neuroscience, 6,* 108–118.

16. Guan et al., 2009, p. 55.

17. Carey, N. (2011). *The epigenetics revolution.* London, England: Icon Books, p. 258.

18. Bredy, T. W., Wu, H., Crego, C., Zellhoefer, J., Sun, Y. E., & Barad, M. (2007). Histone modifications around individual BDNF gene promoters in prefrontal cortex are associated with extinction of conditioned fear. *Learning and Memory, 14,* 268–276.

19a. Carey, 2011.

19b. Guan et al., 2009.

20. Alarcón et al., 2004.

21. Dulac, 2010.

22. Guan et al., 2009.

23. Carey, 2011.

24. Gräff et al., 2012, p. 222.

25. Cruz, J. C., Tseng, H.-C., Goldman, J. A., Shih, H., & Tsai, L.-H. (2003). Aberrant Cdk5 activation by p25 triggers pathological events leading to neurodegeneration and neurofibrillary tangles. *Neuron, 40,* 471–483.

26. Fischer, A., Sananbenesi, F., Wang, X., Dobbin, M., & Tsai, L.-H. (2007). Recovery of learning and memory is associated with chromatin remodeling. *Nature, 447,* 178–182.

27a. See, for example, Branchi, I., D'Andrea, I., Fiore, M., Di Fausto, V., Aloe, L., & Alleva, E. (2006). Early social enrichment shapes social behavior and nerve growth factor and brain-derived neurotrophic factor levels in the adult mouse brain. *Biological Psychiatry, 60,* 690–696.

27b. Branchi, I., Karpova, N. N., D'Andrea, I., Castrén, E., & Alleva, E. (2011). Epigenetic modifications induced by early enrichment are associated with changes in timing of induction of BDNF expression. *Neuroscience Letters, 495,* 168–172.

28. Fischer et al., 2007.

29. These findings were not limited to memories formed during contextual fear conditioning; similar results were obtained when the memory test used was a spatial learning task (Fischer et al., 2007).

30. Fischer et al., 2007, p. 180, emphasis added.

31. Fischer et al., 2007, p. 178.

32. Fischer et al., 2007.

33. Sweatt, J. D. (2009). Experience-dependent epigenetic modifications in the central nervous system. *Biological Psychiatry, 65*, p. 195.

34. Here, too, the effects Fischer and colleagues (2007) reported were not limited to memories formed during contextual fear conditioning; long-term *spatial* memories were also recovered after treatment with HDAC inhibitors, much as they were after exposure to an enriched environment.

35. Fischer et al., 2007, p. 182.

36. Fischer et al., 2007, p. 182.

37. Gräff et al., 2012.

38. Gräff et al., 2012.

39. Gräff et al., 2012, p. 222.

40. Gräff et al., 2012.

41. Gräff et al., 2012, p. 226.

42. This is typical of complex systems; there are always more ways to influence the functioning of a system with 100 working parts than there are to influence the functioning of a system with only a few working parts.

43. Friedman, R. A. (2002, August 27). Like drugs, talk therapy can change brain chemistry. *New York Times.*

44. Kandel, E. R. (2013, September 5). The new science of mind. *New York Times.*

45. Wilson, R. S., Mendes de Leon, C. F., Barnes, L. L., Schneider, J. A., Bienias, J. L., Evans, D. A., & Bennett, D. A. (2002). Participation in cognitively stimulating activities and risk of incident Alzheimer disease. *Journal of the American Medical Association, 287*, 742–748.

46a. Geda, Y. E., Roberts, R. O., Knopman, D. S., Christianson, T. J. H., Pankratz, V. S., Ivnik, R. J., . . . Rocca, W. A. (2010). Physical exercise and mild cognitive impairment: A population-based study. *Archives of Neurology, 67*, 80–86.

46b. Larson, E. B., Wang, L., Bowen, J. D., McCormick, W. C., Teri, L., Crane, P., & Kukull, W. (2006). Exercise is associated with reduced risk for incident dementia among persons 65 years of age and older. *Annals of Internal Medicine, 144*, 73–81.

47. Yaffe, K., Barnes, D., Nevitt, M., Lui, L.-Y., & Covinsky, K. (2001). A prospective study of physical activity and cognitive decline in elderly women: Women who walk. *Archives of Internal Medicine, 161*, 1703–1708.

48. The quote in the heading is from Cary, J. (1944). *The horse's mouth.* New York: Harper & Brothers.

49. Day, J. J., & Sweatt, J. D. (2010). DNA methylation and memory formation. *Nature Neuroscience, 13*, p. 1320.

50. Bredy et al., 2007.

51. Bredy et al., 2007, p. 271.

52. Levenson et al., 2004.

53. Bredy et al., 2007, p. 268.

54. Bredy et al., 2007.

55a. Day, J. J., & Sweatt, J. D. (2011). Epigenetic mechanisms in cognition. *Neuron, 70*, 813–829.

55b. Hyman, S. E., Malenka, R. C., & Nestler, E. J. (2006). Neural mechanisms of addiction: The role of reward-related learning and memory. *Annual Review of Neuroscience, 29*, 565–598.

56. Zovkic, I. B., & Sweatt, J. D. (2012). Epigenetic mechanisms in learned fear: Implications for PTSD. *Neuropsychopharmacology Reviews*. Advance online publication. doi:10.1038/npp.2012.79

57. Campbell, I. C., Mill, J., Uher, R., & Schmidt, U. (2011). Eating disorders, gene–environment interactions and epigenetics. *Neuroscience and Biobehavioral Reviews*, 35, 784–793.

58a. Mill, J., & Petronis, A. (2007). Molecular studies of major depressive disorder: The epigenetic perspective. *Molecular Psychiatry*, 12, 799–814.

58b. Poulter, M. O., Du, L., Weaver, I. C. G., Palkovits, M., Faludi, G., Merali, Z., . . . Anisman, H. (2008). GABAA receptor promoter hypermethylation in suicide brain: Implications for the involvement of epigenetic processes. *Biological Psychiatry*, 64, 645–652.

59a. Dempster, E. L., Pidsley, R., Schalkwyk, L. C., Owens, S., Georgiades, A., Kane, F., . . . Mill, J. (2011). Disease-associated epigenetic changes in monozygotic twins discordant for schizophrenia and bipolar disorder. *Human Molecular Genetics*, 20, 4786–4796.

59b. Labrie, V., Pai, S., & Petronis, A. (2012). Epigenetics of major psychosis: Progress, problems and perspectives. *Trends in Genetics*, 28, 427–435.

15. Nutrition

1. Jones, A. P., & Friedman, M. I. (1982). Obesity and adipocyte abnormalities in offspring of rats undernourished during pregnancy. *Science*, 215, 1518–1519.

2. Carey, N. (2011). *The epigenetics revolution*. London, England: Icon Books.

3a. Hoek, H. W., Brown, A. S., & Susser, E. (1998). The Dutch Famine and schizophrenia spectrum disorders. *Social Psychiatry and Psychiatric Epidemiology*, 33, 373–379.

3b. Susser, E. S., & Lin, S. P. (1992). Schizophrenia after prenatal exposure to the Dutch Hunger Winter of 1944–1945. *Archives of General Psychiatry*, 49, 983–988.

4. Ravelli, G. P., Stein, Z. A., & Susser, M. W. (1976). Obesity in young men after famine exposure *in utero* and early pregnancy. *New England Journal of Medicine*, 295, 349–353.

5. Jones, A. P., & Dayries, M. (1990). Maternal hormone manipulations and the development of obesity in rats. *Physiology and Behavior*, 47, 1107–1110.

6a. Barker, D. J. P. (1992). The fetal origins of diseases of old age. *European Journal of Clinical Nutrition*, 46, S3–S9.

6b. Barker, D. J. P. (2004). The developmental origins of adult disease. *Journal of the American College of Nutrition*, 23, 588S–595S.

7. For a more thorough history of the emergence of this field, see Gluckman, P. D., Hanson, M. A., & Bukljas, T. (2010). A conceptual framework for the developmental origins of health and disease. *Journal of Developmental Origins of Health and Disease*, 1, 6–18.

8. Barker, 2004, p. 588S.

9. Barker, 2004, p. 589S.

10. Ravelli et al., 1976.

11a. Davenport, M. H., & Cabrero, M. R. (2009). Maternal nutritional history predicts obesity in adult offspring independent of postnatal diet. *Journal of Physiology*, 587, 3423–3424.

11b. Howie, G. J., Sloboda, D. M., Kamal, T., & Vickers, M. H. (2009). Maternal nutritional history predicts obesity in adult offspring independent of postnatal diet. *Journal of Physiology*, 587, 905–915.

12a. Barker, 2004.

12b. Junien, C. (2006). Impact of diets and nutrients/drugs on early epigenetic programming. *Journal of Inherited Metabolic Disease*, 29, 359–365.

13a. Hanson, M. A., Low, F. M., & Gluckman, P. D. (2011). Epigenetic epidemiology: The rebirth of soft inheritance. *Annals of Nutrition and Metabolism*, 58 (suppl 2), 8–15.

13b. Lillycrop, K. A., & Burdge, G. C. (2011). The effect of nutrition during early life on the epigenetic regulation of transcription and implications for human diseases. *Journal of Nutrigenetics and Nutrigenomics, 4*, 248–260.

14. Hanson et al., 2011, p. 10.

15a. Barker, D. J. P., & Clark, P. M. (1997). Fetal undernutrition and disease in later life. *Reviews of Reproduction, 2*, 105–112.

15b. Junien, 2006.

15c. Kuzawa, C. W., & Sweet, E. (2009). Epigenetics and the embodiment of race: Developmental origins of US racial disparities in cardiovascular health. *American Journal of Human Biology, 21*, 2–15.

16. Hanson et al., 2011, p. 9.

17. Gluckman et al., 2010, p. 6.

18. Gluckman et al., 2010, p. 12; see also Lillycrop & Burdge, 2011.

19. Zeisel, S. H. (2009). Importance of methyl donors during reproduction. *American Journal of Clinical Nutrition, 89*, 673S–677S.

20. Singh, S. M., Murphy, B., & O'Reilly, R. L. (2003). Involvement of gene–diet/drug interaction in DNA methylation and its contribution to complex diseases: From cancer to schizophrenia. *Clinical Genetics, 64*, 451–460.

21. Zeisel, 2009.

22. Zeisel, 2009.

23. Cropley, J. E., Suter, C. M., Beckman, K. B., & Martin, D. I. I. (2006). Germ-line epigenetic modification of the murine Avy allele by nutritional supplementation. *Proceedings of the National Academy of Sciences of the USA, 103*, 17308–17312.

24. Lillycrop, K. A., Phillips, E. S., Jackson, A. A., Hanson, M. A., & Burdge, G. C. (2005). Dietary protein restriction of pregnant rats induces and folic acid supplementation prevents epigenetic modification of hepatic gene expression in the offspring. *Journal of Nutrition, 135*, 1382–1386.

25. Sinclair, K. D., Allegrucci, C., Singh, R., Gardner, D. S., Sebastian, S., Bispham, J., . . . Young, L. E. (2007). DNA methylation, insulin resistance, and blood pressure in offspring determined by maternal periconceptional B vitamin and methionine status. *Proceedings of the National Academy of Sciences USA, 104*, 19351–19356.

26. Sinclair et al., 2007.

27. Sinclair et al., 2007, p. 19354.

28. See page 13 in Gluckman et al., 2010.

29. Zeisel, 2009.

30. Meck, W. H., & Williams, C. L. (1999). Choline supplementation during prenatal development reduces proactive interference in spatial memory. *Developmental Brain Research, 118*, 51–59.

31. Albright, C. D., Tsai, A. Y., Friedrich, C. B., Mar, M.-H., & Zeisel, S. H. (1999). Choline availability alters embryonic development of the hippocampus and septum in the rat. *Developmental Brain Research, 113*, 13–20.

32. Craciunescu, C. N., Albright, C. D., Mar, M.-H., Song, J., & Zeisel, S. H. (2003). Choline availability during embryonic development alters progenitor cell mitosis in developing mouse hippocampus. *Journal of Nutrition, 133*, 3614–3618.

33. McGowan, P. O., Meaney, M. J., & Szyf, M. (2008). Diet and the epigenetic (re)programming of phenotypic differences in behavior. *Brain Research, 1237*, 12–24.

34. It should be noted that some researchers who have investigated the hypothesis that prenatal choline affects infant memory have found the topic to be very complicated; for example, see Cheatham, C. L., Goldman, B. D., Fischer, L. M., do Costa, K-A., Reznick, J. S., & Zeisel, S. H. (2012). Phosphatidylcholine supplementation in pregnant women consuming moderate-choline diets does not enhance infant cognitive function: A randomized, double-blind, placebo-controlled trial. *American Journal of Clinical Nutrition, 96*, 1465–1472.

35. Heijmans, B. T., Tobi, E. W., Stein, A. D., Putter, H., Blauw, G. J., Susser, E. S., . . . Lumey, L. H. (2008). Persistent epigenetic differences associated with prenatal exposure to famine in humans. *Proceedings of the National Academy of Sciences USA, 105,* 17046–17049.

36. Heijmans et al., 2008, p. 17047–17048.

37. Tobi, E. W., Lumey, L. H., Talens, R. P., Kremer, D., Putter, H., Stein, A. D., . . . Heijmans, B. T. (2009). DNA methylation differences after exposure to prenatal famine are common and timing- and sex-specific. *Human Molecular Genetics, 18,* 4046–4053.

38. Junien, C., & Nathanielsz, P. (2007). Report on the IASO Stock Conference 2006: Early and lifelong environmental epigenomic programming of metabolic syndrome, obesity and type II diabetes. *Obesity Reviews, 8,* p. 487.

39. Lumey, L. H., Stein, A. D., & Susser, E. (2011). Prenatal famine and adult health. *Annual Review of Public Health, 32,* 237–262.

40. Szyf, M., & Bick, J. (2013). DNA methylation: A mechanism for embedding early life experiences in the genome. *Child Development, 84,* 49–57.

41. Heijmans, B. T., Tobi, E. W., Lumey, L. H., & Slagboom, P. E. (2009). The epigenome: Archive of the prenatal environment. *Epigenetics, 4,* 526–531.

42. Landecker, H. (2011). Food as exposure: Nutritional epigenetics and the new metabolism. *BioSocieties, 6,* 167–194.

43. Choi, S.-W., & Friso, S. (2010). Epigenetics: A new bridge between nutrition and health. *Advances in Nutrition, 1,* 8–16.

44. McGowan et al., 2008.

45. Kaminen-Ahola, N., Ahola, A., Maga, M., Mallitt, K.-A., Fahey, P., Cox, T. C., . . . Chong, S. (2010). Maternal ethanol consumption alters the epigenotype and the phenotype of offspring in a mouse model. *PLoS Genetics, 6*(1), e1000811. doi:10.1371/journal.pgen.1000811

46. Gallou-Kabani, C., Vigé, A., Gross, M.-S., & Junien, C. (2007). Nutri-epigenomics: Lifelong remodelling of our epigenomes by nutritional and metabolic factors and beyond. *Clinical Chemistry and Laboratory Medicine, 45,* 321–327.

47. Anderson, O. S., Sant, K. E., & Dolinoy, D. C. (2012). Nutrition and epigenetics: An interplay of dietary methyl donors, one-carbon metabolism and DNA methylation. *Journal of Nutritional Biochemistry, 23,* 853–859.

48. Another line of research has examined the effects of hormone treatments. For example, studies of prenatal undernutrition in rats have discovered that the obesity in adulthood that results from this kind of experience can be eliminated with a hormone treatment administered shortly after the rats are born (Vickers et al., 2005). By injecting undernourished infant rats with the hormone leptin once a day for 10 days beginning when they were 3 days old, researchers produced rats that ate less as they grew up and ultimately avoided the obesity that would otherwise have developed (but see also Granado, Fuente-Martín, García-Cáceres, Argente, & Chowen, 2012). Subsequent studies of the epigenetics underlying this effect (Gluckman et al., 2007) revealed that the neonatal leptin treatment normalized "both the [gene] expression and methylation changes" associated with prenatal undernutrition (Gluckman et al., 2010, p. 12). Thus, in this case, an effect that had "generally been considered . . . irreversible" (Vickers et al., 2005, p. 4211) has now been found to be open to treatment, particularly if that treatment is administered early in development.

49. Choi & Friso, 2010.

50. Dashwood, R. H., & Ho, E. (2007). Dietary histone deacetylase inhibitors: From cells to mice to man. *Seminars in Cancer Biology, 17,* 363–369.

51. Dashwood & Ho, 2007.

52. McGowan et al., 2008, p. 18.

53. Carey, 2011, p. 310.

54. McGowan et al., 2008.

55a. Papakostas, G. I., Alpert, J. E., & Fava, M. (2003). S-adenosyl-methionine in depression: A comprehensive review of the literature. *Current Psychiatry Reports, 5,* 460–466.

55b. Papakostas, G. I., Mischoulon, D., Shyu, I., Alpert, J. E., & Fava, M. (2010). S-adenosyl-methionine (SAMe) augmentation of serotonin reuptake inhibitors for antidepressant nonresponders with major depressive disorder: A double-blind, randomized clinical trial. *American Journal of Psychiatry, 167,* 942–948.

56. Najm, W. I., Reinsch, S., Hoehler, F., Tobis, J. S., & Harvey, P. W. (2004). S-adenosyl methionine (SAMe) versus celecoxib for the treatment of osteoarthritis symptoms: A double-blind cross-over trial. *BMC Musculoskeletal Disorders, 5,* 6–20.

57. McGowan et al., 2008, p. 13.

58. Anderson et al., 2012.

59a. Anderson, L. M., Riffle, L., Wilson, R., Travlos, G. S., Lubomirski, M. S., & Alvord, W. G. (2006). Preconceptional fasting of fathers alters serum glucose in offspring of mice. *Nutrition, 22,* 327–331.

59b. Chen, T. H.-H., Chiu, Y.-H., & Boucher, B. J. (2006). Transgenerational effects of betel-quid chewing on the development of the metabolic syndrome in the Keelung Community-based Integrated Screening Program. *American Journal of Clinical Nutrition, 83,* 688–692.

59c. Kaati, G., Bygren, L. O., & Edvinsson, S. (2002). Cardiovascular and diabetes mortality determined by nutrition during parents' and grandparents' slow growth period. *European Journal of Human Genetics, 10,* 682–688.

59d. Ng, S.-F., Lin, R. C. Y., Laybutt, D. R., Barres, R., Owens, J. A., & Morris, M. J. (2010). Chronic high-fat diet in fathers programs β-cell dysfunction in female rat offspring. *Nature, 467,* 963–966.

16. Zooming In On Nutrition

1. Moore, D. S. (2013c). Current thinking about nature and nurture. In K. Kampourakis (Ed.), *The philosophy of biology: A companion for educators* (pp. 629–652). New York: Springer.

2. Clayman, C. B. (Ed.). (1989). *American Medical Association Encyclopedia of Medicine.* New York: Random House.

3. Moore, D. S. (2002). *The dependent gene: The fallacy of nature vs. nurture.* New York: W.H. Freeman.

4. Petris, M. J., Strausak, D., & Mercer, J. F. B. (2000). The Menkes copper transporter is required for the activation of tyrosinase. *Human Molecular Genetics, 9,* 2845–2851.

5. McKenzie, C. A., Wakamatsu, K., Hanchard, N. A., Forrester, T., & Ito, S. (2007). Childhood malnutrition is associated with a reduction in the total melanin content of scalp hair. *British Journal of Nutrition, 98,* 159–164.

6. McKenzie et al., 2007.

7. Cole, M., & Cole, S. R. (1993). *The development of children* (2nd ed.). New York: Freeman.

8. Duhl, D. M. J., Vrieling, H., Miller, K. A., Wolff, G. L., & Barsh, G. S. (1994). Neomorphic *agouti* mutations in obese yellow mice. *Nature Genetics, 8,* 59–65.

9a. Cropley, J. E., Suter, C. M., Beckman, K. B., & Martin, D. I. I. (2006). Germ-line epigenetic modification of the murine Avy allele by nutritional supplementation. *Proceedings of the National Academy of Sciences of the USA, 103,* 17308–17312.

9b. Cropley, J. E., Dang, T. H. Y., Martin, D. I. K., & Suter, C. M. (2012). The penetrance of an epigenetic trait in mice is progressively yet reversibly increased by selection and environment. *Proceedings of the Royal Society B, 279,* 2347–2353.

9c. Martin, D. I. K., Cropley, J. E., & Suter, C. M. (2008). Environmental influence on epigenetic inheritance at the Avy allele. *Nutrition Reviews, 66,* S12–S14.

10a. Heijmans, B. T., Tobi, E. W., Stein, A. D., Putter, H., Blauw, G. J., Susser, E. S., . . . Lumey, L. H. (2008). Persistent epigenetic differences associated with prenatal exposure to famine in humans. *Proceedings of the National Academy of Sciences USA, 105,* 17046–17049.

10b. Heijmans, B. T., Tobi, E. W., Lumey, L. H., & Slagboom, P. E. (2009). The epigenome: Archive of the prenatal environment. *Epigenetics, 4,* 526–531.

10c. Junien, C., & Nathanielsz, P. (2007). Report on the IASO Stock Conference 2006: Early and lifelong environmental epigenomic programming of metabolic syndrome, obesity and type II diabetes. *Obesity Reviews, 8,* 487–502.

10d. Tobi, E. W., Lumey, L. H., Talens, R. P., Kremer, D., Putter, H., Stein, A. D., . . . Heijmans, B. T. (2009). DNA methylation differences after exposure to prenatal famine are common and timing- and sex-specific. *Human Molecular Genetics, 18,* 4046–4053.

11. Carey, N. (2011). *The epigenetics revolution.* London, England: Icon Books.

12a. Morgan, H. D., Sutherland, H. G. E., Martin, D. I. K., & Whitelaw, E. (1999). Epigenetic inheritance at the agouti locus in the mouse. *Nature Genetics, 23,* 314–318.

12b. Waterland, R. A., & Jirtle, R. L. (2003). Transposable elements: Targets for early nutritional effects on epigenetic gene regulation. *Molecular and Cellular Biology, 23,* 5293–5300.

13. Morgan et al., 1999.

14. It is worth noting that Mendel's conception of genes is strikingly different in several respects from the classical molecular gene concept I have used in this book (Griffiths & Neumann-Held, 1999). In fact, the genes Mendel envisioned have not been found to exist in DNA. As Neumann-Held has written, "there is no fundamental way by which the classical . . . gene concept could be applied to DNA segments" (1998, p. 125). Thus, molecular genes in our DNA do not correspond with the merely theoretical "genes" identified by Mendelian geneticists (Moore, 2013b).

15. The agouti gene is present in most mammals (Francis, 2011), although it has been difficult to find in human beings (Carey, 2011). In addition to contributing to the agouti color of wild mice, the action of this gene contributes to the color of horses described as "bay" and of dogs described as "sable."

16. The word "viable" in its name reflects the fact that yet another allele found at this spot in the genome also produces offspring with yellow coats, but the mutation associated with this allele is lethal—the offspring are yellow, but not "viable."

17. Duhl et al., 1994.

18. Rakyan, V. K., & Beck, S. (2006). Epigenetic variation and inheritance in mammals. *Current Opinion in Genetics and Development, 16,* 573–577.

19. Waterland & Jirtle, 2003.

20. Such mice can be considered genetically identical because they have been produced by letting siblings mate for 30 generations (Morgan et al., 1999).

21. Morgan et al., 1999.

22. Carey, 2011.

23. The mottled mice are actually mosaics like the calico cats discussed in chapter 7, "Zooming in on Regulation"; they have highly methylated retrotransposons in some cells and relatively unmethylated retrotransposons in other cells, giving rise to browner regions of fur amid yellower regions of fur.

24. Rakyan & Beck, 2006.

25. Daxinger, L., & Whitelaw, E. (2012). Understanding transgenerational epigenetic inheritance via the gametes in mammals. *Nature Reviews: Genetics, 13,* 153–162.

26. Richards, E. J. (2006). Inherited epigenetic variation—Revisiting soft inheritance. *Nature Reviews: Genetics, 7,* 395–401.

27. In fact, some amount of the epigenetic effects discussed earlier in this book can probably be attributed to random processes. For example, the epigenomes of identical twins can be expected to diverge with age simply as a function of this kind of randomness. As a result, any epigenetic effects of experience must be shown to exist above and beyond random epigenetic effects; this is why it was important for the researchers at the Spanish National Cancer Centre (Fraga et al., 2005)—those researchers who studied epigenetic changes across the life spans of identical twins—to show *more* divergence in identical twins who spent most of their lives apart than there was in identical twins who spent most of their lives together.

28. Waterland & Jirtle, 2003.

29. Waterland & Jirtle, 2003.
30. Waterland & Jirtle, 2003, p. 5297.
31. Waterland & Jirtle, 2003.
32. Together with related DNA segments called transposons, retrotransposons make up more than 35% of our genome (Waterland & Jirtle, 2003).
33. Kaminen-Ahola, N., Ahola, A., Maga, M., Mallitt, K.-A., Fahey, P., Cox, T. C., . . . Chong, S. (2010). Maternal ethanol consumption alters the epigenotype and the phenotype of off-spring in a mouse model. *PLoS Genetics, 6*(1), e1000811. doi:10.1371/journal.pgen.1000811
34. McGowan, P. O., Meaney, M. J., & Szyf, M. (2008). Diet and the epigenetic (re)program-ming of phenotypic differences in behavior. *Brain Research, 1237,* 12–24.
35. Kaminen-Ahola et al., 2010, p. e1000811.
36. Calafat, A. M., Kuklenyik, Z., Reidy, J. A., Caudill, S. P., Ekong, J., & Needham, L. L. (2005). Urinary concentrations of bisphenol A and 4-nonylphenol in a human reference population. *Environmental Health Perspectives, 113,* 391–395.
37. Dolinoy, D. C., Huang, D., & Jirtle, R. L. (2007). Maternal nutrient supplementation coun-teracts bisphenol A-induced DNA hypomethylation in early development. *Proceedings of the National Academy of Sciences of the USA, 104,* p. 13056.
38. Dolinoy et al., 2007.
39. Bernal, A. J., & Jirtle, R. L. (2010). Epigenomic disruption: The effects of early develop-mental exposures. *Birth Defects Research (Part A), 88,* p. 942.
40. Waterland & Jirtle, 2003.
41a. Cropley et al., 2006.
41b. Cropley et al., 2012.
41c. Martin et al., 2008.
42a. Anderson, L. M., Riffle, L., Wilson, R., Travlos, G. S., Lubomirski, M. S., & Alvord, W. G. (2006). Preconceptional fasting of fathers alters serum glucose in offspring of mice. *Nutrition, 22,* 327–331.
42b. Chen, T. H.-H., Chiu, Y.-H., & Boucher, B. J. (2006). Transgenerational effects of betel-quid chewing on the development of the metabolic syndrome in the Keelung Community-based Integrated Screening Program. *American Journal of Clinical Nutrition, 83,* 688–692.
42c. Kaati, G., Bygren, L. O., & Edvinsson, S. (2002). Cardiovascular and diabetes mortality determined by nutrition during parents' and grandparents' slow growth period. *European Journal of Human Genetics, 10,* 682–688.
42d. Ng, S.-F., Lin, R. C. Y., Laybutt, D. R., Barres, R., Owens, J. A., & Morris, M. J. (2010). Chronic high-fat diet in fathers programs β-cell dysfunction in female rat offspring. *Nature, 467,* 963–966.
43a. See, for example, this and the next four references: Danchin, É., Charmantier, A., Champagne, F. A., Mesoudi, A., Pujol, B., & Blanchet, S. (2011). Beyond DNA: Integrating inclusive inheritance into an extended theory of evolution. *Nature Reviews: Genetics, 12,* 475–486.
43b. Jablonka, E., & Lamb, M. J. (2005). *Evolution in four dimensions: Genetic, epigenetic, behavioral, and symbolic variation in the history of life.* Cambridge, MA: MIT Press.
43c. Jablonka, E., & Lamb, M. J. (2007). Précis of evolution in four dimensions. *Behavioral and Brain Sciences, 30,* 353–392.
43d. Moore, D. S. (2008b). Individuals and populations: How biology's theory and data have interfered with the integration of development and evolution. *New Ideas in Psychology, 26,* 370–386.
43e. Varmuza, S. (2003). Epigenetics and the renaissance of heresy. *Genome, 46,* 963–967.

17. Inheritance

1. Mayr, E. (1980). Prologue: Some thoughts on the history of the evolutionary synthesis. In E. Mayr & W. B. Provine (Eds.), *The evolutionary synthesis: Perspectives on the unification of biology* (pp. 1–48). Cambridge, MA: Harvard University Press.

2a. Maderspacher, F. (2010). Lysenko rising. *Current Biology, 20,* R835–R837.

2b. Madhani, H. D., Francis, N. J., Kingston, R. E., Kornberg, R. D., Moazed, D., Narlikar, G. J., . . . Struhl, K. (2008). Epigenomics: A roadmap, but to where? *Science, 322,* 43–44.

2c. Miller, G. (2010). The seductive allure of behavioral epigenetics. *Science, 329,* 24–27.

2d. Ptashne, M. (2010). Questions over the scientific basis of epigenome project. *Nature, 464,* 487.

3. Johannsen, W. (1911). The genotype conception of heredity. *American Naturalist, 45,* 129–159.

4. Johannsen, 1911, p. 129.

5. Johannsen, 1911, p. 129.

6. Johannsen, 1911, p. 130.

7. Gould, S. J. (1980). *The panda's thumb: More reflections in natural history.* New York: Norton.

8. Barker, G. (1993). Models of biological change: Implications of three studies of "Lamarckian" change. In P. P. G. Bateson, P. H. Klopfer, & N. S. Thompson (Eds.), *Perspectives in ethology (Vol. 10): Behavior and evolution.* New York: Plenum Press.

9. Weismann, A. (1889). *Essays upon heredity and kindred biological problems.* London: Frowde.

10. Weismann, 1889.

11. Robert, J. S. (2002). How developmental is evolutionary developmental biology? *Biology and Philosophy, 17,* 591–611.

12. Weismann, 1889, p. 422.

13. Wei, G., & Mahowald, A. P. (1994). The germline: Familiar and newly uncovered properties. *Annual Review of Genetics, 28,* 309–324.

14. Richards, E. J. (2006). Inherited epigenetic variation—Revisiting soft inheritance. *Nature Reviews: Genetics, 7,* 395–401.

15. Pigliucci, M. (2010). Genotype–phenotype mapping and the end of the "genes as blueprint" metaphor. *Philosophical Transactions of the Royal Society B, 365,* 557–566.

16a. Danchin, É., Charmantier, A., Champagne, F. A., Mesoudi, A., Pujol, B., & Blanchet, S. (2011). Beyond DNA: Integrating inclusive inheritance into an extended theory of evolution. *Nature Reviews: Genetics, 12,* 475–486.

16b. Lickliter, R. (2009). The fallacy of partitioning: Epigenetics' validation of the organism-environment system. *Ecological Psychology, 21,* 138–146.

16c. Lickliter, R., & Honeycutt, H. (2013). A developmental evolutionary framework for psychology. *Review of General Psychology, 17,* 184–189.

17a. Coyne, J. A. (2009). Evolution's challenge to genetics. *Nature, 457,* 382–383.

17b. Mayr, E. (2001). *What evolution is.* New York: Basic Books.

18. Ellegren, H., & Sheldon, B. C. (2008). Genetic basis of fitness differences in natural populations. *Nature, 452,* 169–175.

19. I am using the word "inheritable" here (and subsequently) to mean "able to be inherited." In contrast, the word "heritable" is a technical word that refers to a statistic that measures the extent to which genetic variation in a population is related to phenotypic variation in that population. This statistic was developed in the 19th century in an effort to measure the extent to which a phenotype can be inherited, hence its name. However, because it does not actually measure what it was intended to measure, its name is confusing; this is why I prefer to use the word "inheritable" when discussing the ability of phenotypes to be reliably transmitted across generations. Other writers sometimes use these words interchangeably, so the word "heritable" will appear in some of the quotations found in this book. For more information on the distinction between "heritability" and "inheritability"—and the shortcomings of the former concept—see any of the following three publications: Moore, D. S. (2002). *The dependent gene: The fallacy of nature vs. nurture.* New York: W.H. Freeman; Moore, D. S. (2006). A very little bit of knowledge: Re-evaluating the meaning of the heritability of IQ. *Human Development, 49,* 347–353; or Moore, D. S. (2013c). Current thinking about nature and nurture. In K. Kampourakis (Ed.), *The philosophy of biology: A companion for educators* (pp. 629–652). New York: Springer.

20a. Anway, M. D., Cupp, A. S., Uzumcu, M., & Skinner, M. K. (2005). Epigenetic transgenerational actions of endocrine disruptors and male fertility. *Science, 308,* 1466–1469.

20b. Franklin, T. B., Russig, H., Weiss, I. C., Graff, J., Linder, N., Michalon, A., . . . Mansuy, I. M. (2010). Epigenetic transmission of the impact of early stress across generations. *Biological Psychiatry, 68,* 408–415.

20c. Rakyan, V. K., Chong, S., Champ, M. E., Cuthbert, P. C., Morgan, H. D., Luu, K. V. K., & Whitelaw, E. (2003). Transgenerational inheritance of epigenetic states at the murine *AxinFu* allele occurs after maternal and paternal transmission. *Proceedings of the National Academy of Sciences USA, 100,* 2538–2543.

21a. Bateson, P., & Gluckman, P. (2011). *Plasticity, robustness, development and evolution.* Cambridge, England: Cambridge University Press.

21b. Blumberg, M. S. (2005). *Basic instinct: The genesis of behavior.* New York: Thunder's Mouth Press.

21c. Gottlieb, G. (2007). Probabilistic epigenesis. *Developmental Science, 10,* 1–11.

21d. Jablonka, E., & Lamb, M. J. (2005). *Evolution in four dimensions: Genetic, epigenetic, behavioral, and symbolic variation in the history of life.* Cambridge, MA: The MIT Press.

21e. Lewkowicz, D. J. (2011). The biological implausibility of the nature–nurture dichotomy and what it means for the study of infancy. *Infancy, 16,* 331–367.

21f. Lewontin, R. C. (2000). *The triple helix: Gene, organism, and environment.* Cambridge, MA: Harvard University Press.

21g. Lickliter, R. (2008). The growth of developmental thought: Implications for a new evolutionary psychology. *New Ideas in Psychology, 26,* 353–369.

21h. Lickliter, 2009.

21i. Meaney, M. J. (2010). Epigenetics and the biological definition of gene × environment interactions. *Child Development, 81,* 41–79.

21j. Moore, 2002.

21k. Noble, D. (2006). *The music of life: Biology beyond genes.* New York: Oxford University Press.

21l. Oyama, S. (1985/2000). *The ontogeny of information.* Durham, NC: Duke University Press.

21m. Robert, J. S. (2004). *Embryology, epigenesis, and evolution: Taking development seriously.* New York: Cambridge University Press.

21n. Spencer, J. P., Blumberg, M. S., McMurray, B., Robinson, S. R., Samuelson, L. K., & Tomblin, J. B. (2009). Short arms and talking eggs: Why we should no longer abide the nativist–empiricist debate. *Child Development Perspectives, 3,* 79–87.

22. Gilbert, S. F. (2005). Mechanisms for the environmental regulation of gene expression: Ecological aspects of animal development. *Journal of Biosciences, 30,* p. 65.

23. Development also sometimes unfolds in *extremely* specific environments, and it is sometimes in these environments alone that offspring can develop characteristics like their parents. Consider just one illustrative example of how extremely specific some organisms' normal developmental contexts are: There is a kind of fly that develops only in the mouth of a specific kind of land crab that is found only on a particular Caribbean island! For more information, see Stensmyr, M. C., Stieber, R., & Hansson, B. S. (2008). The Cayman crab fly revisited—Phylogeny and biology of *Drosophila endobranchia. PLoS ONE, 3*(4), e1942. doi:10.1371/journal.pone.0001942

24. Gottlieb, 2007.

25. Laland, K. N., Odling-Smee, J., & Myles, S. (2010). How culture shaped the human genome: Bringing genetics and the human sciences together. *Nature Reviews: Genetics, 11,* 137–148.

26. Xu, J., & Gordon, J. I. (2003). Honor thy symbionts. *Proceedings of the National Academy of Sciences USA, 100,* 10452–10459.

27. Evelyn Fox Keller has done theorists a service by disambiguating several different meanings of "DST" that have appeared in the literatures of developmental psychology, philosophy of biology, and developmental psychobiology. Using her nomenclature, the sense of DST I have in mind here is DST-1, which "emphasizes the multiplicity of resources employed in

heredity, development, and evolution." See Keller, E. F. (2005). DDS: Dynamics of developmental systems. *Biology and Philosophy, 20*, p. 412.

28. Of course, in writing her 1985 book, Oyama drew on significant theoretical work completed in earlier decades (e.g., by Zing-Yang Kuo, Gilbert Gottlieb, T. C. Schneirla, Patrick Bateson, and others). Likewise, between the publication of Oyama's book and Griffiths and Gray's article, theoretical work continued in this area, for instance by Donald Ford and Richard Lerner (1992).

29. Griffiths, P. E., & Gray, R. D. (1994). Developmental systems and evolutionary explanation. *Journal of Philosophy, 91*, p. 283.

30. Lickliter, R., & Honeycutt, H. (2003). Developmental dynamics: Toward a biologically plausible evolutionary psychology. *Psychological Bulletin, 129*, 819–835.

31. Griffiths & Gray, 1994.

32. Oyama, S., Griffiths, P. E., & Gray, R. D. (2001). *Cycles of contingency: Developmental systems and evolution.* Cambridge, MA: MIT Press.

33a. Itard, J. G. (1962). *The wild boy of Aveyron.* Norwalk, CT: Appleton & Lange.

33b. Curtiss, S. (1977). *Genie: A psycholinguistic study of a modern-day "wild child."* Boston, MA: Academic Press.

34. Mayr, 1980, p. 4.

35. See notes 21a through 21n, above.

36a. Hanson, M. A., Low, F. M., & Gluckman, P. D. (2011). Epigenetic epidemiology: The rebirth of soft inheritance. *Annals of Nutrition and Metabolism, 58* (suppl 2), 8–15.

36b. Petronis, A. (2010). Epigenetics as a unifying principle in the aetiology of complex traits and diseases. *Nature, 465*, 721–727.

36c. Richards, 2006.

37. Richards, 2006.

38. Hanson et al., 2011, p. 12.

39. Lickliter, R., & Berry, T. D. (1990). The phylogeny fallacy: Developmental psychology's misapplication of evolutionary theory. *Developmental Review, 10*, 348–364.

40. Of course, concluding that acquired characteristics can be inherited does not mean modern Darwinians have overestimated the importance of natural selection; as biologists have recognized for the last 50 years, natural selection is an extremely important evolutionary mechanism. Natural selection is likely to remain important even for the evolution of the quasi-Lamarckian systems we now find in the world; see Haig, D. (2007). Weismann rules! OK? Epigenetics and the Lamarckian temptation. *Biology and Philosophy, 22*, 415–428.

41. One of the primary reasons biologists have objected to the idea that acquired characteristics can be inherited is because this phenomenon suggests that evolution might be directed, rather than influenced strictly by the natural selection of *random* alterations to our traits (Mayr, 1980). Also, some biologists are loathe to see characteristics that depend on environmental factors like culture as being relevant to biological evolution, because these are characteristics that can disappear quickly from populations that develop in novel environments (relative to the environments in which their ancestors developed; Haig, 2007). These remain important questions, of course, but they are beyond the scope of this book. Jablonka and Lamb's (2005) excellent book, *Evolution in four dimensions*, considers these questions in detail.

42a. Anway et al., 2005.

42b. Franklin et al., 2010.

42c. Rakyan et al., 2003.

18. Multiplicity

1. Gilbert, S. F. (2005). Mechanisms for the environmental regulation of gene expression: Ecological aspects of animal development. *Journal of Biosciences, 30*, 65–74.

2. Xu, J., & Gordon, J. I. (2003). Honor thy symbionts. *Proceedings of the National Academy of Sciences USA, 100*, 10452–10459.

3. Turnbaugh, P. J., Ley, R. E., Hamady, M., Fraser-Liggett, C. M., Knight, R., & Gordon, J. I. (2007). The human microbiome project. *Nature, 449*, 804–810.

4. Frank, D. N., & Pace, N. R. (2008). Gastrointestinal microbiology enters the metagenomics era. *Current Opinion in Gastroenterology, 24*, 4–10.

5. Mullard, A. (2008). The inside story. *Nature, 453*, 578–580.

6. Xu & Gordon, 2003.

7. Mullard, 2008, p. 578.

8a. Gilbert, 2005.

8b. Xu & Gordon, 2003.

9a. Gilbert, 2005.

9b. Xu & Gordon, 2003.

10. Gilbert, 2005, p. 69.

11. Jablonka, E., & Lamb, M. J. (2005). *Evolution in four dimensions: Genetic, epigenetic, behavioral, and symbolic variation in the history of life.* Cambridge, MA: MIT Press.

12. Jablonka, E., & Lamb, M. J. (2007). Précis of evolution in four dimensions. *Behavioral and Brain Sciences, 30*, p. 362.

13. Jablonka & Lamb, 2005, p. 161.

14. Jablonka & Lamb, 2007.

15. Hirata, S., Watanabe, K., & Kawai, M. (2001). "Sweet-potato washing" revisited. In T. Matsuzawa (Ed.), *Primate origins of human cognition and behavior* (pp. 487–508). Tokyo: Springer-Verlag.

16. Hirata et al., 2001, p. 502 and p. 507.

17. Avital, E., & Jablonka, E. (2000). *Animal traditions: Behavioural inheritance in evolution.* New Cambridge, England: Cambridge University Press, p. 355.

18. Mennella, J. A., Jagnow, C. P., & Beauchamp, G. K. (2001). Prenatal and postnatal flavor learning by human infants. *Pediatrics, 107*(6), e88.

19a. Jablonka & Lamb, 2005.

19b. Jablonka & Lamb, 2007.

20. Mennella et al., 2001.

21. Hoek, H. W., Brown, A. S., & Susser, E. (1998). The Dutch Famine and schizophrenia spectrum disorders. *Social Psychiatry and Psychiatric Epidemiology, 33*, 373–379.

22. Ravelli, G. P., Stein, Z. A., & Susser, M. W. (1976). Obesity in young men after famine exposure *in utero* and early pregnancy. *New England Journal of Medicine, 295*, 349–353.

23a. DeCasper, A. J., & Fifer, W. P. (1980). Of human bonding: Newborns prefer their mothers' voices. *Science, 208*, 1174–1176.

23b. DeCasper, A. J., & Spence, M. J. (1986). Prenatal maternal speech influences newborns' perception of speech sound. *Infant Behavior and Development, 9*, 133–150.

24. Francis, D., Diorio, J., Liu, D., & Meaney, M. J. (1999b). Nongenomic transmission across generations of maternal behavior and stress responses in the rat. *Science, 286*, 1155–1158.

25. Meaney, M. J. (2010). Epigenetics and the biological definition of gene × environment interactions. *Child Development, 81*, 41–79.

26. Champagne, F. A., Weaver, I. C. G., Diorio, J., Dymov, S., Szyf, M., & Meaney, M. J. (2006). Maternal care associated with methylation of the estrogen receptor-α1b promoter and estrogen receptor-α expression in the medial preoptic area of female offspring. *Endocrinology, 147*, 2909–2915.

27. Danchin, É., Charmantier, A., Champagne, F. A., Mesoudi, A., Pujol, B., & Blanchet, S. (2011). Beyond DNA: Integrating inclusive inheritance into an extended theory of evolution. *Nature Reviews: Genetics, 12*, 475–486.

28. Champagne et al., 2006.

29. Pedersen, C. A. (1997). Oxytocin control of maternal behavior: Regulation by sex steroids and offspring stimuli. *Annals of the New York Academy of Sciences, 807*, 126–145.

30a. Champagne et al., 2006.

30b. Champagne, F. A. (2013). Epigenetics and developmental plasticity across species. *Developmental Psychobiology, 55,* 31–41.

31. Champagne et al., 2006.

32. Daxinger, L., & Whitelaw, E. (2012). Understanding transgenerational epigenetic inheritance via the gametes in mammals. *Nature Reviews: Genetics, 13,* 153–162.

33. Roth, T. L., Lubin, F. D., Funk, A. J., & Sweatt, J. D. (2009). Lasting epigenetic influence of early-life adversity on the BDNF gene. *Biological Psychiatry, 65,* 760–769.

34. Roth et al., 2009.

35. Because cross-fostering the grandpups to normal mothers did not completely eliminate the altered methylation patterns in the grandpups' brains, the epigenetic effect appears to have been influenced both by the postnatal experience of abuse *and* by the prenatal experience of developing as a fetus in an abnormally anxious mother; see Roth et al., 2009.

36. Champagne, F. A. (2008). Epigenetic mechanisms and the transgenerational effects of maternal care. *Frontiers in Neuroendocrinology, 29,* 386–397.

37. The same could be said of some other primate species as well; for data from a study on a transgenerational effect in monkeys, see Maestripieri, D. (2005). Early experience affects the intergenerational transmission of infant abuse in rhesus monkeys. *Proceedings of the National Academy of Sciences USA, 102,* 9726–9729.

38. Champagne, 2008, p. 387.

39. Weaver, I. C. G., Meaney, M. J., & Szyf, M. (2006). Maternal care effects on the hippocampal transcriptome and anxiety-mediated behaviors in the offspring that are reversible in adulthood. *Proceedings of the National Academy of Sciences USA, 103,* 3480–3485.

40a. Fischer, A., Sananbenesi, F., Wang, X., Dobbin, M., & Tsai, L.-H. (2007). Recovery of learning and memory is associated with chromatin remodeling. *Nature, 447,* 178–182.

40b. Peña, C. L. J., & Champagne, F. A. (2012). Epigenetic and neurodevelopmental perspectives on variation in parenting behavior. *Parenting: Science and Practice, 12,* 202–211.

41. Peña & Champagne, 2012, p. 209.

42. Jablonka & Lamb, 2005.

43. Jablonka & Lamb, 2007.

44. In addition to containing DNA and cytoplasm, mammalian eggs contain RNA, proteins, and other cellular structures. The role that inherited RNAs play in very early embryonic development has been drawing increasing attention from researchers lately, and it is now clear that mature mammalian sperm, like mammalian eggs, contain RNA, that this RNA can be detected in newly formed zygotes after fertilization (see Daxinger & Whitelaw, 2012), and that such molecules can have important effects on phenotypic development, effects that can be transmitted across generations; for more information, see Franklin, T. B., & Mansuy, I. M. (2010). Epigenetic inheritance in mammals: Evidence for the impact of adverse environmental effects. *Neurobiology of Disease, 39,* 61–65.

45. Daxinger & Whitelaw, 2012.

46. Roemer, I., Reik, W., Dean, W., & Klose, J. (1997). Epigenetic inheritance in the mouse. *Current Biology, 7,* 277–280.

47. Roemer et al., 1997, p. 277.

48. There were, however, epigenetic marks on your mother's genome that specified *which* grandparent provided *which* chromosomes, and these marks survived this reprogramming process; sparing such marks from "erasure" allows embryos to keep track of which chromosomes came from its male parent and which came from its female parent.

49. The epigenetic reprogramming that occurs in the primordial germ cells removes all epigenetic marks, including those that specify which grandparent the DNA originally came from. This is critical, because when a zygote receives a chromosome that its mother received from her father, it is coming from the zygote's female parent, so it must be stripped of any epigenetic marks designating it as having come originally from a male parent.

50. Roemer et al., 1997.

51. Daxinger & Whitelaw, 2012.

52a. Blewitt, M. E., Vickaryous, N. K., Paldi, A., Koseki, H., & Whitelaw, E. (2006). Dynamic reprogramming of DNA methylation at an epigenetically sensitive allele in mice. *PLoS Genetics 2*(4), e49. doi:10.1371/journal.pgen.0020049

52b. Daxinger & Whitelaw, 2012.

53. Daxinger & Whitelaw, 2012, p. 160.

54. Jablonka & Lamb, 2005, p. 359.

55. Jablonka, E., & Raz, G. (2009). Transgenerational epigenetic inheritance: Prevalence, mechanisms, and implications for the study of heredity and evolution. *Quarterly Review of Biology, 84*, p. 131.

56. Waterland, R. A., & Jirtle, R. L. (2003). Transposable elements: Targets for early nutritional effects on epigenetic gene regulation. *Molecular and Cellular Biology, 23*, 5293–5300.

57a. Morgan, H. D., Sutherland, H. G. E., Martin, D. I. K., & Whitelaw, E. (1999). Epigenetic inheritance at the agouti locus in the mouse. *Nature Genetics, 23*, 314–318.

57b. Rakyan, V. K., Chong, S., Champ, M. E., Cuthbert, P. C., Morgan, H. D., Luu, K. V. K., & Whitelaw, E. (2003). Transgenerational inheritance of epigenetic states at the murine *AxinFu* allele occurs after maternal and paternal transmission. *Proceedings of the National Academy of Sciences USA, 100*, 2538–2543.

58a. Hanson, M. A., Low, F. M., & Gluckman, P. D. (2011). Epigenetic epidemiology: The rebirth of soft inheritance. *Annals of Nutrition and Metabolism, 58*(suppl 2), 8–15.

58b. Richards, E. J. (2006). Inherited epigenetic variation—Revisiting soft inheritance. *Nature Reviews: Genetics, 7*, 395–401.

59. Dawkins, R. (1987). *The blind watchmaker.* New York: Norton, p. 290.

60. Haig, D. (2007). Weismann rules! OK? Epigenetics and the Lamarckian temptation. *Biology and Philosophy, 22*, 415–428.

61a. Haig, 2007.

61b. Jablonka & Lamb, 2007.

62a. Haig, 2007.

62b. Jablonka & Lamb, 2005.

62c. Maderspacher, F. (2010). Lysenko rising. *Current Biology, 20*, R835–R837.

62d. Varmuza, S. (2003). Epigenetics and the renaissance of heresy. *Genome, 46*, 963–967.

19. *Evidence*

1. Spiegelman, A. (1986). *Maus: A survivor's tale.* New York: Pantheon.

2. Waterland, R. A., & Jirtle, R. L. (2003). Transposable elements: Targets for early nutritional effects on epigenetic gene regulation. *Molecular and Cellular Biology, 23*, 5293–5300.

3. Wolff, G. L. (1978). Influence of maternal phenotype on metabolic differentiation of agouti locus mutants in the mouse. *Genetics, 88*, 529–539.

4. Morgan, H. D., Sutherland, H. G. E., Martin, D. I. K., & Whitelaw, E. (1999). Epigenetic inheritance at the agouti locus in the mouse. *Nature Genetics, 23*, 314–318.

5. Wolff, 1978.

6. Morgan et al., 1999.

7. Morgan et al., 1999, p. 316.

8. Morgan et al., 1999.

9. Morgan et al., 1999, p. 316.

10. Rakyan, V. K., Chong, S., Champ, M. E., Cuthbert, P. C., Morgan, H. D., Luu, K. V. K., & Whitelaw, E. (2003). Transgenerational inheritance of epigenetic states at the murine *AxinFu* allele occurs after maternal and paternal transmission. *Proceedings of the National Academy of Sciences USA, 100*, 2538–2543.

11. Rakyan et al., 2003, p. 2538.

12a. Morgan et al., 1999.

12b. Rakyan et al., 2003.

13. For example, Waterland & Jirtle, 2003.

14. Waterland & Jirtle, 2003.

15a. Daxinger, L., & Whitelaw, E. (2012). Understanding transgenerational epigenetic inheritance via the gametes in mammals. *Nature Reviews: Genetics, 13,* 153–162.

15b. Rakyan et al., 2003.

16. Anderson, L. M., Riffle, L., Wilson, R., Travlos, G. S., Lubomirski, M. S., & Alvord, W. G. (2006). Preconceptional fasting of fathers alters serum glucose in offspring of mice. *Nutrition, 22,* 327–331.

17. Ng, S.-F., Lin, R. C. Y., Laybutt, D. R., Barres, R., Owens, J. A., & Morris, M. J. (2010). Chronic high-fat diet in fathers programs β-cell dysfunction in female rat offspring. *Nature, 467,* 963–966.

18. Carone, B. R., Fauquier, L., Habib, N., Shea, J. M., Hart, C. E., Li, R., . . . Rando, O. J. (2010). Paternally induced transgenerational environmental reprogramming of metabolic gene expression in mammals. *Cell, 143,* 1084–1096.

19. Cropley, J. E., Suter, C. M., Beckman, K. B., & Martin, D. I. I. (2006). Germ-line epigenetic modification of the murine Avy allele by nutritional supplementation. *Proceedings of the National Academy of Sciences of the USA, 103,* 17308–17312.

20. Cropley et al., 2006.

21. Cropley et al., 2006, p. 17310.

22. Martin, D. I. K., Cropley, J. E., & Suter, C. M. (2008). Environmental influence on epigenetic inheritance at the Avy allele. *Nutrition Reviews, 66,* p. S13.

23. It is important to consider the results of another study that was designed to explore this phenomenon further: see Waterland, R. A., Travisano, M., & Tahiliani, K. G. (2007). Diet-induced hypermethylation at *agouti viable yellow* is not inherited transgenerationally through the female. *FASEB Journal, 21,* 3380–3385. The results of this study suggested that the brownish fur of the daughters should not be considered an *acquired* characteristic, because even though the daughters' coat-colors reflect their experiences, their mothers had brownish fur as well, and not because they had eaten any sort of a special diet. Thus, rather than understanding the dietary supplementation as having added new epigenetic information, we should perhaps understand the dietary manipulations as having merely *maintained* existing information that might otherwise have been lost in descendant generations. But regardless of whether we should consider this to be a genuine case of the inheritance of an acquired trait, the fact remains that the grandmothers' experiences influenced their daughters' epigenetic states in a way that could be detected in the granddaughters. This sort of effect should be enough to make us rethink the assumption that characteristics can only be transmitted from generation to generation via "hard" inheritance mechanisms (for more information, see Daxinger & Whitelaw, 2010).

24. Franklin, T. B., & Mansuy, I. M. (2010). Epigenetic inheritance in mammals: Evidence for the impact of adverse environmental effects. *Neurobiology of Disease, 39,* p. 64.

25. Benyshek, D. C., Johnston, C. S., & Martin, J. F. (2006). Glucose metabolism is altered in the adequately-nourished grand-offspring (F3 generation) of rats malnourished during gestation and perinatal life. *Dibetologia, 49,* 1117–1119.

26. Dunn, G. A., & Bale, T. L. (2011). Maternal high-fat diet effects on third-generation female body size via the paternal lineage. *Endocrinology, 152,* 2228–2236.

27. Dunn & Bale, 2011, p. 2228.

28. Franklin, T. B., Russig, H., Weiss, I. C., Graff, J., Linder, N., Michalon, A., . . . Mansuy, I. M. (2010). Epigenetic transmission of the impact of early stress across generations. *Biological Psychiatry, 68,* 408–415.

29. Murgatroyd, C., Patchev, A. V., Wu, Y., Micale, V., Bockmühl, Y., Fischer, D., . . . Spengler, D. (2009). Dynamic DNA methylation programs persistent adverse effects of early-life stress. *Nature Neuroscience, 12,* 1559–1566.

30. Franklin et al., 2010, p. 409.

31. Franklin et al., 2010.

32. The discovery that some epigenetic effects can be transmitted through paternal germ-lines will no doubt continue to draw researchers' attention, particularly now that we know that most of a man's individual sperm cells carry "unique DNA methylation profiles" (Flanagan et al., 2006, p. 67); this finding means that the differing *epigenetic* information in different sperm cells could potentially contribute to variability among offspring just as the differing *genetic* information in different sperm cells contributes to such variability.

33. Gottlieb, G. (1992). *Individual development and evolution: The genesis of novel behavior.* New York: Oxford University Press.

34. Cropley, J. E., Dang, T. H. Y., Martin, D. I. K., & Suter, C. M. (2012). The penetrance of an epigenetic trait in mice is progressively yet reversibly increased by selection and environment. *Proceedings of the Royal Society B, 279,* 2347–2353.

35. Cropley et al., 2012, p. 2351.

36. Anway, M. D., Cupp, A. S., Uzumcu, M., & Skinner, M. K. (2005). Epigenetic transgenerational actions of endocrine disruptors and male fertility. *Science, 308,* 1466–1469.

37. Jablonka, E., & Raz, G. (2009). Transgenerational epigenetic inheritance: Prevalence, mechanisms, and implications for the study of heredity and evolution. *Quarterly Review of Biology, 84,* 131–176.

38. Skinner, M. K. (2011). Role of epigenetics in developmental biology and transgenerational inheritance. *Birth Defects Research (Part C), 93,* 51–55.

39. Jablonka & Raz, 2009.

40. Daxinger & Whitelaw, 2012.

41. Crews, D., Gore, A. C., Hsu, T. S., Dangleben, N. L., Spinetta, M., Schallert, T., . . . Skinner, M. K. (2007). Transgenerational epigenetic imprints on mate preference. *Proceedings of the National Academy of Sciences of the USA, 104,* 5942–5946.

42. Crews et al., 2007, p. 5942.

43. Crews et al., 2007, p. 5945.

44. Kaiser, J. (2014). The epigenetics heretic. *Science, 343,* 361–363.

45. Skinner, M. K., Savenkova, M. I., Zhang, B., Gore, A. C., & Crews, D. (2014). Gene bio-networks involved in the epigenetic transgenerational inheritance of altered mate preference: Environmental epigenetics and evolutionary biology. *BMC Genomics, 15,* 377. doi:10.1186/1471-2164-15-377

46. Franklin & Mansuy, 2010.

47. For experimental data exploring the mechanisms by which DES produces its transgenerational effects in mice, see Newbold, R. R., Padilla-Banks, E., & Jefferson, W. N. (2006). Adverse effects of the model environmental estrogen diethylstilbestrol are transmitted to subsequent generations. *Endocrinology, 147,* S11–S17.

20. *Grandparents*

1. Ellis, E. C. (2013, September 13). Overpopulation is not the problem. *New York Times.*

2a. Hoek, H. W., Brown, A. S., & Susser, E. (1998). The Dutch Famine and schizophrenia spectrum disorders. *Social Psychiatry and Psychiatric Epidemiology, 33,* 373–379.

2b. Lumey, L. H., Stein, A. D., & Susser, E. (2011). Prenatal famine and adult health. *Annual Review of Public Health, 32,* 237–262.

2c. Susser, M., & Stein, Z. (1994). Timing in prenatal nutrition: A reprise of the Dutch famine study. *Nutrition Reviews, 52,* 84–94.

3. Ravelli, G. P., Stein, Z. A., & Susser, M. W. (1976). Obesity in young men after famine exposure in utero and early pregnancy. *New England Journal of Medicine, 295,* 349–353.

4a. Lumey, L. H., Stein, A. D., Kahn, H. S., & Romijn, J. A. (2009). Lipid profiles in middle-aged men and women after famine exposure during gestation: The Dutch Hunger Winter Families Study. *American Journal of Clinical Nutrition, 89,* 1737–1743.

4b. Lumey et al., 2011.

5. Heijmans, B. T., Tobi, E. W., Stein, A. D., Putter, H., Blauw, G. J., Susser, E. S., . . . Lumey, L. H. (2008). Persistent epigenetic differences associated with prenatal exposure to famine in humans. *Proceedings of the National Academy of Sciences USA, 105,* 17046–17049.

6. Tobi, E. W., Lumey, L. H., Talens, R. P., Kremer, D., Putter, H., Stein, A. D., . . . Heijmans, B. T. (2009). DNA methylation differences after exposure to prenatal famine are common and timing- and sex-specific. *Human Molecular Genetics, 18,* 4046–4053.

7. As interesting as these effects are, we currently do not know whether these methylation patterns cause—or are merely associated with—the kinds of phenotypes that emerge in people exposed to famine in utero; for more information on this issue, see Daxinger, L., & Whitelaw, E. (2012). Understanding transgenerational epigenetic inheritance via the gametes in mammals. *Nature Reviews: Genetics, 13,* 153–162.

8a. Lumey, L. H. (1992). Decreased birthweights in infants after maternal *in utero* exposure to the Dutch famine of 1944–1945. *Paediatric and Perinatal Epidemiology, 6,* 240–253.

8b. Susser & Stein, 1994.

9. Franklin, T. B., & Mansuy, I. M. (2010). Epigenetic inheritance in mammals: Evidence for the impact of adverse environmental effects. *Neurobiology of Disease, 39,* 61–65.

10. Painter, R. C., Osmond, C., Gluckman, P., Hanson, M., Phillips, D. I. W., & Roseboom, T. J. (2008). Transgenerational effects of prenatal exposure to the Dutch famine on neonatal adiposity and health in later life. *BJOG, 115,* 1243–1249.

11. Lumey et al., 2011, pp. 252–256.

12a. Kaati, G., Bygren, L. O., Pembrey, M., & Sjöström, M. (2007). Transgenerational response to nutrition, early life circumstances and longevity. *European Journal of Human Genetics, 15,* 784–790.

12b. Pembrey, M. E. (2002). Time to take epigenetic inheritance seriously. *European Journal of Human Genetics, 10,* 669–671.

12c. Rakyan, V. K., & Beck, S. (2006). Epigenetic variation and inheritance in mammals. *Current Opinion in Genetics and Development, 16,* 573–577.

13. Radiolab (Producer). (2012b, November 19). *You are what your grandpa eats* [Audio podcast]. Retrieved from http://www.radiolab.org/2012/nov/19/you-are-what-your-grandpa-eats/

14. Pembrey, M. (2008). Human inheritance, differences and diseases: Putting genes in their place. Part II. *Paediatric and Perinatal Epidemiology, 22,* 507–513.

15. Kaati, G., Bygren, L. O., & Edvinsson, S. (2002). Cardiovascular and diabetes mortality determined by nutrition during parents' and grandparents' slow growth period. *European Journal of Human Genetics, 10,* p. 684.

16. Kaati et al., 2002, p. 684.

17. Radiolab, 2012b.

18. Kaati et al., 2002, p. 687.

19. Kaati et al., 2002.

20. Kaati et al., 2002.

21. Kaati et al., 2002.

22. Kaati et al., 2007.

23. Pembrey, 2002, p. 670.

24a. Kaati et al., 2002.

24b. Pembrey, 2002.

24c. Pembrey, 2008.

24d. Pembrey, M. E. (2010). Male-line transgenerational responses in humans. *Human Fertility, 13,* 268–271.

25. Pembrey, 2002, p. 670.

26. Pembrey, M. E., Bygren, L. O., Kaati, G., Edvinsson, S., Northstone, K., Sjöström, M., . . . The ALSPAC study team (2006). Sex-specific, male-line transgenerational responses in humans. *European Journal of Human Genetics, 14,* 159–166.

27. Pembrey, 2008.

28. Pembrey et al., 2006.

29. Radiolab, 2012b.

30. Pembrey et al., 2006.

31. Pembrey, 2010.

32. Pembrey, 2008.

33. Pembrey et al., 2006, p. 164.

34. Pembrey et al., 2006, p. 165.

35. Radiolab, 2012b.

36. World Health Organization, International Agency for Research on Cancer (2004). Betel-quid and areca-nut chewing and some areca-nut-derived nitrosamines. *IARC Monographs on the Evaluation of Carcinogenic Risks to Humans, 85,* p. 33.

37. World Health Organization IARC, 2004.

38. Chen, T. H.-H., Chiu, Y.-H., & Boucher, B. J. (2006). Transgenerational effects of betel-quid chewing on the development of the metabolic syndrome in the Keelung Community-based Integrated Screening Program. *American Journal of Clinical Nutrition, 83,* 688–692.

39. Pembrey, 2008.

40. Chen, et al., 2006, p. 688.

41. Chen, et al., 2006.

42a. Chen et al., 2006.

42b. Pembrey, 2008.

43. Chen, et al., 2006, p. 692.

44. At the very least, *something* can be carried through the germline that can *re*create parental epigenetic marks in offspring.

45. Maestripieri, D. (2005). Early experience affects the intergenerational transmission of infant abuse in rhesus monkeys. *Proceedings of the National Academy of Sciences USA, 102,* 9726–9729.

46. Champagne, F. A. (2008). Epigenetic mechanisms and the transgenerational effects of maternal care. *Frontiers in Neuroendocrinology, 29,* 386–397.

47a. Gottlieb, G. (1992). *Individual development and evolution: The genesis of novel behavior.* New York: Oxford University Press.

47b. Laland, K. N., Odling-Smee, J., & Myles, S. (2010). How culture shaped the human genome: Bringing genetics and the human sciences together. *Nature Reviews: Genetics, 11,* 137–148.

48. Michel, G. F., & Moore, C. L. (1995). *Developmental psychobiology: An interdisciplinary science.* Cambridge, MA: MIT.

49a. Dobzhansky, T. (1937). *Genetics and the origin of species.* New York: Columbia University Press.

49b. Mayr, E. (1963). *Animal species and evolution.* Cambridge, MA: Harvard University Press.

21. Caution

1. Hu, V. W. (2013). From genes to environment: Using integrative genomics to build a "systems level" understanding of autism spectrum disorders. *Child Development, 84,* 89–103.

2. Connolly, J. J., Glessner, J. T., & Hakonarson, H. (2013). A genome-wide association study of autism incorporating autism diagnostic interview–revised, autism diagnostic observation schedule, and social responsiveness scale. *Child Development, 84,* 17–33.

3. Joseph, J. (2006). *The missing gene: Psychiatry, heredity, and the fruitless search for genes.* New York: Algora Publishing.

4. Cloud, J. (2010, January 6). Why your DNA isn't your destiny. *Time Magazine*. Retrieved from www.time.com/time/magazine/

5. Blech, J. (2010, August 9). Der sieg über die gene: Das gedächtnis des körpers [Victory over the genes: The memory of the body]. *Der Spiegel*. Retrieved from http://www.spiegel.de/spiegel/print/d-73109479.html

6a. Lewontin, R. C. (2000). *The triple helix: Gene, organism, and environment*. Cambridge, MA: Harvard University Press.

6b. Moore, D. S. (2002). *The dependent gene: The fallacy of nature vs. nurture*. New York: W.H. Freeman.

6c. Robert, J. S. (2004). *Embryology, epigenesis, and evolution: Taking development seriously*. New York: Cambridge University Press.

7. Moore, 2002.

8. Weaver, I. C. G., Cervoni, N., Champagne, F. A., D'Alessio, A. C., Sharma, S., Seckl, J. R., . . . Meaney, M. J. (2004a). Epigenetic programming by maternal behavior. *Nature Neuroscience, 7*, 847–854.

9a. Vickers, M. H., Gluckman, P. D., Coveny, A. H., Hofman, P. L., Cutfield, W. S., Gertler, A., . . . Harris, M. (2005). Neonatal leptin treatment reverses developmental programming. *Endocrinology, 146*, 4211–4216.

9b. Weaver, I. C. G., Champagne, F. A., Brown, S. E., Dymov, S., Sharma, S., Meaney, M. J., & Szyf, M. (2005). Reversal of maternal programming of stress responses in adult offspring through methyl supplementation: Altering epigenetic marking later in life. *Journal of Neuroscience, 25*, 11045–11054.

9c. Weaver, I. C. G., Meaney, M. J., & Szyf, M. (2006). Maternal care effects on the hippocampal transcriptome and anxiety-mediated behaviors in the offspring that are reversible in adulthood. *Proceedings of the National Academy of Sciences USA, 103*, 3480–3485.

10. For hints about ways in which research on the epigenetics of memory could contribute to the development of future treatments for post-traumatic stress disorders, see Bredy, T. W., Wu, H., Crego, C., Zellhoefer, J., Sun, Y. E., & Barad, M. (2007). Histone modifications around individual BDNF gene promoters in prefrontal cortex are associated with extinction of conditioned fear. *Learning and Memory, 14*, 268–276.

11. Murgatroyd, C., Patchev, A. V., Wu, Y., Micale, V., Bockmühl, Y., Fischer, D., . . . Spengler, D. (2009). Dynamic DNA methylation programs persistent adverse effects of early-life stress. *Nature Neuroscience, 12*, 1559–1566.

12. Eyer, D. E. (1992). *Mother-infant bonding: A scientific fiction*. New Haven, CT: Yale University Press.

13. Mack, G. S. (2010). To selectivity and beyond. *Nature Biotechnology, 28*, p. 1262.

14. Shulevitz, J. (2012, September 8). Why fathers really matter. *New York Times*. Retrieved from http://www.nytimes.com/2012/09/09/opinion/sunday/why-fathers-really-matter.html?pagewanted=all&_r=0

15a. Carvajal, D. (2012, August 17). On the trail of inherited memories. *New York Times*.

15b. Kellermann, N. P. F. (2013). Epigenetic transmission of holocaust trauma: Can nightmares be inherited? *Israel Journal of Psychiatry and Related Sciences, 50*, 33–39.

16. Dias, B. G., & Ressler, K. J. (2014). Parental olfactory experience influences behavior and neural structure in subsequent generations. *Nature Neuroscience, 17*, 89–96.

17. Levenson, J. M., & Sweatt, J. D. (2005). Epigenetic mechanisms in memory formation. *Nature Reviews: Neuroscience, 6*, 108–118.

22. Hope

1a. Rothstein, M. A., Cai, Y., & Marchant, G. E. (2009). The ghost in our genes: Legal and ethical implications of epigenetics. *Health Matrix, 19*, 1–62.

1b. Gore, A. C., Balthazart, J., Bikle, D. D., Carpenter, D. O., Crews, D., Czernichow, P., . . . Watson, C. S. (2013). Policy decisions on endocrine disruptors should be based on science across disciplines: A response to Dietrich et al. *Endocrine Disruptors, 1*, e26644. doi:10.4161/endo.26644

2. Rothstein et al., 2009.

3. Lester, B. M., Tronick, E., Nestler, E., Abel, T., Kosofsky, B., Kuzawa, C. W., . . . Wood, M. A. (2011). Behavioral epigenetics. *Annals of the New York Academy of Sciences, 1226*, 14–33.

4. Lester et al., 2011.

5. For a comprehensive review, see Feinberg, A. P. (2007). Phenotypic plasticity and the epigenetics of human disease. *Nature, 447*, 433–440.

6. Gaudet, F., Hodgson, J. G., Eden, A., Jackson-Grusby, L., Dausman, J., Gray, J. W., . . . Jaenisch, R. (2003). Induction of tumors in mice by genomic hypomethylation. *Science, 300*, 489–492.

7. Feinberg, A. P., Ohlsson, R., & Henikoff, S. (2006). The epigenetic progenitor origin of human cancer. *Nature Reviews: Genetics, 7*, p. 22.

8. Feinberg, 2007.

9. Feinberg et al., 2006.

10. Francis, R. C. (2011). *Epigenetics: The ultimate mystery of inheritance.* New York: Norton, p. 150.

11. Carey, N. (2011). *The epigenetics revolution.* London, England: Icon Books.

12. Anand, P., Kunnumakara, A. B., Sundaram, C., Harikumar, K. B., Tharakan, S. T., Lai, O. S., . . . Aggarwal, B. B. (2008). Cancer is a preventable disease that requires major lifestyle changes. *Pharmaceutical Research, 25*, 2097–2116.

13. Bjornsson, H. T., Sigurdsson, M. I., Fallin, M. D., Irizarry, R. A., Aspelund, T., Cui, H., . . . Feinberg, A. P. (2008). Intra-individual change over time in DNA methylation with familial clustering. *Journal of the American Medical Association, 299*, 2877–2883.

14. Bjornsson et al., 2008.

15. For example, see De Grey, A., & Rae, M. (2007). *Ending aging: The rejuvenation breakthroughs that could reverse human aging in our lifetime.* New York: St. Martin's Press.

16. Of course, this is not necessarily desirable, but I will leave it to other writers to address this issue; see for example, Illes, J. (2007). Blurring our edges. *Nature, 450*, 351–352.

17. Carey, 2011.

18a. Carey, 2011.

18b. Kanfi, Y., Naiman, S., Amir, G., Peshti, V., Zinman, G., Nahum, L., . . . Cohen, H. Y. (2012). The sirtuin SIRT6 regulates lifespan in male mice. *Nature, 483*, 218–221.

18c. Mostoslavsky, R., Chua, K. F., Lombard, D. B., Pang, W. W., Fischer, M. R., Gellon, L., . . . Alt, F. W. (2006). Genomic instability and aging-like phenotype in the absence of mammalian SIRT6. *Cell, 124*, 315–329.

19. Genetic Science Learning Center (2012, August 6). Are telomeres the key to aging and cancer? *Learn.Genetics.* Retrieved January 9, 2013, from http://learn.genetics.utah.edu/content/begin/traits/telomeres/

20. Of course, telomere lengths alone are not the sole determinants of life span. In fact, some species have longer telomeres than people do, but shorter life spans (Genetic Science Learning Center, 2012). Moreover, cancer cells produce a protein that allows them to divide indefinitely, without ever getting to a point where their telomeres have become too short to support further division; although such cancer cells are immortal, a body containing them would certainly not be considered healthy!

21. Genetic Science Learning Center, 2012.

22. Although telomeres cannot be methylated, DNA regions *close* to telomeres *can* be methylated, and recent research has revealed that DNA methylation levels in these regions are associated with telomere lengths in human white blood cells. For more information, see Buxton, J. L., Suderman, M., Pappas, J. J., Borghol, N., McArdle, W., Blakemore, A. I. F., . . . Pembrey, M. (2014). Human leukocyte telomere length is associated with DNA methylation levels in multiple subtelomeric and imprinted loci. *Scientific Reports, 4*, 4954. doi:10.1038/srep04954

23. Carey, 2011.

24. Carey, 2011.

25. Michishita, E., McCord, R. A., Berber, E., Kioi, M., Padilla-Nash, H., Damian, M., . . . Chua, K. F. (2008). SIRT6 is a histone H3 lysine 9 deacetylase that modulates telomeric chromatin. *Nature, 452,* 492–496.

26. Mostoslavsky et al., 2006.

27. Kanfi et al., 2012, p. 218.

28. It is important to note that some researchers have cautioned that life span extension in this study should not be understood to necessarily "imply an effect on ageing [per se, because] . . . interventions unrelated to ageing, such as giving insulin to a person with type I diabetes, can increase . . . lifespan" (Lombard & Miller, 2012, p. 166).

29. Michishita et al., 2008.

30a. Gluckman, P. D., Hanson, M. A., & Beedle, A. S. (2007). Non-genomic transgenerational inheritance of disease risk. *BioEssays, 29,* 145–154.

30b. Rothstein et al., 2009.

31. Gluckman, P. D., Hanson, M. A., & Buklijas, T. (2010). A conceptual framework for the developmental origins of health and disease. *Journal of Developmental Origins of Health and Disease, 1,* 6–18.

32. Gluckman et al., 2010, p. 14.

33. For example, see Nestler, E. J. (2009). Epigenetic mechanisms in psychiatry. *Biological Psychiatry, 65,* 189–190.

34. Akbarian, S., & Nestler, E. J. (Eds.). (2013). Epigenetic mechanisms in psychiatry [Special issue]. *Neuropsychopharmacology, 38*(1).

35. Groleau, P., Joober, R., Israel, M., Zeramdini, N., DeGuzman, R., & Steiger, H. (2014). Methylation of the dopamine D2 receptor (DRD2) gene promoter in women with a bulimia-spectrum disorder: Associations with borderline personality disorder and exposure to childhood abuse. *Journal of Psychiatric Research, 48,* 121–127.

36a. Provençal, N., Suderman, M. J., Caramaschi, D., Wang, D., Hallett, M., Vitaro, F., . . . Szyf, M. (2013). Differential DNA methylation regions in cytokine and transcription factor genomic loci associate with childhood physical aggression. *PLoS ONE, 8*(8), e71691. doi:10.1371/journal.pone.0071691

36b. Guillemin, C., Provençal, N., Suderman, M., Côte, S. M., Vitaro, F., Hallett, M., . . . Szyf, M. (2014). DNA methylation signature of childhood chronic physical aggression in T cells of both men and women. *PLoS ONE, 9*(1), e86822. doi:10.1371/journal.pone.0086822

36c. Provençal, N., Suderman, M. J., Guillemin, C., Vitaro, F., Côte, S. M., Hallett, M., . . . Szyf, M. (2014). Association of childhood chronic physical aggression with a DNA methylation signature in adult human T cells. *PLoS ONE, 9*(4), e89839. doi:10.1371/journal. pone.0089839

37. Tsankova, N., Renthal, W., Kumar, A., & Nestler, E. J. (2007). Epigenetic regulation in psychiatric disorders. *Nature Reviews: Neuroscience, 8,* 355–367.

38. When one reads the current scientific literature on the epigenetics of psychopathology, it can seem as if the big news (for instance, see Nestler, 2009) is that theories that explain abnormal behavior in terms of genes and environments *alone* are bound to fail. Consider, for example, the conclusion drawn by one research team: "it seems worthwhile to add methylation to the G [genes] × E [environment] equation . . . the findings of our [studies might best] be cast in terms of G × M × E where M stands for methylation status" (Van IJzendoorn et al., 2011, p. 308). But the truth is, it is *not* news that "G × E"-style equations—which take into account only genes and environments—fail to explain psychopathology; the study of normal development made it obvious years ago that such equations are of limited value (Moore, 2013a). And merely adding a new term to such equations— whether it is an "M" for methylation or an "E" for epigenetic factors more generally—will not overcome these limitations. At best, these kinds of equations reveal only statistical interactions between factors, not the real "causal-mechanical" (Griffiths & Tabery, 2008, p. 341) interactions between genes and their environments, which are what actually create

phenotypes (see also Moore, 2013c). Nonetheless, despite some researchers' continued use of these sorts of simplistic "models" (e.g., Danchin et al., 2011; van IJzendoorn et al., 2011), increasing awareness of epigenetics is almost sure to help mental health professionals recognize the complexity that characterizes the real interactions by which genetic, environmental, and epigenetic factors influence abnormal behavior.

39. Labrie, V., Pai, S., & Petronis, A. (2012). Epigenetics of major psychosis: Progress, problems and perspectives. *Trends in Genetics, 28*, 427–435.

40a. Keller, S., Sarchiapone, M., Zarrilli, F., Videtič, A., Ferraro, A., Carli, V., ... Chiariotti, L. (2010). Increased *BDNF* promoter methylation in the Wernicke area of suicide subjects. *Archives of General Psychiatry, 67*, 258–267.

40b. Poulter, M. O., Du, L., Weaver, I. C. G., Palkovits, M., Faludi, G., Merali, Z., ... Anisman, H. (2008). GABAA receptor promoter hypermethylation in suicide brain: Implications for the involvement of epigenetic processes. *Biological Psychiatry, 64*, 645–652.

41a. Alarcón, J. M., Malleret, G., Touzani, K., Vronskaya, S., Ishii, S., Kandel, E. R., & Barco, A. (2004). Chromatin acetylation, memory, and LTP are impaired in CBP+/- mice: A model for the cognitive deficit in Rubinstein-Taybi syndrome and its amelioration. *Neuron, 42*, 947–959.

41b. Borrelli, E., Nestler, E. J., Allis, C. D., & Sassone-Corsi, P. (2008). Decoding the epigenetic language of neuronal plasticity. *Neuron, 60*, 961–974.

41c. Guan, J.-S., Haggarty, S. J., Giacometti, E., Dannenberg, J.-H., Joseph, N., Gao, J., ... Tsai, L.-H. (2009). HDAC2 negatively regulates memory formation and synaptic plasticity. *Nature, 459*, 55–60.

41d. Levenson, J. M., O'Riordan, K. J., Brown, K. D., Trinh, M. A., Molfese, D. L., & Sweatt, J. D. (2004). Regulation of histone acetylation during memory formation in the hippocampus. *Journal of Biological Chemistry, 279*, 40545–40559.

41e. Levenson, J. M., & Sweatt, J. D. (2005). Epigenetic mechanisms in memory formation. *Nature Reviews: Neuroscience, 6*, 108–118.

42. Fischer, A., Sananbenesi, F., Wang, X., Dobbin, M., & Tsai, L.-H. (2007). Recovery of learning and memory is associated with chromatin remodeling. *Nature, 447*, 178–182.

43. Gräff, J., Rei, D., Guan, J.-S., Wang, W.-Y., Seo, J., Hennig, K. M., ... Tsai, L.-H. (2012). An epigenetic blockade of cognitive functions in the neurodegenerating brain. *Nature, 483*, 222–226.

44. Zovkic, I. B., & Sweatt, J. D. (2012). Epigenetic mechanisms in learned fear: Implications for PTSD. *Neuropsychopharmacology Reviews*. Advance online publication. doi:10.1038/npp.2012.79, p. 1.

45. Yehuda, R., & Bierer, L. M. (2009). The relevance of epigenetics to PTSD: Implications for the DSM-V. *Journal of Traumatic Stress, 22*, p. 427.

46a. Maze, I., & Nestler, E. J. (2011). The epigenetic landscape of addiction. *Annals of the New York Academy of Sciences, 1216*, 99–113.

46b. Tsankova et al., 2007.

46c. Wong, C. C. Y., Mill, J., & Fernandes, C. (2011). Drugs and addiction: An introduction to epigenetics. *Addiction, 106*, 480–489.

47. Bönsch, D., Lenz, B., Reulbach, U., Kornhuber, J., & Bleich, S. (2004). Homocysteine associated genomic DNA hypermethylation in patients with chronic alcoholism. *Journal of Neural Transmission, 111*, 1611–1616.

48. Launay, J.-M., Del Pino, M., Chironi, G., Callebert, J., Peoc'h, K., Mégnien, J., ... Rendu, F. (2009). Smoking induces long-lasting effects through a monoamine-oxidase epigenetic regulation. *PLoS ONE, 4*(11), e7959. doi:10.1371/journal.pone.0007959

49a. Maze, I., Covington, H. E. III, Dietz, D. M., LaPlant, Q., Renthal, W., Russo, S. J., ... Nestler, E. J. (2010). Essential role of the histone methyltransferase G9a in cocaine-induced plasticity. *Science, 327*, 213–216.

49b. Vassoler, F. M., White, S. L., Schmidt, H. D., Sadri-Vakili, G., & Pierce, R. C. (2013). Epigenetic inheritance of a cocaine-resistance phenotype. *Nature Neuroscience, 16*, 42–47.

50. Wong et al., 2011.

51. Byrnes, J. J., Johnson, N. L., Carini, L. M., & Byrnes, E. M. (2013). Multigenerational effects of adolescent morphine exposure on dopamine D2 receptor function. *Psychopharmacology, 227*, 263–272.

52a. Hyman, S. E., Malenka, R. C., & Nestler, E. J. (2006). Neural mechanisms of addiction: The role of reward-related learning and memory. *Annual Review of Neuroscience, 29*, 565–598.

52b. Day, J. J., & Sweatt, J. D. (2011). Epigenetic mechanisms in cognition. *Neuron, 70*, 813–829.

53. Carey, 2011, p. 259.

54a. Dulac, C. (2010). Brain function and chromatin plasticity. *Nature, 465*, 728–735.

54b. Tsankova et al., 2007.

55. Maze et al., 2010, p. 213.

56. Maze & Nestler, 2011, p. 111.

57. Wong et al., 2011.

58a. Abdolmaleky, H. M., Cheng, K., Faraone, S. V., Wilcox, M., Glatt, S. J., Gao, F., . . . Thiagalingam, S. (2006). Hypomethylation of *MB-COMT* promoter is a major risk factor for schizophrenia and bipolar disorder. *Human Molecular Genetics, 15*, 3132–3145.

58b. Mill, J., Tang, T., Kaminsky, Z., Khare, T., Yazdanpanah, S., Bouchard, L., . . . Petronis, A. (2008). Epigenomic profiling reveals DNA-methylation changes associated with major psychosis. *American Journal of Human Genetics, 82*, 696–711.

58c. Tsankova et al., 2007.

58d. Veldic, M., Guidotti, A., Maloku, E., Davis, J. M., & Costa, E. (2005). In psychosis, cortical interneurons overexpress DNA-methyltransferase 1. *Proceedings of the National Academy of Sciences USA, 102*, 2152–2157.

59. Labrie et al., 2012.

60. Nestler, 2009.

61. Cardno, A. G., & Gottesman, I. I. (2000). Twin studies of schizophrenia: From bow-and-arrow concordances to star wars Mx and functional genomics. *American Journal of Medical Genetics, 97*, 12–17.

62. Feinberg, 2007.

63. Petronis, A., Gottesman, I. I., Kan, P., Kennedy, J. L., Basile, V. S., Paterson, A. D., & Popendikyte, V. (2003). Monozygotic twins exhibit numerous epigenetic differences: Clues to twin discordance? *Schizophrenia Bulletin, 29*, 169–178.

64. Dempster, E. L., Pidsley, R., Schalkwyk, L. C., Owens, S., Georgiades, A., Kane, F., . . . Mill, J. (2011). Disease-associated epigenetic changes in monozygotic twins discordant for schizophrenia and bipolar disorder. *Human Molecular Genetics, 20*, 4786–4796.

65. Labrie et al., 2012.

66. Masterpasqua, F. (2009). Psychology and epigenetics. *Review of General Psychology, 13*, 194–201.

67. Rutten, B. P. F., & Mill, J. (2009). Epigenetic mediation of environmental influences in major psychotic disorders. *Schizophrenia Bulletin, 35*, p. 1051.

68. Rutten & Mill, 2009, p. 1045.

69. Labrie et al., 2012.

70. Labrie et al., 2012, p. 431.

71. Persico, A. M., & Bourgeron, T. (2006). Searching for ways out of the autism maze: Genetic, epigenetic and environmental clues. *Trends in Neurosciences, 29*, 349–358.

72. Persico & Bourgeron, 2006, p. 350.

73. Voineagu, I., Wang, X., Johnston, P., Lowe, J. K., Tian, Y., Horvath, S., . . . Geschwind, D. H. (2011). Transcriptomic analysis of autistic brain reveals convergent molecular pathology. *Nature, 474*, 380–384.

74. For example, Asprey, L., & Asprey, D. (2013). *The better baby book: How to have a healthier, smarter, happier baby*. New York: Wiley.

75. Miyake, K., Hirasawa, T., Koide, T., & Kubota, T. (2012). Epigenetics in autism and other neurodevelopmental diseases. In S. I. Ahmad (Ed.), *Neurodegenerative diseases* (pp. 91–98). New York: Springer Science+Business Media, p. 95.

76. Korade, Ž., & Mirnics, K. (2011). The autism disconnect. *Nature, 474*, 294–295.

77a. Keller et al., 2010.

77b. Poulter et al., 2008.

78. Neigh, G. N., Gillespie, C. F., & Nemeroff, C. B. (2009). The neurobiological toll of child abuse and neglect. *Trauma, Violence, and Abuse 10*, 389–410.

79a. Beach, S. R. H., Brody, G. H., Todorov, A. A., Gunter, T. D., & Philibert, R. A. (2010). Methylation at *SLC6A4* is linked to family history of child abuse: An examination of the Iowa adoptee sample. *American Journal of Medical Genetics Part B, 153B*, 710–713.

79b. McGowan, P. O., Sasaki, A., D'Alessio, A. C., Dymov, S., Labonté, B., Szyf, M., . . . Meaney, M. J. (2009). Epigenetic regulation of the glucocorticoid receptor in human brain associates with childhood abuse. *Nature Neuroscience, 12*, 342–348.

79c. Labonté, B., Suderman, M., Maussion, G., Navaro, L., Yerko, V., Mahar, I., . . . Turecki, G. (2012). Genome-wide epigenetic regulation by early-life trauma. *Archives of General Psychiatry, 69*, 722–731.

79d. Suderman, M., Borghol, N., Pappas, J. J., Pereira, S. M. P., Pembrey, M., Hertzman, C., . . . Szyf, M. (2014). Childhood abuse is associated with methylation of multiple loci in adult DNA. *BMC Medical Genomics, 7*, 13. doi:10.1186/1755-8794-7-13

80a. Tsankova, N. M., Berton, O., Renthal, W., Kumar, A., Neve, R. L., & Nestler, E. J. (2006). Sustained hippocampal chromatin regulation in a mouse model of depression and antidepressant action. *Nature Neuroscience, 9*, 519–525.

80b. Tsankova et al., 2007.

81. Tsankova et al., 2006.

82. Tsankova et al., 2006, p. 523.

83. Elliott, E., Ezra-Nevo, G., Regev, L., Neufeld-Cohen, A., & Chen, A. (2010). Resilience to social stress coincides with functional DNA methylation of the Crf gene in adult mice. *Nature Neuroscience, 13*, 1351–1353.

84. For readers who read "Zooming in on Experience," the hormone affected was CRH, corticotropin-releasing hormone.

85. Elliott et al., 2010, p. 1353.

86a. Elliott et al., 2010.

86b. Tsankova et al., 2006.

87. Elliott et al., 2010.

88. Tsankova et al., 2006, p. 519.

89a. Curley, J. P., Jensen, C. L., Mashoodh, R., & Champagne, F. A. (2011). Social influences on neurobiology and behavior: Epigenetic effects during development. *Psychoneuroendocrinology, 36*, 352–371.

89b. Kenworthy, C. A., Sengupta, A., Luz, S. M., Ver Hoeve, E. S., Meda, K., Bhatnagar, S., & Abel, T. (2014). Social defeat induces changes in histone acetylation and expression of histone modifying enzymes in the ventral hippocampus, prefrontal cortex, and dorsal raphe nucleus. *Neuroscience, 264*, 88–98.

90a. Berger, S. L. (2007). The complex language of chromatin regulation during transcription. *Nature, 447*, 407–412.

90b. Wang, Z., Zang, C., Rosenfeld, J. A., Schones, D. E., Barski, A., Cuddapah, S., . . . Zhao, K. (2008). Combinatorial patterns of histone acetylations and methylations in the human genome. *Nature Genetics, 40*, 897–903.

91a. Fischer et al., 2007.

91b. Gräff et al., 2012.

91c. Levenson et al., 2004.

92. Mack, G. S. (2010). To selectivity and beyond. *Nature Biotechnology, 28*, 1259–1266.

93. Carey, 2011.

94a. Grayson, D. R., Kundakovic, M., & Sharma, R. P. (2010). Is there a future for histone deacetylase inhibitors in the pharmacotherapy of psychiatric disorders? *Molecular Pharmacology, 77*, 126–135.

94b. Gräff, J., & Tsai, L.-H. (2013). The potential of HDAC inhibitors as cognitive enhancers. *Annual Review of Pharmacology and Toxicology, 53*, 311–330.

95. Feinberg, A. P. (2008). Epigenetics at the epicenter of modern medicine. *Journal of the American Medical Association, 299*, 1345–1350.

96. Day & Sweatt, 2011.

97. Mack, 2010.

98. See, for example, Gräff et al., 2012.

99. Grayson et al., 2010.

100. Grayson et al., 2010.

101. Carey, 2011.

102. Gräff & Tsai, 2013.

103. Guan et al., 2009.

104. Alarcón et al., 2004.

105. Peleg, S., Sananbenesi, F., Zovoilis, A., Burhardt, S., Bahari-Javan, S., Agis-Balboa, R. C., . . . Fischer, A. (2010). Altered histone acetylation is associated with age-dependent memory impairment in mice. *Science, 328*, 753–756.

106. Peleg et al., 2010.

107. Bredy, T. W., Wu, H., Crego, C., Zellhoefer, J., Sun, Y. E., & Barad, M. (2007). Histone modifications around individual BDNF gene promoters in prefrontal cortex are associated with extinction of conditioned fear. *Learning and Memory, 14*, 268–276.

108. Day & Sweatt, 2011.

109a. Weaver, I. C. G., Champagne, F. A., Brown, S. E., Dymov, S., Sharma, S., Meaney, M. J., & Szyf, M. (2005). Reversal of maternal programming of stress responses in adult offspring through methyl supplementation: Altering epigenetic marking later in life. *Journal of Neuroscience, 25*, 11045–11054.

109b. Weaver, I. C. G., Meaney, M. J., & Szyf, M. (2006). Maternal care effects on the hippocampal transcriptome and anxiety-mediated behaviors in the offspring that are reversible in adulthood. *Proceedings of the National Academy of Sciences USA, 103*, 3480–3485.

110. Weaver et al., 2006.

111. Weaver, I. C. G., Cervoni, N., Champagne, F. A., D'Alessio, A. C., Sharma, S., Seckl, J. R., . . . Meaney, M. J. (2004a). Epigenetic programming by maternal behavior. *Nature Neuroscience, 7*, 847–854.

112. Covington, H. E. III, Maze, I., LaPlant, Q. C., Vialou, V. F., Ohnishi, Y. N., Berton, O., . . . Nestler, E. J. (2009). Antidepressant actions of histone deacetylase inhibitors. *Journal of Neuroscience, 29*, 11451–11460.

113. Covington et al., 2009.

114. Uchida, S., Hara, K., Kobayashi, A., Otsuki, K., Yamagata, H., Hobara, T., . . . Watanabe, Y. (2011). Epigenetic status of *Gdnf* in the ventral striatum determines susceptibility and adaptation to daily stressful events. *Neuron, 69*, 359–372.

115a. Covington et al., 2009.

115b. Elliott et al., 2010.

115c. Tsankova et al., 2006.

115d. Uchida et al., 2011.

116. Dulac 2010, p. 730.

117. Labrie et al., 2012.

118. Uchida et al., 2011.

119a. Cropley, J. E., Suter, C. M., Beckman, K. B., & Martin, D. I. I. (2006). Germ-line epigenetic modification of the murine Avy allele by nutritional supplementation. *Proceedings of the National Academy of Sciences of the USA, 103*, 17308–17312.

119b. Waterland, R. A., & Jirtle, R. L. (2003). Transposable elements: Targets for early nutritional effects on epigenetic gene regulation. *Molecular and Cellular Biology, 23,* 5293–5300.

120a. Papakostas, G. I., Alpert, J. E., & Fava, M. (2003). S-adenosyl-methionine in depression: A comprehensive review of the literature. *Current Psychiatry Reports, 5,* 460–466.

120b. Papakostas, G. I., Mischoulon, D., Shyu, I., Alpert, J. E., & Fava, M. (2010). S-adenosyl-methionine (SAMe) augmentation of serotonin reuptake inhibitors for antidepressant nonresponders with major depressive disorder: A double-blind, randomized clinical trial. *American Journal of Psychiatry, 167,* 942–948.

121a. Weaver et al., 2005.

121b. Weaver et al., 2006.

122. Sweatt, J. D. (2009). Experience-dependent epigenetic modifications in the central nervous system. *Biological Psychiatry, 65,* 191–197.

123. Fischer et al., 2007.

124. Rothstein et al., 2009.

125. Rothstein et al., 2009.

126. Rothstein et al., 2009, pp. 61–62.

127. Loi, M., Del Savio, L., & Stupka, E. (2013). Social epigenetics and equality of opportunity. *Public Health Ethics, 6,* 142–153.

23. *Conclusions*

1. Lewontin, R. C. (2000). *The triple helix: Gene, organism, and environment.* Cambridge, MA: Harvard University Press.

2. See, for example, Moore, D. S. (2002). *The dependent gene: The fallacy of nature vs. nurture.* New York: W.H. Freeman.

3. Zhang, T.-Y., & Meaney, M. J. (2010). Epigenetics and the environmental regulation of the genome and its function. *Annual Review of Psychology, 61,* 439–466.

4. Weaver, I. C. G., Cervoni, N., Champagne, F. A., D'Alessio, A. C., Sharma, S., Seckl, J. R., . . . Meaney, M. J. (2004a). Epigenetic programming by maternal behavior. *Nature Neuroscience, 7,* 847–854.

5a. Weaver, I. C. G., Champagne, F. A., Brown, S. E., Dymov, S., Sharma, S., Meaney, M. J., & Szyf, M. (2005). Reversal of maternal programming of stress responses in adult offspring through methyl supplementation: Altering epigenetic marking later in life. *Journal of Neuroscience, 25,* 11045–11054.

5b. Weaver, I. C. G., Meaney, M. J., & Szyf, M. (2006). Maternal care effects on the hippocampal transcriptome and anxiety-mediated behaviors in the offspring that are reversible in adulthood. *Proceedings of the National Academy of Sciences USA, 103,* 3480–3485.

5c. Peña, C. L. J., & Champagne, F. A. (2012). Epigenetic and neurodevelopmental perspectives on variation in parenting behavior. *Parenting: Science and Practice, 12,* 202–211.

6a. Weaver et al., 2005.

6b. Weaver et al., 2006.

7a. Peña & Champagne, 2012.

7b. Fischer, A., Sananbenesi, F., Wang, X., Dobbin, M., & Tsai, L.-H. (2007). Recovery of learning and memory is associated with chromatin remodeling. *Nature, 447,* 178–182.

8. Peña & Champagne, 2012, p. 209.

9. For more information, see Moore, D. S. (2008b). Individuals and populations: How biology's theory and data have interfered with the integration of development and evolution. *New Ideas in Psychology, 26,* 370–386.

10. Woodward, T. E., & Gills, J. P. (2012). *The mysterious epigenome: What lies beyond DNA.* Grand Rapids, MI: Kregel Publications.

11. In fact, the available data on behavioral epigenetics supports the opposite claim: Darwin was right to conclude that people share common ancestors with other primates.

12. Behe, M. J. (1996). *Darwin's black box*. New York: Free Press.

13a. Moore, 2002.

13b. Pigliucci, M. (2010). Genotype–phenotype mapping and the end of the "genes as blueprint" metaphor. *Philosophical Transactions of the Royal Society B, 365*, 557–566.

14. Jablonka, E., & Lamb, M. J. (2002). The changing concept of epigenetics. *Annals of the New York Academy of Science, 981*, p. 93.

15. Jablonka & Lamb, 2002, p. 95.

16. Zhang & Meaney, 2010.

17. Roth, T. L. (2012). Epigenetics of neurobiology and behavior during development and adulthood. *Developmental Psychobiology, 54*, 590–597.

18. Roth, 2012, p. 595.

19. Van IJzendoorn, M. H., Bakermans-Kranenburg, M. J., & Ebstein, R. P. (2011). Methylation matters in child development: Toward developmental behavioral epigenetics. *Child Development Perspectives, 5*, p. 308.

20. Zhang & Meaney, 2010, p. 440.

21. Zhang & Meaney, 2010.

22. Zhang & Meaney, 2010, p. 441.

23. Jirtle, R. L., & Skinner, M. K. (2007). Environmental epigenomics and disease susceptibility. *Nature Reviews: Genetics, 8*, p. 260.

24. Johnston, T. D. (1987). The persistence of dichotomies in the study of behavioral development. *Developmental Review, 7*, p. 150.

25. Johnston, 1987, p. 160.

26. Johnston, 1987, p. 160.

27. Recent (and typical) examples of the deployment of the blueprint metaphor by scientists can be found in a 2008 paper by Shoguchi and colleagues, a 2008 symposium by Larsen, and a 2011 book by Carey.

28a. Jablonka, E., & Lamb, M. J. (2005). *Evolution in four dimensions: Genetic, epigenetic, behavioral, and symbolic variation in the history of life*. Cambridge, MA: The MIT Press.

28b. Nijhout, H. F. (1990). Metaphors and the role of genes in development. *BioEssays, 12*, 441–446.

28c. Noble, D. (2006). *The music of life: Biology beyond genes*. New York: Oxford University Press.

29. Pigliucci, 2010, p. 557.

30. Fisher, S. E. (2006). Tangled webs: Tracing the connections between genes and cognition. *Cognition, 101*, p. 273.

31a. Lickliter, R., & Berry, T. D. (1990). The phylogeny fallacy: Developmental psychology's misapplication of evolutionary theory. *Developmental Review, 10*, 348–364.

31b. Lickliter, R. (2008). The growth of developmental thought: Implications for a new evolutionary psychology. *New Ideas in Psychology, 26*, 353–369.

32a. Nijhout, 1990.

32b. Noble, D. (2008). Genes and causation. *Philosophical Transactions of the Royal Society A, 366*, 3001–3015.

32c. Pigliucci, M., & Boudry, M. (2011). Why machine-information metaphors are bad for science and science education. *Science and Education, 20*, 453–471.

33. Gerstein, M. B., Bruce, C., Rozowsky, J. S., Zheng, D., Du, J., Korbel, J. O., . . . Snyder, M. (2007). What is a gene, post-ENCODE? History and updated definition. *Genome Research, 17*, p. 671.

34. Gerstein et al., 2007, p. 675.

35. Carey, N. (2011). *The epigenetics revolution*. London, England: Icon Books.

36. Carey, 2011, p. 2.

37a. Johnston, 1987.

37b. Oyama, S. (1985/2000). *The ontogeny of information*. Durham, NC: Duke University Press.

37c. Pigliucci & Boudry, 2011.

38. Van IJzendoorn et al., 2011, p. 305.

39. Kolata, G. (2012, September 5). Bits of mystery DNA, far from "junk," play crucial role. *New York Times.*

40. Noble, 2006.

41. Noble, 2006, pp. 14–15.

42. Noble, 2008, p. 3012.

43. Moore, D. S. (2013a). Behavioral genetics, genetics, and epigenetics. In P. D. Zelazo (Ed.), *Oxford handbook of developmental psychology* (pp. 91–128). New York: Oxford University Press.

44. Powledge, T. M. (2011). Behavioral epigenetics: How nurture shapes nature. *BioScience, 61,* p. 588, emphasis added.

45. Aspinwall, L. G., Brown, T. R., & Tabery, J. (2012). The double-edged sword: Does bio-mechanism increase or decrease judges' sentencing of psychopaths? *Science, 337,* 846–849.

REFERENCES

Abdolmaleky, H. M., Cheng, K., Faraone, S. V., Wilcox, M., Glatt, S. J., Gao, F., . . . Thiagalingam, S. (2006). Hypomethylation of *MB-COMT* promoter is a major risk factor for schizophrenia and bipolar disorder. *Human Molecular Genetics, 15,* 3132–3145.

Abel, J. L., & Rissman, E. F. (2013). Running-induced epigenetic and gene expression changes in the adolescent brain. *International Journal of Developmental Neuroscience, 31,* 382–390.

Akbarian, S., & Nestler, E. J. (Eds.). (2013). Epigenetic mechanisms in psychiatry [Special issue]. *Neuropsychopharmacology, 38*(1).

Alarcón, J. M., Malleret, G., Touzani, K., Vronskaya, S., Ishii, S., Kandel, E. R., & Barco, A. (2004). Chromatin acetylation, memory, and LTP are impaired in CBP$^{+/-}$ mice: A model for the cognitive deficit in Rubinstein-Taybi syndrome and its amelioration. *Neuron, 42,* 947–959.

Albert, P. R. (2010). Epigenetics in mental illness: Hope or hype? *Journal of Psychiatry and Neuroscience, 35,* 366–368.

Albright, C. D., Tsai, A. Y., Friedrich, C. B., Mar, M.-H., & Zeisel, S. H. (1999). Choline availability alters embryonic development of the hippocampus and septum in the rat. *Developmental Brain Research, 113,* 13–20.

Alvarado, S., Fernald, R. D., Storey, K. B., & Szyf, M. (2014). The dynamic nature of DNA methylation: A role in response to social and seasonal variation. *Integrative and Comparative Biology, 54,* 68–76.

Alvarez-Breckenridge, C. A., Yu, J., Price, R., Wei, M., Wang, Y., Nowicki, M. O., . . . Chiocca, E. A. (2012). The histone deacetylase inhibitor valproic acid lessens NK cell action against oncolytic virus-infected glioblastoma cells by inhibition of STAT5/T-BET signaling and generation of gamma interferon. *Journal of Virology, 86,* 4566–4577.

Amara, S. G., Jonas, V., Rosenfeld, M. B., Ong, E. S., & Evans, R. M. (1982). Alternative RNA processing in calcitonin gene expression generates mRNAs encoding different polypeptide products. *Nature, 298,* 240–244.

Anand, P., Kunnumakara, A. B., Sundaram, C., Harikumar, K. B., Tharakan, S. T., Lai, O. S., . . . Aggarwal, B. B. (2008). Cancer is a preventable disease that requires major lifestyle changes. *Pharmaceutical Research, 25,* 2097–2116.

Anderson, L. M., Riffle, L., Wilson, R., Travlos, G. S., Lubomirski, M. S., & Alvord, W. G. (2006). Preconceptional fasting of fathers alters serum glucose in offspring of mice. *Nutrition, 22,* 327–331.

Anderson, O. S., Sant, K. E., & Dolinoy, D. C. (2012). Nutrition and epigenetics: An interplay of dietary methyl donors, one-carbon metabolism and DNA methylation. *Journal of Nutritional Biochemistry, 23,* 853–859.

Ansorge, M. S., Zhou, M., Lira, A., Hen, R., & Gingrich, J. A. (2004). Early-life blockade of the 5-HT transporter alters emotional behavior in adult mice. *Science, 306*, 879–881.

Anway, M. D., Cupp, A. S., Uzumcu, M., & Skinner, M. K. (2005). Epigenetic transgenerational actions of endocrine disruptors and male fertility. *Science, 308*, 1466–1469.

Aspinwall, L. G., Brown, T. R., & Tabery, J. (2012). The double-edged sword: Does biomechanism increase or decrease judges' sentencing of psychopaths? *Science, 337*, 846–849.

Asprey, L., & Asprey, D. (2013). *The better baby book: How to have a healthier, smarter, happier baby.* New York: Wiley.

Atkinson, R. C., & Shiffrin, R. M. (1968). Human memory: A proposed system and its control processes. In K. W. Spence, (Ed.), *The psychology of learning and motivation: Advances in research and theory* (pp. 89–195). New York, NY: Academic Press.

Avital, E., & Jablonka, E. (2000). *Animal traditions: Behavioural inheritance in evolution.* New Cambridge, England: Cambridge University Press.

Bailey, C. H., & Chen, M. (1988). Long-term memory in *Aplysia* modulates the total number of varicosities of single identified sensory neurons. *Proceedings of the National Academy of Sciences USA, 85*, 2373–2377.

Ballantyne, C. (2007, October 24). Fact or fiction? Stress causes gray hair. *Scientific American.* Retrieved from http://www.scientificamerican.com

Baranzini, S. E., Mudge, J., van Velkinburgh, J. C., Khankhanian, P., Khrebtukova, I., Miller, N. A., . . . Kingsmore, S. F. (2010). Genome, epigenome and RNA sequences of monozygotic twins discordant for multiple sclerosis. *Nature, 464*, 1351–1356.

Barker, D. J. P. (1992). The fetal origins of diseases of old age. *European Journal of Clinical Nutrition, 46*, S3–S9.

Barker, D. J. P. (2004). The developmental origins of adult disease. *Journal of the American College of Nutrition, 23*, 588S–595S.

Barker, D. J. P., & Clark, P. M. (1997). Fetal undernutrition and disease in later life. *Reviews of Reproduction, 2*, 105–112.

Barker, G. (1993). Models of biological change: Implications of three studies of "Lamarckian" change. In P. P. G. Bateson, P. H. Klopfer, & N. S. Thompson (Eds.), *Perspectives in ethology (Vol. 10): Behavior and evolution* (pp. 229–248). New York: Plenum Press.

Baron, D. (2000, February 11). *Clones may not be identical* [Audio podcast]. Retrieved from http://www.npr.org/templates/story/story.php?storyId=1070242

Bateson, P., & Gluckman, P. (2011). *Plasticity, robustness, development and evolution.* Cambridge, England: Cambridge University Press.

Beach, F. A. (1955). The descent of instinct. *Psychological Review, 62*, 401–410.

Beach, S. R. H., Brody, G. H., Todorov, A. A., Gunter, T. D., & Philibert, R. A. (2010). Methylation at SLC6A4 is linked to family history of child abuse: An examination of the Iowa adoptee sample. *American Journal of Medical Genetics Part B, 153B*, 710–713.

Begley, S. (2010, October 30). Sins of the grandfathers. *Newsweek Magazine.* Retrieved from http://www.thedailybeast.com/newsweek/2010/10/30/how-your-experiences-change-your-sperm-and-eggs.html

Behe, M. J. (1996). *Darwin's black box.* New York: Free Press.

Benyshek, D. C., Johnston, C. S., & Martin, J. F. (2006). Glucose metabolism is altered in the adequately-nourished grand-offspring (F_3 generation) of rats malnourished during gestation and perinatal life. *Dibetologia, 49*, 1117–1119.

Berger, S. L. (2007). The complex language of chromatin regulation during transcription. *Nature, 447*, 407–412.

Berget, S. M., Moore, C., and Sharp, P. A. (1977). Spliced segments at the 5' terminus of adenovirus 2 late mRNA. *Proceedings of the National Academy of Sciences USA, 74*, 3171–3175.

Bernal, A. J., & Jirtle, R. L. (2010). Epigenomic disruption: The effects of early developmental exposures. *Birth Defects Research (Part A), 88*, 938–944.

Beutler, E., Yeh, M., & Fairbanks, V. F. (1962). The normal human female as a mosaic of X-chromosome activity: Studies using the gene for G-6-PD deficiency as a marker. *Proceedings of the National Academy of Sciences of the USA, 48*, 9–16.

Bjornsson, H. T., Sigurdsson, M. I., Fallin, M. D., Irizarry, R. A., Aspelund, T., Cui, H., . . . Feinberg, A. P. (2008). Intra-individual change over time in DNA methylation with familial clustering. *Journal of the American Medical Association, 299*, 2877–2883.

Blech, J. (2010, August 9). Der sieg über die gene: Das gedächtnis des körpers [Victory over the genes: The memory of the body]. *Der Spiegel*. Retrieved from http://www.spiegel.de/spiegel/print/d-73109479.html

Blewitt, M. E., Vickaryous, N. K., Paldi, A., Koseki, H., & Whitelaw, E. (2006). Dynamic reprogramming of DNA methylation at an epigenetically sensitive allele in mice. *PLoS Genetics, 2*(4), e49. doi:10.1371/journal.pgen.0020049

Blumberg, M. S. (2005). *Basic instinct: The genesis of behavior*. New York: Thunder's Mouth Press.

Boks, M. P., Derks, E. M., Weisenberger, D. J., Strengman, E., Janson, E., Sommer, I. E., . . . Ophoff, R. A. (2009). The relationship of DNA methylation with age, gender and genotype in twins and healthy controls. *PLoS ONE, 4*(8), e6767. doi:10.1371/journal.pone.0006767

Bönsch, D., Lenz, B., Reulbach, U., Kornhuber, J., & Bleich, S. (2004). Homocysteine associated genomic DNA hypermethylation in patients with chronic alcoholism. *Journal of Neural Transmission, 111*, 1611–1616.

Borghol, N., Suderman, M., McArdle, W., Racine, A., Hallett, M., Pembrey, M., . . . Szyf, M. (2012). Associations with early-life socio-economic position in adult DNA methylation. *International Journal of Epidemiology, 41*, 62–74.

Borrelli, E., Nestler, E. J., Allis, C. D., & Sassone-Corsi, P. (2008). Decoding the epigenetic language of neuronal plasticity. *Neuron, 60*, 961–974.

Branchi, I., D'Andrea, I., Fiore, M., Di Fausto, V., Aloe, L., & Alleva, E. (2006). Early social enrichment shapes social behavior and nerve growth factor and brain-derived neurotrophic factor levels in the adult mouse brain. *Biological Psychiatry, 60*, 690–696.

Branchi, I., Karpova, N. N., D'Andrea, I., Castrén, E., & Alleva, E. (2011). Epigenetic modifications induced by early enrichment are associated with changes in timing of induction of BDNF expression. *Neuroscience Letters, 495*, 168–172.

Bredy, T. W., Wu, H., Crego, C., Zellhoefer, J., Sun, Y. E., & Barad, M. (2007). Histone modifications around individual BDNF gene promoters in prefrontal cortex are associated with extinction of conditioned fear. *Learning and Memory, 14*, 268–276.

Brena, R. M., Huang, T. H-M., & Plass, C. (2006). Toward a human epigenome. *Nature Genetics, 38*, 1359–1360.

Brown, C. J., Ballabio, A., Rupert, J. L., Lafreniere, R. G., Grompe, M., Tonlorenzi, R., & Willard, H. F. (1991). A gene from the region of the human X inactivation centre is expressed exclusively from the inactive X chromosome. *Nature, 349*, 38–44.

Buchen, L. (2010). In their nurture. *Nature, 467*, 146–148.

Buckingham, J. C. (2006). Glucocorticoids: Exemplars of multi-tasking. *British Journal of Pharmacology, 147*, S258–S268.

Buxton, J. L., Suderman, M., Pappas, J. J., Borghol, N., McArdle, W., Blakemore, A. I. F., . . . Pembrey, M. (2014). Human leukocyte telomere length is associated with DNA methylation levels in multiple subtelomeric and imprinted loci. *Scientific Reports, 4*, 4954. doi:10.1038/srep04954

Byrnes, J. J., Johnson, N. L., Carini, L. M., & Byrnes, E. M. (2013). Multigenerational effects of adolescent morphine exposure on dopamine D2 receptor function. *Psychopharmacology, 227*, 263–272.

Calafat, A. M., Kuklenyik, Z., Reidy, J. A., Caudill, S. P., Ekong, J., & Needham, L. L. (2005). Urinary concentrations of bisphenol A and 4-nonylphenol in a human reference population. *Environmental Health Perspectives, 113*, 391–395.

References

Caldji, C., Tannenbaum, B., Sharma, S., Francis, D., Plotsky, P. M., & Meaney, M. J. (1998). Maternal care during infancy regulates the development of neural systems mediating the expression of fearfulness in the rat. *Proceedings of the National Academy of Sciences of the USA, 95,* 5335–5340.

Campbell, I. C., Mill, J., Uher, R., & Schmidt, U. (2011). Eating disorders, gene–environment interactions and epigenetics. *Neuroscience and Biobehavioral Reviews, 35,* 784–793.

Canli, T., Qiu, M., Omura, K., Congdon, E., Haas, B. W., Amin, Z., . . . Lesch, K. P. (2006). Neural correlates of epigenesis. *Proceedings of the National Academy of Sciences USA, 103,* 16033–16038.

Cardno, A. G., & Gottesman, I. I. (2000). Twin studies of schizophrenia: From bow-and-arrow concordances to star wars Mx and functional genomics. *American Journal of Medical Genetics, 97,* 12–17.

Carey, N. (2011). *The epigenetics revolution.* London, England: Icon Books.

Carone, B. R., Fauquier, L., Habib, N., Shea, J. M., Hart, C. E., Li, R., . . . Rando, O. J. (2010). Paternally induced transgenerational environmental reprogramming of metabolic gene expression in mammals. *Cell, 143,* 1084–1096.

Carvajal, D. (2012, August 17). On the trail of inherited memories. *New York Times.*

Cary, J. (1944). *The horse's mouth.* New York: Harper & Brothers.

Cassidy, S. B. (1997). Prader-Willi syndrome. *Journal of Medical Genetics, 34,* 917–923.

Castellucci, V. F., Blumenfeld, H., Goelet, P., Kandel, E. R. (1989). Inhibitor of protein synthesis blocks longterm behavioral sensitization in the isolated gill-withdrawal reflex of *Aplysia. Journal of Neurobiology, 20,* 1–9.

Castéra, J., Abrougui, M., Nisiforou, O., Turcinaviciene, J., Sarapuu, T., Agorram, B., Calado, F., & Carvalho, G. (2008). Genetic determinism in school textbooks: A comparative study conducted among sixteen countries. *Science Education International, 19,* 163–184.

Cattanach, B. M., & Isaacson, J. H. (1967). Controlling elements in the mouse X chromosome. *Genetics, 57,* 331–346.

Champagne, F. A. (2008). Epigenetic mechanisms and the transgenerational effects of maternal care. *Frontiers in Neuroendocrinology, 29,* 386–397.

Champagne, F. A. (2013). Epigenetics and developmental plasticity across species. *Developmental Psychobiology, 55,* 31–41.

Champagne, F. A., Weaver, I. C. G., Diorio, J., Dymov, S., Szyf, M., & Meaney, M. J. (2006). Maternal care associated with methylation of the estrogen receptor-α1b promoter and estrogen receptor-α expression in the medial preoptic area of female offspring. *Endocrinology, 147,* 2909–2915.

Cheatham, C. L., Goldman, B. D., Fischer, L. M., do Costa, K-A., Reznick, J. S., & Zeisel, S. H. (2012). Phosphatidylcholine supplementation in pregnant women consuming moderate-choline diets does not enhance infant cognitive function: A randomized, double-blind, placebo-controlled trial. *American Journal of Clinical Nutrition, 96,* 1465–1472.

Chen, T. H.-H., Chiu, Y.-H., & Boucher, B. J. (2006). Transgenerational effects of betel-quid chewing on the development of the metabolic syndrome in the Keelung Community-based Integrated Screening Program. *American Journal of Clinical Nutrition, 83,* 688–692.

Cheng, M. K., & Disteche, C. M. (2004). Silence of the fathers: Early X inactivation. *BioEssays, 26,* 821–824.

Choi, S.-W., & Friso, S. (2010). Epigenetics: A new bridge between nutrition and health. *Advances in Nutrition, 1,* 8–16.

Choi, J. D., & Lee, J.-S. (2013). Interplay between epigenetics and genetics in cancer. *Genomics and Informatics, 11,* 164–173.

Chow, L. T., Gelinas, R. E., Broker, T. R., & Roberts, R. J. (1977). An amazing sequence arrangement at the 5′ ends of adenovirus 2 messenger RNA. *Cell, 12,* 1–8.

Christensen, B. C., Houseman, E. A., Marsit, C. J., Zheng, S., Wrensch, M. R., Wiemels, J. L., . . . Kelsey, K. T. (2009). Aging and environmental exposures alter tissue-specific DNA methylation dependent upon CpG island context. *PLoS Genetics, 5*(8), e1000602. doi:10.1371/journal.pgen.1000602

Chrousos, G. P. (2009). Stress and disorders of the stress system. *Nature Reviews: Endocrinology, 5*, 374–381.

Chrousos, G. P., Schuermeyer, T. H., Doppman, J., Oldfield, E. H., Schulte, H. M., Gold, P. W., & Loriaux, D. L. (1985). NIH conference: Clinical applications of corticotropin-releasing factor. *Annals of Internal Medicine, 102*, 344–358.

Clayman, C. B. (Ed.). (1989). *American Medical Association Encyclopedia of Medicine.* New York: Random House.

Clayton, D. F. (2000). The genomic action potential. *Neurobiology of Learning and Memory, 74*, 185–216.

Cloud, J. (2010, January 6). Why your DNA isn't your destiny. *Time Magazine.* Retrieved from www.time.com/time/magazine/

Cole, M., & Cole, S. R. (1993). *The development of children* (2nd ed.). New York: Freeman.

Cole, S. W., Hawkley, L. C., Arevalo, J. M., Sung. C. Y., Rose, R. M., & Cacioppo, J. T. (2007). Social regulation of gene expression in human leukocytes. *Genome Biology, 8*, R189.

Connolly, J. J., Glessner, J. T., & Hakonarson, H. (2013). A genome-wide association study of autism incorporating autism diagnostic interview–revised, autism diagnostic observation schedule, and social responsiveness scale. *Child Development, 84*, 17–33.

Coplan, J. D., Andrews, M. W., Rosenblum, L. A., Owens, M. J., Friedman, S., Gorman, J. M., & Nemeroff, C. B. (1996). Persistent elevations of cerebrospinal fluid concentrations of corticotropin-releasing factor in adult nonhuman primates exposed to early-life stressors: Implications for the pathophysiology of mood and anxiety disorders. *Proceedings of the National Academy of Sciences of the USA, 93*, 1619–1623.

Covington, H. E. III, Maze, I., LaPlant, Q. C., Vialou, V. F., Ohnishi, Y. N., Berton, O., . . . Nestler, E. J. (2009). Antidepressant actions of histone deacetylase inhibitors. *Journal of Neuroscience, 29*, 11451–11460.

Coyne, J. A. (2009). Evolution's challenge to genetics. *Nature, 457*, 382–383.

Craciunescu, C. N., Albright, C. D., Mar, M.-H., Song, J., & Zeisel, S. H. (2003). Choline availability during embryonic development alters progenitor cell mitosis in developing mouse hippocampus. *Journal of Nutrition, 133*, 3614–3618.

Crews, D. (2010). Epigenetics, brain, behavior, and the environment. *Hormones, 9*, 41–50.

Crews, D., Gore, A. C., Hsu, T. S., Dangleben, N. L., Spinetta, M., Schallert, T., . . . Skinner, M. K. (2007). Transgenerational epigenetic imprints on mate preference. *Proceedings of the National Academy of Sciences of the USA, 104*, 5942–5946.

Cropley, J. E., Dang, T. H. Y., Martin, D. I. K., & Suter, C. M. (2012). The penetrance of an epigenetic trait in mice is progressively yet reversibly increased by selection and environment. *Proceedings of the Royal Society B, 279*, 2347–2353.

Cropley, J. E., Suter, C. M., Beckman, K. B., & Martin, D. I. K. (2006). Germ-line epigenetic modification of the murine A^{vy} allele by nutritional supplementation. *Proceedings of the National Academy of Sciences of the USA, 103*, 17308–17312.

Cruz, J. C., Tseng, H.-C., Goldman, J. A., Shih, H., & Tsai, L.-H. (2003). Aberrant Cdk5 activation by p25 triggers pathological events leading to neurodegeneration and neurofibrillary tangles. *Neuron, 40*, 471–483.

Cubas, P., Vincent, C., & Coen, E. (1999). An epigenetic mutation responsible for natural variation in floral symmetry. *Nature, 401*, 157–161.

Curley, J. P., Jensen, C. L., Mashoodh, R., & Champagne, F. A. (2011). Social influences on neurobiology and behavior: Epigenetic effects during development. *Psychoneuroendocrinology, 36*, 352–371.

Curtiss, S. (1977). *Genie: A psycholinguistic study of a modern-day "wild child."* Boston, MA: Academic Press.

Danchin, É., Charmantier, A., Champagne, F. A., Mesoudi, A., Pujol, B., & Blanchet, S. (2011). Beyond DNA: Integrating inclusive inheritance into an extended theory of evolution. *Nature Reviews: Genetics, 12*, 475–486.

Darwin, C. (1859/1991). *On the origin of species by means of natural selection.* Amherst, NY: Prometheus Books.

Dashwood, R. H., & Ho, E. (2007). Dietary histone deacetylase inhibitors: From cells to mice to man. *Seminars in Cancer Biology, 17*, 363–369.

Davenport, M. H., & Cabrero, M. R. (2009). Maternal nutritional history predicts obesity in adult offspring independent of postnatal diet. *Journal of Physiology, 587*, 3423–3424.

Dawkins, R. (1987). *The blind watchmaker.* New York: Norton.

Dawkins, R. (1999). *The extended phenotype: The long reach of the gene* (Rev. ed.). Oxford, England: Oxford University Press.

Dawkins, R. (2004). *The ancestor's tale: A pilgrimage to the dawn of evolution.* New York: Houghton Mifflin.

Daxinger, L., & Whitelaw, E. (2010). Transgenerational epigenetic inheritance: More questions than answers. *Genome Research, 20*, 1623–1628.

Daxinger, L., & Whitelaw, E. (2012). Understanding transgenerational epigenetic inheritance via the gametes in mammals. *Nature Reviews: Genetics, 13*, 153–162.

Day, J. J., & Sweatt, J. D. (2010). DNA methylation and memory formation. *Nature Neuroscience, 13*, 1319–1323.

Day, J. J., & Sweatt, J. D. (2011). Epigenetic mechanisms in cognition. *Neuron, 70*, 813–829.

Dębiec, J., Doyère, V., Nader, K., & LeDoux, J. E. (2006). Directly reactivated, but not indirectly reactivated, memories undergo reconsolidation in the amygdala. *Proceedings of the National Academy of Sciences of the USA, 102*, 3428–3433.

DeCasper, A. J., & Fifer, W. P. (1980). Of human bonding: Newborns prefer their mothers' voices. *Science, 208*, 1174–1176.

DeCasper, A. J., & Spence, M. J. (1986). Prenatal maternal speech influences newborns' perception of speech sound. *Infant Behavior and Development, 9*, 133–150.

De Grey, A., & Rae, M. (2007). *Ending aging: The rejuvenation breakthroughs that could reverse human aging in our lifetime.* New York: St. Martin's Press.

Dempster, E. L., Pidsley, R., Schalkwyk, L. C., Owens, S., Georgiades, A., Kane, F., . . . Mill, J. (2011). Disease-associated epigenetic changes in monozygotic twins discordant for schizophrenia and bipolar disorder. *Human Molecular Genetics, 20*, 4786–4796.

Devlin, A. M., Brain, U., Austin, J., & Oberlander, T. F. (2010). Prenatal exposure to maternal depressed mood and the *MTHFR* C677T variant affect *SLC6A4* methylation in infants at birth. *PLoS ONE, 5*(8), e12201. doi:10.1371/journal.pone.0012201

Dewsbury, D. A. (1991). Psychobiology. *American Psychologist, 46*, 198–205.

Dias, B. G., & Ressler, K. J. (2014). Parental olfactory experience influences behavior and neural structure in subsequent generations. *Nature Neuroscience, 17*, 89–96.

Diego, M. A., Field, T., & Hernandez-Reif, M. (2009). Procedural pain heart rate responses in massaged preterm infants. *Infant Behavior and Development, 32*, 226–229.

Dimsdale, J. E. (2008). Psychological stress and cardiovascular disease. *Journal of the American College of Cardiology, 51*, 1237–1246.

Dinger, M. E., Pang, K. C., Mercer, T. R., & Mattick, J. S. (2008). Differentiating protein-coding and noncoding RNA: Challenges and ambiguities. *PLoS Computational Biology, 4*, 1–5 (e1000176).

Dobzhansky, T. (1937). *Genetics and the origin of species.* New York: Columbia University Press.

Dolinoy, D. C., Huang, D., & Jirtle, R. L. (2007). Maternal nutrient supplementation counteracts bisphenol A-induced DNA hypomethylation in early development. *Proceedings of the National Academy of Sciences of the USA, 104*, 13056–13061.

dos Santos, V. C., Joaquim, L. M., & El-Hani, C. N. (2012). Hybrid deterministic views about genes in biology textbooks: A key problem in genetics teaching. *Science and Education, 21*, 543–578. doi:10.1007/s11191-011-9348-1

Dowd, M. (2013, May 14). Cascading confessions. *New York Times.*

Doyère, V., Dębiec, J., Monfils, M., Schafe, G. E., & LeDoux, J. E. (2007). Synapse-specific reconsolidation of distinct fear memories in the lateral amygdala. *Nature Neuroscience, 10*, 414–416.

Driesch, H. A. E. (1910). Physiology of development. In *The Encyclopaedia Britannica*, (11th ed., Vol. 9, pp. 329–331). London, England: Cambridge University Press.

Duhl, D. M. J., Vrieling, H., Miller, K. A., Wolff, G. L., & Barsh, G. S. (1994). Neomorphic *agouti* mutations in obese yellow mice. *Nature Genetics, 8*, 59–65.

Dulac, C. (2010). Brain function and chromatin plasticity. *Nature, 465*, 728–735.

Dunn, G. A., & Bale, T. L. (2011). Maternal high-fat diet effects on third-generation female body size via the paternal lineage. *Endocrinology, 152*, 2228–2236.

Eckhardt, F., Lewin, J., Cortese, R., Rakyan, V. K., Attwood, J., Burger, M., . . . Beck, S. (2006). DNA methylation profiling of human chromosomes 6, 20 and 22. *Nature Genetics, 38*, 1378–1385.

Ellegren, H., & Sheldon, B. C. (2008). Genetic basis of fitness differences in natural populations. *Nature, 452*, 169–175.

Elliott, E., Ezra-Nevo, G., Regev, L., Neufeld-Cohen, A., & Chen, A. (2010). Resilience to social stress coincides with functional DNA methylation of the *Crf* gene in adult mice. *Nature Neuroscience, 13*, 1351–1353.

Ellis, E. C. (2013, September 13). Overpopulation is not the problem. *New York Times.*

Essex, M. J., Boyce, W. T., Hertzman, C., Lam, L. L., Armstrong, J. M., Neumann, S. M. A., & Kobor, M. S. (2013). Epigenetic vestiges of early developmental adversity: Childhood stress exposure and DNA methylation in adolescence. *Child Development, 84*, 58–75.

Evans, J. D., & Wheeler, D. E. (2001). Gene expression and the evolution of insect polyphenisms. *BioEssays, 23*, 62–68.

Eyer, D. E. (1992). *Mother-infant bonding: A scientific fiction.* New Haven, CT: Yale University Press.

Faghihi, M. A., Modarresi, F., Khalil, A. M., Wood, D. E., Sahagan, B. G., Morgan, T., . . . Wahlestedt, C. (2008). Expression of a noncoding RNA is elevated in Alzheimer's disease and drives rapid feed-forward regulation of β-secretase. *Nature Medicine, 14*, 723–730.

Feinberg, A. P. (2007). Phenotypic plasticity and the epigenetics of human disease. *Nature, 447*, 433–440.

Feinberg, A. P. (2008). Epigenetics at the epicenter of modern medicine. *Journal of the American Medical Association, 299*, 1345–1350.

Feinberg, A. P., Ohlsson, R., & Henikoff, S. (2006). The epigenetic progenitor origin of human cancer. *Nature Reviews: Genetics, 7*, 21–33.

Fiering, S., Whitelaw, E., & Martin, D. I. K. (2000). To be or not to be active: The stochastic nature of enhancer action. *BioEssays, 22*, 381–387.

Fischer, A., Sananbenesi, F., Wang, X., Dobbin, M., & Tsai, L.-H. (2007). Recovery of learning and memory is associated with chromatin remodeling. *Nature, 447*, 178–182.

Fisher, S. E. (2006). Tangled webs: Tracing the connections between genes and cognition. *Cognition, 101*, 270–297.

Flanagan, J. M., Popendikyte, V., Pozdniakovaite, N., Sobolev, M., Assadzadeh, A., Schumacher, A., . . . Petronis, A. (2006). Intra- and interindividual epigenetic variation in human germ cells. *American Journal of Human Genetics, 79*, 67–84.

Flexner, L. B., & Flexner, J. B. (1966). Effect of acetoxycycloheximide and of an acetoxycycloheximide-puromycin mixture on cerebral protein synthesis and memory in mice. *Proceedings of the National Academy of Sciences of the USA, 55*, 369–374.

Ford, D. H., & Lerner, R. M. (1992). *Developmental systems theory: An integrative approach.* Thousand Oaks, CA: Sage.

Fraga, M. F., Ballestar, E., Paz, M. F., Ropero, S., Setien, F., Ballestar, M. L., . . . Esteller, M. (2005). Epigenetic differences arise during the lifetime of monozygotic twins. *Proceedings of the National Academy of Sciences of the USA, 102,* 10604–10609.

Francis, D. D., Caldji, C., Champagne, F., Plotsky, P. M., & Meaney, M. J. (1999a). The role of corticotropin-releasing factor—norepinephrine systems in mediating the effects of early experience on the development of behavioral and endocrine responses to stress. *Biological Psychiatry, 46,* 1153–1166.

Francis, D., Diorio, J., Liu, D., & Meaney, M. J. (1999b). Nongenomic transmission across generations of maternal behavior and stress responses in the rat. *Science, 286,* 1155–1158.

Francis, R. C. (2011). *Epigenetics: The ultimate mystery of inheritance.* New York: Norton.

Frank, D. N., & Pace, N. R. (2008). Gastrointestinal microbiology enters the metagenomics era. *Current Opinion in Gastroenterology, 24,* 4–10.

Franklin, T. B., & Mansuy, I. M. (2010). Epigenetic inheritance in mammals: Evidence for the impact of adverse environmental effects. *Neurobiology of Disease, 39,* 61–65.

Franklin, T. B., Russig, H., Weiss, I. C., Graff, J., Linder, N., Michalon, A., . . . Mansuy, I. M. (2010). Epigenetic transmission of the impact of early stress across generations. *Biological Psychiatry, 68,* 408–415.

Fredrickson, B. L., Grewen, K. M., Coffey, K. A., Algoe, S. B., Firestine, A. M., Arevalo, J. M. G., . . . Cole, S. W. (2013). A functional genomic perspective on human well-being. *Proceedings of the National Academy of Sciences USA, 110,* 13684–13689.

Friedman, R. A. (2002, August 27). Like drugs, talk therapy can change brain chemistry. *New York Times.*

Gallagher, J. (2013, July 19). Pioneering adult stem cell trial approved by Japan. *BBC News.* Retrieved from http://www.bbc.co.uk/news/health-23374622

Gallou-Kabani, C., Vigé, A., Gross, M.-S., & Junien, C. (2007). Nutri-epigenomics: Lifelong remodelling of our epigenomes by nutritional and metabolic factors and beyond. *Clinical Chemistry and Laboratory Medicine, 45,* 321–327.

Gaudet, F., Hodgson, J. G., Eden, A., Jackson-Grusby, L., Dausman, J., Gray, J. W., . . . Jaenisch, R. (2003). Induction of tumors in mice by genomic hypomethylation. *Science, 300,* 489–492.

Geda, Y. E., Roberts, R. O., Knopman, D. S., Christianson, T. J. H., Pankratz, V. S., Ivnik, R. J., . . . Rocca, W. A. (2010). Physical exercise and mild cognitive impairment: A population-based study. *Archives of Neurology, 67,* 80–86.

Genetic Science Learning Center. (2012, August 6). Are Telomeres the Key to Aging and Cancer? *Learn.Genetics.* Retrieved January 9, 2013, from http://learn.genetics.utah.edu/content/begin/traits/telomeres/

Gericke, N. M., & Hagberg, M. (2010). Conceptual variation in the depiction of gene function in upper secondary school textbooks. *Science and Education, 19,* 963–994.

Gerstein, M. B., Bruce, C., Rozowsky, J. S., Zheng, D., Du, J., Korbel, J. O., . . . Snyder, M. (2007). What is a gene, post-ENCODE? History and updated definition. *Genome Research, 17,* 669–681.

Gibbs, W. W. (2003). The unseen genome: Beyond DNA. *Scientific American, 289*(6), 106–113.

Gilbert, S. F. (2000). *Developmental biology* (6th ed.). Sunderland, MA: Sinauer Associates.

Gilbert, S. F. (2001). Ecological developmental biology: Developmental biology meets the real world. *Developmental Biology, 233,* 1–12.

Gilbert, S. F. (2005). Mechanisms for the environmental regulation of gene expression: Ecological aspects of animal development. *Journal of Biosciences, 30,* 65–74.

Gilbert, W. (1978). Why genes in pieces? *Nature, 271,* 501.

Glaser, R., Kennedy, S., Lafuse, W. P., Bonneau, R. H., Speicher, C., Hillhouse, J., & Kiecolt-Glaser, J. K. (1990). Psychological stress-induced modulation of interleukin 2 receptor gene expression and interleukin 2 production in peripheral blood leukocytes. *Archives of General Psychiatry, 47,* 707–712.

Glaser, R., Rice, J., Sheridan, J., Fertel, R., Stout, J., Speicher, C., . . . Kiecolt-Glaser, J. (1987). Stress-related immune suppression: Health implications. *Brain, Behavior, and Immunity, 1,* 7–20.

Globisch, D., Münzel, M., Müller, M., Michalakis, S., Wagner, M., Koch, S., . . . Carell, T. (2010). Tissue distribution of 5-hydroxymethylcytosine and search for active demethylation intermediates. *PLoS ONE, 5*(12), e15367. doi:10.1371/journal.pone.0015367

Gluckman, P. D., Hanson, M. A., & Beedle, A. S. (2007). Non-genomic transgenerational inheritance of disease risk. *BioEssays, 29,* 145–154.

Gluckman, P. D., Hanson, M. A., & Buklijas, T. (2010). A conceptual framework for the developmental origins of health and disease. *Journal of Developmental Origins of Health and Disease, 1,* 6–18.

Gluckman, P. D., Lillycrop, K. A., Vickers, M. H., Pleasants, A. B., Phillips, E. S., Beedle, A. S., . . . Hanson, M. A. (2007). Metabolic plasticity during mammalian development is directionally dependent on early nutritional status. *Proceedings of the National Academy of Sciences USA, 104,* 12796–12800.

Gokhman, D., Lavi, E., Prüfer, K., Fraga, M. F., Riancho, J. A., Kelso, J., . . . Carmel, L. (2014). Reconstructing the DNA methylation maps of the Neandertal and the Denisovan. *Science, 344,* 523–527.

Gomase, V. S., & Tagore, S. (2008). Epigenomics. *Current Drug Metabolism, 9,* 232–237.

Gomez-Pinilla, F., Zhuang, Y., Feng, J., Ying, Z., & Fan, G. (2011). Exercise impacts brain-derived neurotrophic factor plasticity by engaging mechanisms of epigenetic regulation. *European Journal of Neuroscience, 33,* 383–390.

González-Pardo, H., & Álvarez, M. P. (2013). Epigenetics and its implications for psychology. *Psicothema, 25,* 3–12.

Gordon, L., Joo, J. E., Powell, J. E., Ollikainen, M., Novakovic, B., Li, X., . . . Saffery, R. (2012). Neonatal DNA methylation profile in human twins is specified by a complex interplay between intrauterine environmental and genetic factors, subject to tissue-specific influence. *Genome Research, 22,* 1395–1406.

Gore, A. C., Balthazart, J., Bikle, D. D., Carpenter, D. O., Crews, D., Czernichow, P., . . . Watson, C. S. (2013). Policy decisions on endocrine disruptors should be based on science across disciplines: A response to Dietrich et al. *Endocrine Disruptors, 1,* e26644. doi:10.4161/endo.26644

Gottlieb, G. (1991). Experiential canalization of behavioral development: Theory. *Developmental Psychology, 27,* 4–13.

Gottlieb, G. (1992). *Individual development and evolution: The genesis of novel behavior.* New York: Oxford University Press.

Gottlieb, G. (1997). *Synthesizing nature-nurture: Prenatal roots of instinctive behavior.* Mahwah, NJ: Erlbaum.

Gottlieb, G. (1998). Normally occurring environmental and behavioral influences on gene activity: From central dogma to probabilistic epigenesis. *Psychological Review, 105,* 792–802.

Gottlieb, G. (2007). Probabilistic epigenesis. *Developmental Science, 10,* 1–11.

Gottlieb, G., & Lickliter, R. (2004). The various roles of animal models in understanding human development. *Social Development, 13,* 311–325.

Gould, S. J. (1977). *Ontogeny and phylogeny.* Cambridge, MA: Belknap Press of Harvard University Press.

Gould, S. J. (1980). *The panda's thumb: More reflections in natural history.* New York: Norton.

Gould, S. J., & Vrba, E. S. (1982). Exaptation—A missing term in the science of form. *Paleobiology, 8,* 4–15.

Grady, D., Parker-Pope, T., & Belluck, P. (2013, May 14). Jolie's disclosure of preventive mastectomy highlights dilemma. *New York Times.*

Gräff, J., Rei, D., Guan, J.-S., Wang, W.-Y., Seo, J., Hennig, K. M., . . . Tsai, L.-H. (2012). An epigenetic blockade of cognitive functions in the neurodegenerating brain. *Nature, 483,* 222–226.

Gräff, J., & Tsai, L.-H. (2013). The potential of HDAC inhibitors as cognitive enhancers. *Annual Review of Pharmacology and Toxicology, 53,* 311–330.

Granado, M., Fuente-Martín, E., García-Cáceres, C., Argente, J., & Chowen, J. A. (2012). Leptin in early life: A key factor for the development of the adult metabolic profile. *Obesity Facts, 5,* 138–150.

Grayson, D. R., Kundakovic, M., & Sharma, R. P. (2010). Is there a future for histone deacetylase inhibitors in the pharmacotherapy of psychiatric disorders? *Molecular Pharmacology, 77,* 126–135.

Gregg, C., Zhang, J., Weissbourd, B., Luo, S., Schroth, G. P., Haig, D., & Dulac, C. (2010). High-resolution analysis of parent-of-origin allelic expression in the mouse brain. *Science, 329,* 643–648.

Griffiths, P. E., & Gray, R. D. (1994). Developmental systems and evolutionary explanation. *Journal of Philosophy, XCI,* 277–304.

Griffiths, P. E., & Neumann-Held, E. M. (1999). The many faces of the gene. *BioScience, 49,* 656–662.

Griffiths, P. E., & Tabery, J. (2008). Behavioral genetics and development: Historical and conceptual causes of controversy. *New Ideas in Psychology, 26,* 332–352.

Groleau, P., Joober, R., Israel, M., Zeramdini, N., DeGuzman, R., & Steiger, H. (2014). Methylation of the dopamine D2 receptor (DRD2) gene promoter in women with a bulimia-spectrum disorder: Associations with borderline personality disorder and exposure to childhood abuse. *Journal of Psychiatric Research, 48,* 121–127.

Guan, J.-S., Haggarty, S. J., Giacometti, E., Dannenberg, J.-H., Joseph, N., Gao, J., . . . Tsai, L.-H. (2009). HDAC2 negatively regulates memory formation and synaptic plasticity. *Nature, 459,* 55–60.

Guan, Z., Giustetto, M., Lomvardas, S., Kim, J.-H., Miniaci, M. C., Schwartz, J. H., . . . Kandel, E. R. (2002). Integration of long-term-memory-related synaptic plasticity involves bidirectional regulation of gene expression and chromatin structure. *Cell, 111,* 483–493.

Guillemin, C., Provençal, N., Suderman, M., Côte, S. M., Vitaro, F., Hallett, M., . . . Szyf, M. (2014). DNA methylation signature of childhood chronic physical aggression in T cells of both men and women. *PLoS ONE, 9*(1), e86822. doi:10.1371/journal.pone.0086822

Guo, J. U., Su, Y., Zhong, C., Ming, G.-L., & Song, H. (2011). Emerging roles of TET proteins and 5-hydroxymethylcytosines in active DNA demethylation and beyond. *Cell Cycle, 10,* 2662–2668.

Guo, J. U., Su, Y., Zhong, C., Ming, G.-L., & Song, H. (2011). Hydroxylation of 5-methylcytosine by Tet1 promotes active DNA demethylation in the adult brain. *Cell, 145,* 423–434.

Gupta, S., Kim, S. Y., Artis, S., Molfese, D. L., Schumacher, A., Sweatt, J. D., . . . Lubin, F. D. (2010). Histone methylation regulates memory formation. *Journal of Neuroscience, 30,* 3589–3599.

Gurdon, J. B., Laskey, R. A., & Reeves, O. R. (1975). The developmental capacity of nuclei transplanted from keratinized skin cells of adult frogs. *Journal of Embryology and Experimental Morphology, 34,* 93–112.

Hackman, D. A., Farah, M. J., & Meaney, M. J. (2010). Socioeconomic status and the brain: Mechanistic insights from human and animal research. *Nature Reviews: Neuroscience, 11,* 651–659.

Haig, D. (2007). Weismann rules! OK? Epigenetics and the Lamarckian temptation. *Biology and Philosophy, 22,* 415–428.

Hall, B. K. (1988). The embryonic development of bone. *American Scientist, 76*(2), 174–181.

Hanson, M. A., Low, F. M., & Gluckman, P. D. (2011). Epigenetic epidemiology: The rebirth of soft inheritance. *Annals of Nutrition and Metabolism, 58* (suppl 2), 8–15.

Hardin, P. E., Hall, J. C., & Rosbash, M. (1990). Feedback of the *Drosophila* period gene product on circadian cycling of its messenger RNA levels. *Nature, 343,* 536–540.

Harlow, H. F. (1958). The nature of love. *American Psychologist, 13,* 673–685.

Harlow, H. F., Dodsworth, R. O., & Harlow, M. K. (1965). Total social isolation in monkeys. *Proceedings of the National Academy of Sciences USA, 54,* 90–97.

Heard, E. (2004). Recent advances in X-chromosome inactivation. *Current Opinion in Cell Biology, 16,* 247–255.

Heijmans, B. T., Tobi, E. W., Lumey, L. H., & Slagboom, P. E. (2009). The epigenome: Archive of the prenatal environment. *Epigenetics, 4,* 526–531.

Heijmans, B. T., Tobi, E. W., Stein, A. D., Putter, H., Blauw, G. J., Susser, E. S., . . . Lumey, L. H. (2008). Persistent epigenetic differences associated with prenatal exposure to famine in humans. *Proceedings of the National Academy of Sciences USA, 105,* 17046–17049.

Hernandez-Reif, M., Diego, M., & Field, T. (2007). Preterm infants show reduced stress behaviors and activity after 5 days of massage therapy. *Infant Behavior and Development, 30,* 557–561.

Hirata, S., Watanabe, K., Kawai, M. (2001). "Sweet-potato washing" revisited. In T. Matsuzawa (Ed.), *Primate origins of human cognition and behavior* (pp. 487–508). Tokyo: Springer-Verlag.

Ho, M. (1984). Environment and heredity in development and evolution. In M. Ho & P. T. Saunders (Eds.), *Beyond neo-Darwinism: An introduction to the new evolutionary paradigm* (pp. 267–289). London: Academic Press.

Hoek, H. W., Brown, A. S., & Susser, E. (1998). The Dutch Famine and schizophrenia spectrum disorders. *Social Psychiatry and Psychiatric Epidemiology, 33,* 373–379.

Holden, C. (2002). Carbon-Copy clone is the real thing. *Science, 295,* 1443–1444.

Holm, V. A., Cassidy, S. B., Butler, M. G., Hanchett, J. M., Greenswag, L. R., Whitman, B. Y., & Greenberg, F. (1993). Prader-Willi syndrome: Consensus diagnostic criteria. *Pediatrics, 91,* 398–402.

House, J. S., Landis, K. R., & Umberson, D. (1988). Social relationships and health. *Science, 241,* 540–545.

Howie, G. J., Sloboda, D. M., Kamal, T., & Vickers, M. H. (2009). Maternal nutritional history predicts obesity in adult offspring independent of postnatal diet. *Journal of Physiology, 587,* 905–915.

Hu, V. W. (2013). From genes to environment: Using integrative genomics to build a "systems level" understanding of autism spectrum disorders. *Child Development, 84,* 89–103.

Human Epigenome Consortium. (2013). *The Human Epigenome Project.* Retrieved from http://www.epigenome.org/index.php?page=project

Hyman, S. E., Malenka, R. C., & Nestler, E. J. (2006). Neural mechanisms of addiction: The role of reward-related learning and memory. *Annual Review of Neuroscience, 29,* 565–598.

Illes, J. (2007). Blurring our edges. *Nature, 450,* 351–352.

Itard, J. G. (1962). *The wild boy of Aveyron.* Norwalk, CT: Appleton & Lange.

Jablonka, E., & Lamb, M. J. (2002). The changing concept of epigenetics. *Annals of the New York Academy of Science, 981,* 82–96.

Jablonka, E., & Lamb, M. J. (2005). *Evolution in four dimensions: Genetic, epigenetic, behavioral, and symbolic variation in the history of life.* Cambridge, MA: MIT Press.

Jablonka, E., & Lamb, M. J. (2007). Précis of evolution in four dimensions. *Behavioral and Brain Sciences, 30,* 353–392.

Jablonka, E., & Raz, G. (2009). Transgenerational epigenetic inheritance: Prevalence, mechanisms, and implications for the study of heredity and evolution. *Quarterly Review of Biology, 84,* 131–176.

Jacob, F. (1977). Evolution and tinkering. *Science, 196,* 1161–1166.

Jacob, F., Perrin, D., Sanchez, C., & Monod, J. (1960). [Operon: A group of genes with the expression coordinated by an operator]. *Comptes Rendus Hebdomadaires des Séances de l'Académie des Sciences, 250,* 1727–1729.

Jacob, F., & Monod, J. (1961). Genetic regulatory mechanisms in the synthesis of proteins. *Journal of Molecular Biology, 3,* 318–356.

Jaenisch, R., & Bird, A. (2003). Epigenetic regulation of gene expression: How the genome integrates intrinsic and environmental signals. *Nature Genetics Supplement, 33,* 245–254.

Jirtle, R. L., & Skinner, M. K. (2007). Environmental epigenomics and disease susceptibility. *Nature Reviews: Genetics, 8,* 253–262.

Johannsen, W. (1911). The genotype conception of heredity. *American Naturalist, 45,* 129–159.

Johnson, J. M., Castle, J., Garrett-Engele, P., Kan, Z., Loerch, P. M., Armour, C. D., . . . Shoemaker, D. D. (2003). Genome-wide survey of human alternative pre-mRNA splicing with exon junction microarrays. *Science, 302,* 2141–2144.

Johnson, M. H. (2010). *Developmental cognitive neuroscience* (3rd ed.). Malden, MA: Wiley-Blackwell.

Johnston, T. D. (1987). The persistence of dichotomies in the study of behavioral development. *Developmental Review, 7,* 149–182.

Jolie, A. (2013, May 14). My medical choice. *New York Times.*

Jones, A. P., & Dayries, M. (1990). Maternal hormone manipulations and the development of obesity in rats. *Physiology and Behavior, 47,* 1107–1110.

Jones, A. P., & Friedman, M. I. (1982). Obesity and adipocyte abnormalities in offspring of rats undernourished during pregnancy. *Science, 215,* 1518–1519.

Jones, E. E., & Harris, V. A. (1967). The attribution of attitudes. *Journal of Experimental Social Psychology, 3,* 1–24.

Joseph, J. (2006). *The missing gene: Psychiatry, heredity, and the fruitless search for genes.* New York: Algora Publishing.

Junien, C. (2006). Impact of diets and nutrients/drugs on early epigenetic programming. *Journal of Inherited Metabolic Disease, 29,* 359–365.

Junien, C., & Nathanielsz, P. (2007). Report on the IASO Stock Conference 2006: Early and lifelong environmental epigenomic programming of metabolic syndrome, obesity and type II diabetes. *Obesity Reviews, 8,* 487–502.

Kaati, G., Bygren, L. O., & Edvinsson, S. (2002). Cardiovascular and diabetes mortality determined by nutrition during parents' and grandparents' slow growth period. *European Journal of Human Genetics, 10,* 682–688.

Kaati, G., Bygren, L. O., Pembrey, M., & Sjöström, M. (2007). Transgenerational response to nutrition, early life circumstances and longevity. *European Journal of Human Genetics, 15,* 784–790.

Kaiser, J. (2014). The epigenetics heretic. *Science, 343,* 361–363.

Kamakura, M. (2011). Royalactin induces queen differentiation in honeybees. *Nature, 473,* 478–483.

Kaminen-Ahola, N., Ahola, A., Maga, M., Mallitt, K.-A., Fahey, P., Cox, T. C., . . . Chong, S. (2010). Maternal ethanol consumption alters the epigenotype and the phenotype of offspring in a mouse model. *PLoS Genetics, 6*(1), e1000811. doi:10.1371/journal.pgen.1000811

Kandel, E. R. (2001). The molecular biology of memory storage: A dialogue between genes and synapses. *Science, 294,* 1030–1038.

Kandel, E. R. (2013, September 5). The new science of mind. *New York Times.*

Kanfi, Y., Naiman, S., Amir, G., Peshti, V., Zinman, G., Nahum, L., . . . Cohen, H. Y. (2012). The sirtuin SIRT6 regulates lifespan in male mice. *Nature, 483,* 218–221.

Karp, G. (2008). *Cell and molecular biology: Concepts and experiments* (5th ed.). New York: Wiley.

Kasl, S. V., Evans, A. S., & Niederman, J. C. (1979). Psychosocial risk factors in the development of infectious mononucleosis. *Psychosomatic Medicine, 41,* 445–466.

Katada, S., & Sassone-Corsi, P. (2010). The histone methyltransferase MLL1 permits the oscillation of circadian gene expression. *Nature Structural and Molecular Biology, 17,* 1414–1421.

Keeley, B. L. (2004). Anthropomorphism, primatomorphism, mammalomorphism: Understanding cross-species comparisons. *Biology and Philosophy, 19,* 521–540.

Keller, E. F. (2000). *The century of the gene.* Cambridge: Harvard University Press.

Keller, E. F. (2005). DDS: Dynamics of developmental systems. *Biology and Philosophy, 20,* 409–416.

Keller, E. F. (2014). From gene action to reactive genomes. *Journal of Physiology, 592,* 2423–2429.

Keller, S., Sarchiapone, M., Zarrilli, F., Videtič, A., Ferraro, A., Carli, V., ... Chiariotti, L. (2010). Increased BDNF promoter methylation in the Wernicke area of suicide subjects. *Archives of General Psychiatry, 67,* 258–267.

Kellermann, N. P. F. (2013). Epigenetic transmission of holocaust trauma: Can nightmares be inherited? *Israel Journal of Psychiatry and Related Sciences, 50,* 33–39.

Kenworthy, C. A., Sengupta, A., Luz, S. M., Ver Hoeve, E. S., Meda, K., Bhatnagar, S., & Abel, T. (2014). Social defeat induces changes in histone acetylation and expression of histone modifying enzymes in the ventral hippocampus, prefrontal cortex, and dorsal raphe nucleus. *Neuroscience, 264,* 88–98.

Kerkel, K., Spadola, A., Yuan, E., Kosek, J., Jiang, L., Hod, E., ... Tycko, B. (2008). Genomic surveys by methylation-sensitive SNP analysis identify sequence-dependent allele-specific DNA methylation. *Nature Genetics, 40,* 904–908.

Kim, J. B., Zaehres, H., Wu, G., Gentile, L., Ko, K., Sebastiano, V., ... Schöler, H. R. (2008). Pluripotent stem cells induced from adult neural stem cells by reprogramming with two factors. *Nature, 454,* 646–650.

Klengel, T., Pape, J., Binder, E. B., & Mehta, D. (2014). The role of DNA methylation in stress-related psychiatric disorders. *Neuropharmacology, 80,* 115–132.

Knoll, J. H. M., Nicholls, R. D., Magenis, R. E., Graham, J. M., Lalande, M., Latt, S. A., ... Reynolds, J. F. (1989). Angelman and Prader-Willi syndromes share a common chromosome 15 deletion but differ in parental origin of the deletion. *American Journal of Medical Genetics, 32,* 285–290.

Kolata, G. (2012, September 5). Bits of mystery DNA, far from "junk," play crucial role. *New York Times.*

Kolata, G. (2013, July 18, 2:02 p.m. ET). Overweight? Maybe your genes really are at fault. *New York Times.*

Konopka, R. J., & Benzer, S. (1971). Clock mutants of *Drosophila melanogaster. Proceedings of the National Academy of Sciences USA, 68,* 2112–2116.

Korade, Ž., & Mirnics, K. (2011). The autism disconnect. *Nature, 474,* 294–295.

Kriaucionis, S., & Heintz, N. (2009). The nuclear DNA base 5-hydroxymethylcytosine is present in Purkinje neurons and the brain. *Science, 324,* 929–930.

Kucharski, R., Maleszka, J., Foret, S., & Maleszka, R. (2008). Nutritional control of reproductive status in honeybees via DNA methylation. *Science, 319,* 1827–1830.

Kupperman, K. O. (1984). *Roanoke: The abandoned colony.* Lanham, MD: Rowman & Littlefield.

Kuzawa, C. W., & Sweet, E. (2009). Epigenetics and the embodiment of race: Developmental origins of US racial disparities in cardiovascular health. *American Journal of Human Biology, 21,* 2–15.

Labonté, B., Suderman, M., Maussion, G., Navaro, L., Yerko, V., Mahar, I., ... Turecki, G. (2012). Genome-wide epigenetic regulation by early-life trauma. *Archives of General Psychiatry, 69,* 722–731.

Labrie, V., Pai, S., & Petronis, A. (2012). Epigenetics of major psychosis: Progress, problems and perspectives. *Trends in Genetics, 28,* 427–435.

Laland, K. N., Odling-Smee, J., & Myles, S. (2010). How culture shaped the human genome: Bringing genetics and the human sciences together. *Nature Reviews: Genetics, 11,* 137–148.

Landecker, H. (2011). Food as exposure: Nutritional epigenetics and the new metabolism. *BioSocieties, 6,* 167–194.

Larsen, P. L. (2008, November). *Presidential symposium: Genetic blueprint and environment—Which has the bigger impact?* Symposium conducted at the 61st annual scientific meeting of The Gerontological Society of America, National Harbor, Maryland.

Larson, E. B., Wang, L., Bowen, J. D., McCormick, W. C., Teri, L., Crane, P., & Kukull, W. (2006). Exercise is associated with reduced risk for incident dementia among persons 65 years of age and older. *Annals of Internal Medicine, 144*, 73–81.

Launay, J.-M., Del Pino, M., Chironi, G., Callebert, J., Peoc'h, K., Mégnien, J., . . . Rendu, F. (2009). Smoking induces long-lasting effects through a monoamine-oxidase epigenetic regulation. *PLoS ONE, 4*(11), e7959. doi:10.1371/journal.pone.0007959

Lee, K. K., & Workman, J. L. (2007). Histone acetyltransferase complexes: One size doesn't fit all. *Nature Reviews: Molecular Cell Biology, 8*, 284–295.

Lee, R., Geracioti, T. D., Kasckow, J. W., & Coccaro, E. F. (2005). Childhood trauma and personality disorder: Positive correlation with adult CSF corticotropin-releasing factor concentrations. *American Journal of Psychiatry, 162*, 995–997.

Lehrman, D. S. (1953). A critique of Konrad Lorenz's theory of instinctive behavior. *Quarterly Review of Biology, 28*, 337–363.

Lester, B. M., Tronick, E., Nestler, E., Abel, T., Kosofsky, B., Kuzawa, C. W., . . . Wood, M. A. (2011). Behavioral epigenetics. *Annals of the New York Academy of Sciences, 1226*, 14–33.

Levenberg, S., Golub, J. S., Amit, M., Itskovitz-Eldor, J., & Langer, R. (2002). Endothelial cells derived from human embryonic stem cells. *Proceedings of the National Academy of Sciences USA, 99*, 4391–4396.

Levenson, J. M., O'Riordan, K. J., Brown, K. D., Trinh, M. A., Molfese, D. L., & Sweatt, J. D. (2004). Regulation of histone acetylation during memory formation in the hippocampus. *Journal of Biological Chemistry, 279*, 40545–40559.

Levenson, J. M., Roth, T. L., Lubin, F. D., Miller, C. A., Huang, I.-C., Desai, P., . . . Sweatt, J. D. (2006). Evidence that DNA (cytosine-5) methyltransferase regulates synaptic plasticity in the hippocampus. *Journal of Biological Chemistry, 281*, 15763–15773.

Levenson, J. M., & Sweatt, J. D. (2005). Epigenetic mechanisms in memory formation. *Nature Reviews: Neuroscience, 6*, 108–118.

Lewkowicz, D. J. (2011). The biological implausibility of the nature–nurture dichotomy and what it means for the study of infancy. *Infancy, 16*, 331–367.

Lewontin, R. C. (2000). *The triple helix: Gene, organism, and environment.* Cambridge, MA: Harvard University Press.

Li, E., Beard, C., & Jaenisch, R. (1993). Role for DNA methylation in genomic imprinting. *Nature, 366*, 362–365.

Li, W., & Liu, M. (2011). Distribution of 5-hydroxymethylcytosine in different human tissues. *Journal of Nucleic Acids, 2011*, 870726. doi:10.4061/2011/870726

Lichtenstein, P., Holm, N. V., Verkasalo, P. K., Iliadou, A., Kaprio, J., Koskenvuo, M., . . . Hemminki, K. (2000). Environmental and heritable factors in the causation of cancer— Analyses of cohorts of twins from Sweden, Denmark, and Finland. *New England Journal of Medicine, 343*, 78–85.

Lickliter, R. (2008). The growth of developmental thought: Implications for a new evolutionary psychology. *New Ideas in Psychology, 26*, 353–369.

Lickliter, R. (2009). The fallacy of partitioning: Epigenetics' validation of the organism-environment system. *Ecological Psychology, 21*, 138–146.

Lickliter, R., & Berry, T. D. (1990). The phylogeny fallacy: Developmental psychology's misapplication of evolutionary theory. *Developmental Review, 10*, 348–364.

Lickliter, R., & Honeycutt, H. (2003). Developmental dynamics: Toward a biologically plausible evolutionary psychology. *Psychological Bulletin, 129*, 819–835.

Lickliter, R., & Honeycutt, H. (2010). Rethinking epigenesis and evolution in light of developmental science. In M. S. Blumberg, J. H. Freeman, & S. R. Robinson (Eds.), *Oxford handbook of developmental behavioral neuroscience* (pp. 30–47). New York: Oxford University Press.

Lickliter, R., & Honeycutt, H. (2013). A developmental evolutionary framework for psychology. *Review of General Psychology, 17,* 184–189.

Lillycrop, K. A., & Burdge, G. C. (2011). The effect of nutrition during early life on the epigenetic regulation of transcription and implications for human diseases. *Journal of Nutrigenetics and Nutrigenomics, 4,* 248–260.

Lillycrop, K. A., Phillips, E. S., Jackson, A. A., Hanson, M. A., & Burdge, G. C. (2005). Dietary protein restriction of pregnant rats induces and folic acid supplementation prevents epigenetic modification of hepatic gene expression in the offspring. *Journal of Nutrition, 135,* 1382–1386.

Lister, R., Mukamel, E. A., Nery, J. R., Urich, M., Puddifoot, C. A., Johnson, N. D., . . . Ecker, J. R. (2013). Global epigenomic reconfiguration during mammalian brain development. *Science, 341,* 1237905. doi:10.1126/science.1237905

Liu, D., Diorio, J., Day, J. C., Francis, D. D., & Meaney, M. J. (2000). Maternal care, hippocampal synaptogenesis and cognitive development in rats. *Nature Neuroscience, 3,* 799–806.

Liu, D., Diorio, J., Tannenbaum, B., Caldji, C., Francis, D., Freedman, A., . . . Meaney, M. J. (1997). Maternal care, hippocampal glucocorticoid receptors and hypothalamic-pituitary-adrenal responses to stress. *Science, 277,* 1659–1662.

Loi, M., Del Savio, L., & Stupka, E. (2013). Social epigenetics and equality of opportunity. *Public Health Ethics, 6,* 142–153.

Lombard, D. B., & Miller, R. A. (2012). Sorting out the sirtuins. *Nature, 483,* 166–167.

Lovatel, G. A., Elsner, V. R., Bertoldi, K., Vanzella, C., Moysés, F. D. S., Vizuete, A., . . . Siqueira, I. R. (2013). Treadmill exercise induces age-related changes in aversive memory, neuroinflammatory and epigenetic processes in the rat hippocampus. *Neurobiology of Learning and Memory, 101,* 94–102.

Lubin, F. D., Roth, T. L., & Sweatt, J. D. (2008). Epigenetic regulation of bdnf gene transcription in the consolidation of fear memory. *Journal of Neuroscience, 28,* 10576–10586.

Lum, T. E., & Merritt, T. J. S. (2011). Nonclassical regulation of transcription: Interchromosomal interactions at the *Malic enzyme* locus of *Drosophila melanogaster. Genetics, 189,* 837–849.

Lumey, L. H. (1992). Decreased birthweights in infants after maternal *in utero* exposure to the Dutch famine of 1944–1945. *Paediatric and Perinatal Epidemiology, 6,* 240–253.

Lumey, L. H., Stein, A. D., Kahn, H. S., & Romijn, J. A. (2009). Lipid profiles in middle-aged men and women after famine exposure during gestation: The Dutch Hunger Winter Families Study. *American Journal of Clinical Nutrition, 89,* 1737–1743.

Lumey, L. H., Stein, A. D., & Susser, E. (2011). Prenatal famine and adult health. *Annual Review of Public Health, 32,* 237–262.

Lutz, P.-E., & Turecki, G. (2014). DNA methylation and childhood maltreatment: From animal models to human studies. *Neuroscience, 264,* 142–156.

Lyon, M. F. (1961). Gene action in the X-chromosome of the mouse (*Mus musculus* L.). *Nature, 190,* 372–373.

Lyon, M. F. (1962). Sex chromatin and gene action in the mammalian X-chromosome. *American Journal of Human Genetics, 14,* 135–148.

Mack, G. S. (2010). To selectivity and beyond. *Nature Biotechnology, 28,* 1259–1266.

Maderspacher, F. (2010). Lysenko rising. *Current Biology, 20,* R835–R837.

Madhani, H. D., Francis, N. J., Kingston, R. E., Kornberg, R. D., Moazed, D., Narlikar, G. J., Panning, B., & Struhl, K. (2008). Epigenomics: A roadmap, but to where? *Science, 322,* 43–44.

Maestripieri, D. (2005). Early experience affects the intergenerational transmission of infant abuse in rhesus monkeys. *Proceedings of the National Academy of Sciences USA, 102,* 9726–9729.

Maher, B. (2012). The human encyclopaedia. *Nature, 489,* 46–48.

Martin, C., & Zhang, Y. (2007). Mechanisms of epigenetic inheritance. *Current Opinion in Cell Biology, 19,* 266–272.

Martin, D. I. K., Cropley, J. E., & Suter, C. M. (2008). Environmental influence on epigenetic inheritance at the A^{vy} allele. *Nutrition Reviews, 66,* S12–S14.

Massart, R., Suderman, M., Provencal, N., Yi, C., Bennett, A. J., Suomi, S., & Szyf, M. (2014). Hydroxymethylation and DNA methylation profiles in the prefrontal cortex of the non-human primate rhesus macaque and the impact of maternal deprivation on hydroxy-methylation. *Neuroscience, 268,* 139–148.

Masten, A. S. (2001). Ordinary magic: Resilience processes in development. *American Psychologist, 56,* 227–238.

Masterpasqua, F. (2009). Psychology and epigenetics. *Review of General Psychology, 13,* 194–201.

Mattick, J. S. (2005). The functional genomics of noncoding RNA. *Science, 309,* 1527–1528.

Mattick, J. S. (2010). RNA as the substrate for epigenome-environment interactions. *BioEssays, 32,* 548–552.

Mattick, J. S., & Makunin, I. V. (2006). Non-coding RNA. *Human Molecular Genetics, 15,* R17–R29.

Mayer, W., Niveleau, A., Walter, J., Fundele, R., & Haaf, T. (2000). Demethylation of the zygotic paternal genome. *Nature, 403,* 501–502.

Mayr, E. (1963). *Animal species and evolution.* Cambridge, MA: Harvard University Press.

Mayr, E. (1980). Prologue: Some thoughts on the history of the evolutionary synthesis. In E. Mayr & W. B. Provine (Eds.), *The evolutionary synthesis: Perspectives on the unification of biology* (pp. 1–48). Cambridge, MA: Harvard University Press.

Mayr, E. (2001). *What evolution is.* New York: Basic Books.

Maze, I., Covington, H. E. III, Dietz, D. M., LaPlant, Q., Renthal, W., Russo, S. J., . . . Nestler, E. J. (2010). Essential role of the histone methyltransferase G9a in cocaine-induced plasticity. *Science, 327,* 213–216.

Maze, I., & Nestler, E. J. (2011). The epigenetic landscape of addiction. *Annals of the New York Academy of Sciences, 1216,* 99–113.

McCarthy, M. M., Auger, A. P., Bale, T. L., De Vries, G. J., Dunn, G. A., Forger, N. G., . . . Wilson, M. E. (2009). The epigenetics of sex differences in the brain. *Journal of Neuroscience, 29,* 12815–12823.

McDaniel, I. E., Lee, J. M., Berger, M. S., Hanagami, C. K., & Armstrong, J. A. (2008). Investigations of CHD1 function in transcription and development of *Drosophila melano-gaster. Genetics, 178,* 583–587.

McEwen, B. S. (2008). Central effects of stress hormones in health and disease: Understanding the protective and damaging effects of stress and stress mediators. *European Journal of Pharmacology, 583,* 174–185.

McGee, S. L., Fairlie, E., Garnham, A. P., & Hargreaves, M. (2009). Exercise-induced histone modifications in human skeletal muscle. *Journal of Physiology, 587,* 5951–5958.

McGowan, P. O., Meaney, M. J., & Szyf, M. (2008). Diet and the epigenetic (re)programming of phenotypic differences in behavior. *Brain Research, 1237,* 12–24.

McGowan, P. O., Sasaki, A., D'Alessio, A. C., Dymov, S., Labonté, B., Szyf, M., . . . Meaney, M. J. (2009). Epigenetic regulation of the glucocorticoid receptor in human brain associates with childhood abuse. *Nature Neuroscience, 12,* 342–348.

McKenzie, C. A., Wakamatsu, K., Hanchard, N. A., Forrester, T., & Ito, S. (2007). Childhood malnutrition is associated with a reduction in the total melanin content of scalp hair. *British Journal of Nutrition, 98,* 159–164.

Meaney, M. J. (2001). Maternal care, gene expression, and the transmission of individual differences in stress reactivity across generations. *Annual Review of Neuroscience, 24,* 1161–1192.

Meaney, M. J. (2010). Epigenetics and the biological definition of gene × environment interactions. *Child Development, 81,* 41–79.

Meaney, M. J., & Szyf, M. (2005). Maternal care as a model for experience-dependent chromatin plasticity? *Trends in Neurosciences, 28,* 456–463.

Meck, W. H., & Williams, C. L. (1999). Choline supplementation during prenatal development reduces proactive interference in spatial memory. *Developmental Brain Research, 118,* 51–59.

Mennella, J. A., Jagnow, C. P., & Beauchamp, G. K. (2001). Prenatal and postnatal flavor learning by human infants. *Pediatrics, 107*(6), e88.

Michel, G. F., & Moore, C. L. (1995). *Developmental psychobiology: An interdisciplinary science.* Cambridge, MA: MIT Press.

Michishita, E., McCord, R. A., Berber, E., Kioi, M., Padilla-Nash, H., Damian, M., . . . Chua, K. F. (2008). SIRT6 is a histone H3 lysine 9 deacetylase that modulates telomeric chromatin. *Nature, 452,* 492–496.

Mill, J., & Petronis, A. (2007). Molecular studies of major depressive disorder: The epigenetic perspective. *Molecular Psychiatry, 12,* 799–814.

Mill, J., Tang, T., Kaminsky, Z., Khare, T., Yazdanpanah, S., Bouchard, L., . . . Petronis, A. (2008). Epigenomic profiling reveals DNA-methylation changes associated with major psychosis. *American Journal of Human Genetics, 82,* 696–711.

Miller, C. A., Gavin, C. F., White, J. A., Parrish, R. R., Honasoge, A., Yancey, C. R., . . . Sweatt, J. D. (2010). Cortical DNA methylation maintains remote memory. *Nature Neuroscience, 13,* 664–666.

Miller, C. A., & Sweatt, J. D. (2006). Amnesia or retrieval deficit? Implications of a molecular approach to the question of reconsolidation. *Learning and Memory, 13,* 498–505.

Miller, G. (2010). The seductive allure of behavioral epigenetics. *Science, 329,* 24–27.

Miller, G. E., Chen, E., Fok, A. K., Walker, H., Lim, A., Nicholls, E. F., . . . Kobor, M. S. (2009). Low early-life social class leaves a biological residue manifested by decreased glucocorticoid and increased proinflammatory signaling. *Proceedings of the National Academy of Sciences USA, 106,* 14716–14721.

Miyake, K., Hirasawa, T., Koide, T., & Kubota, T. (2012). Epigenetics in autism and other neurodevelopmental diseases. In S. I. Ahmad (Ed.), *Neurodegenerative diseases* (pp. 91–98). New York: Springer Science+Business Media.

Moore, D. S. (2002). *The dependent gene: The fallacy of nature vs. nurture.* New York: W.H. Freeman.

Moore, D. S. (2006). A very little bit of knowledge: Re-evaluating the meaning of the heritability of IQ. *Human Development, 49,* 347–353.

Moore, D. S. (2008a). Espousing interactions and fielding reactions: Addressing laypeople's beliefs about genetic determinism. *Philosophical Psychology, 21,* 331–348.

Moore, D. S. (2008b). Individuals and populations: How biology's theory and data have interfered with the integration of development and evolution. *New Ideas in Psychology, 26,* 370–386.

Moore, D. S. (2013a). Behavioral genetics, genetics, and epigenetics. In P. D. Zelazo (Ed.), *Oxford handbook of developmental psychology* (pp. 91–128). New York: Oxford University Press.

Moore, D. S. (2013b). Big B, little b: Myth #1 is that Mendelian genes actually exist. In S. Krimsky & J. Gruber (Eds.), *Genetic explanations: Sense and nonsense* (pp. 43–50). Cambridge, MA: Harvard University Press.

Moore, D. S. (2013c). Current thinking about nature and nurture. In K. Kampourakis (Ed.), *The philosophy of biology: A companion for educators* (pp. 629–652). New York: Springer.

Morgan, H. D., Sutherland, H. G. E., Martin, D. I. K., & Whitelaw, E. (1999). Epigenetic inheritance at the agouti locus in the mouse. *Nature Genetics, 23,* 314–318.

Mostoslavsky, R., Chua, K. F., Lombard, D. B., Pang, W. W., Fischer, M. R., Gellon, L., . . . Alt, F. W. (2006). Genomic instability and aging-like phenotype in the absence of mammalian SIRT6. *Cell, 124,* 315–329.

Mueller, B. R., & Bale, T. L. (2008). Sex-specific programming of offspring emotionality after stress early in pregnancy. *Journal of Neuroscience, 28,* 9055–9065.

Mullard, A. (2008). The inside story. *Nature, 453,* 578–580.

Murgatroyd, C., Patchev, A. V., Wu, Y., Micale, V., Bockmühl, Y., Fischer, D., . . . Spengler, D. (2009). Dynamic DNA methylation programs persistent adverse effects of early-life stress. *Nature Neuroscience, 12*, 1559–1566.

Myzak, M. C., & Dashwood, R. H. (2006). Histone deacetylases as targets for dietary cancer preventive agents: Lessons learned with butyrate, diallyl disulfide, and sulforaphane. *Current Drug Targets, 7*, 443–452.

Nagoshi, E., Saini, C., Bauer, C., Laroche, T., Naef, F., & Schibler, U. (2004). Circadian gene expression in individual fibroblasts: Cell-autonomous and self-sustained oscillators pass time to daughter cells. *Cell, 119*, 693–705.

Najm, W. I., Reinsch, S., Hoehler, F., Tobis, J. S., & Harvey, P. W. (2004). S-adenosyl methionine (SAMe) versus celecoxib for the treatment of osteoarthritis symptoms: A double-blind cross-over trial. *BMC Musculoskeletal Disorders, 5*, 6–20.

Nakahata, Y., Kaluzova, M., Grimaldi, B., Sahar, S., Hirayama, J., Chen, D., . . . Sassone-Corsi, P. (2008). The NAD^+-dependent deacetylase SIRT1 modulates CLOCK-mediated chromatin remodeling and circadian control. *Cell, 134*, 329–340.

Naruse, Y., Oh-hashi, K., Iijima, N., Naruse, M., Yoshioka, H., & Tanaka, M. (2004). Circadian and light-induced transcription of clock gene *Per1* depends on histone acetylation and deacetylation. *Molecular and Cellular Biology, 24*, 6278–6287.

National Cancer Institute (2009, May 29). BRCA1 and BRCA2: Cancer risk and genetic testing. *National Cancer Institute Fact Sheet.* Retrieved July 13, 2013, from http://www.cancer.gov/cancertopics/factsheet/Risk/BRCA

Needham, B. L., Epel, E. S., Adler, N. E., & Kiefe, C. (2010). Trajectories of change in obesity and symptoms of depression: The CARDIA study. *American Journal of Public Health, 100*, 1040–1046.

Neigh, G. N., Gillespie, C. F., & Nemeroff, C. B. (2009). The neurobiological toll of child abuse and neglect. *Trauma, Violence, and Abuse, 10*, 389–410.

Nestler, E. J. (2009). Epigenetic mechanisms in psychiatry. *Biological Psychiatry, 65*, 189–190.

Neumann-Held, E. M. (1998). The gene is dead—Long live the gene: Conceptualizing genes the constructionist way. In P. Koslowski (Ed.), *Sociobiology and bioeconomics: The theory of evolution in biological and economic theory* (pp. 105–137). Berlin: Springer-Verlag.

Newbold, R. R., Padilla-Banks, E., & Jefferson, W. N. (2006). Adverse effects of the model environmental estrogen diethylstilbestrol are transmitted to subsequent generations. *Endocrinology, 147*, S11–S17.

Ng, S.-F., Lin, R. C. Y., Laybutt, D. R., Barres, R., Owens, J. A., & Morris, M. J. (2010). Chronic high-fat diet in fathers programs β-cell dysfunction in female rat offspring. *Nature, 467*, 963–966.

Nicholls, R. D., Knoll, J. H. M., Butler, M. G., Karam, S., & Lalande, M. (1989). Genetic imprinting suggested by maternal heterodisomy in non-deletion Prader-Willi syndrome. *Nature, 342*, 281–285.

Nijhout, H. F. (1990). Metaphors and the role of genes in development. *BioEssays, 12*, 441–446.

Nikolova, Y. S., Koenen, K. C., Galea, S., Wang, C.-M., Seney, M. L., Sibille, E., . . . Hariri, A. R. (2014). Beyond genotype: Serotonin transporter epigenetic modification predicts human brain function. *Nature Neuroscience.* Advance online publication. doi:10.1038/nn.3778

Noble, D. (2006). *The music of life: Biology beyond genes.* New York: Oxford University Press.

Noble, D. (2008). Genes and causation. *Philosophical Transactions of the Royal Society A, 366*, 3001–3015.

Nüsslein-Volhard, C. (2006). *Coming to life: How genes drive development.* Carlsbad, CA: Kales Press.

Oberlander, T. F., Weinberg, J., Papsdorf, M., Grunau, R., Misri, S., & Devlin, A. M. (2008). Prenatal exposure to maternal depression, neonatal methylation of human glucocorticoid receptor gene (*NR3C1*) and infant cortisol stress responses. *Epigenetics, 3*, 97–106.

Ohno, S. (1972). So much "junk" DNA in our genome. In H. H. Smith (Ed.), *Evolution of genetic systems: Vol. 23. Brookhaven Symposia in Biology* (pp. 366–370). New York: Gordon & Breach.

Ollikainen, M., Smith, K. R., Joo, E. J., Ng, H. K., Andronikos, R., Novakovic, B., . . . Craig, J. M. (2010). DNA methylation analysis of multiple tissues from newborn twins reveals both genetic and intrauterine components to variation in the human neonatal epigenome. *Human Molecular Genetics, 19,* 4176–4188.

Olshansky, S. J. (2011). Aging of US presidents. *Journal of the American Medical Association, 306,* 2328–2329.

Ooi, S. K. T., & Bestor, T. H. (2008). The colorful history of active DNA demethylation. *Cell, 133,* 1145–1148.

Orozco-Solis, R., & Sassone-Corsi, P. (2014). Epigenetic control and the circadian clock: Linking metabolism to neuronal responses. *Neuroscience, 264,* 76–87.

Otu, H. H., Naxerova, K., Ho, K., Can, H., Nesbitt, N., Libermann, T. A., & Karp, S. J. (2007). Restoration of liver mass after injury requires proliferative and not embryonic transcriptional patterns. *Journal of Biological Chemistry, 282,* 11197–11204.

Oyama, S. (1992). Transmission and construction: Levels and the problem of heredity. In E. Tobach & G. Greenberg (Eds.), *Levels of social behavior: Evolutionary and genetic aspects: Award winning papers from the Third T. C. Schneirla Conference: Evolution of social behavior and integrative levels* (pp. 51–60). Wichita, KS: T.C. Schneirla Research Fund.

Oyama, S. (1985/2000). *The ontogeny of information.* Durham, NC: Duke University Press.

Oyama, S., Griffiths, P. E., & Gray, R. D. (2001). *Cycles of contingency: Developmental systems and evolution.* Cambridge, MA: MIT Press.

Painter, R. C., Osmond, C., Gluckman, P., Hanson, M., Phillips, D. I. W., & Roseboom, T. J. (2008). Transgenerational effects of prenatal exposure to the Dutch famine on neonatal adiposity and health in later life. *BJOG, 115,* 1243–1249.

Pan, Q., Shai, O., Lee, L. J., Frey, B. J., & Blencowe, B. J. (2008). Deep surveying of alternative splicing complexity in the human transcriptome by high-throughput sequencing. *Nature Genetics, 40,* 1413–1415.

Pandya, K., Cowhig, J., Brackhan, J., Kim, H. S., Hagaman, J., Rojas, M., . . . Smithies, O. (2008). Discordant on/off switching of gene expression in myocytes during cardiac hypertrophy *in vivo. Proceedings of the National Academy of Sciences USA, 105,* 13063–13068.

Papakostas, G. I., Alpert, J. E., & Fava, M. (2003). S-adenosyl-methionine in depression: A comprehensive review of the literature. *Current Psychiatry Reports, 5,* 460–466.

Papakostas, G. I., Mischoulon, D., Shyu, I., Alpert, J. E., & Fava, M. (2010). S-adenosyl-methionine (SAMe) augmentation of serotonin reuptake inhibitors for antidepressant nonresponders with major depressive disorder: A double-blind, randomized clinical trial. *American Journal of Psychiatry, 167,* 942–948.

Parker-Pope, T. (2009, March 9). Unlocking the secrets of gray hair. *New York Times.*

Pedersen, C. A. (1997). Oxytocin control of maternal behavior: Regulation by sex steroids and offspring stimuli. *Annals of the New York Academy of Sciences, 807,* 126–145.

Peleg, S., Sananbenesi, F., Zovoilis, A., Burhardt, S., Bahari-Javan, S., Agis-Balboa, R. C., . . . Fischer, A. (2010). Altered histone acetylation is associated with age-dependent memory impairment in mice. *Science, 328,* 753–756.

Pembrey, M. (2008). Human inheritance, differences and diseases: Putting genes in their place. Part II. *Paediatric and Perinatal Epidemiology, 22,* 507–513.

Pembrey, M. E. (2002). Time to take epigenetic inheritance seriously. *European Journal of Human Genetics, 10,* 669–671.

Pembrey, M. E. (2010). Male-line transgenerational responses in humans. *Human Fertility, 13,* 268–271.

Pembrey, M. E., Bygren, L. O., Kaati, G., Edvinsson, S., Northstone, K., Sjöström, M., . . . The ALSPAC study team (2006). Sex-specific, male-line transgenerational responses in humans. *European Journal of Human Genetics, 14,* 159–166.

Peña, C. L. J., & Champagne, F. A. (2012). Epigenetic and neurodevelopmental perspectives on variation in parenting behavior. *Parenting: Science and Practice, 12,* 202–211.

Pennisi, E. (2007). DNA study forces rethink of what it means to be a gene. *Science, 316,* 1556–1557.

Perroud, N., Paoloni-Giacobino, A., Prada, P. Olié, E., Salzmann, A., Nicastro, R., ... Malafosse, A. (2011). Increased methylation of glucocorticoid receptor gene (*NR3C1*) in adults with a history of childhood maltreatment: a link with the severity and type of trauma. *Translational Psychiatry, 1,* e59. doi:10.1038/tp.2011.60

Persico, A. M., & Bourgeron, T. (2006). Searching for ways out of the autism maze: Genetic, epigenetic and environmental clues. *Trends in Neurosciences, 29,* 349–358.

Petris, M. J., Strausak, D., & Mercer, J. F. B. (2000). The Menkes copper transporter is required for the activation of tyrosinase. *Human Molecular Genetics, 9,* 2845–2851.

Petronis, A. (2010). Epigenetics as a unifying principle in the aetiology of complex traits and diseases. *Nature, 465,* 721–727.

Petronis, A., Gottesman, I. I., Kan, P., Kennedy, J. L., Basile, V. S., Paterson, A. D., & Popendikyte, V. (2003). Monozygotic twins exhibit numerous epigenetic differences: Clues to twin discordance? *Schizophrenia Bulletin, 29,* 169–178.

Pigliucci, M. (2010). Genotype–phenotype mapping and the end of the "genes as blueprint" metaphor. *Philosophical Transactions of the Royal Society B, 365,* 557–566.

Pigliucci, M., & Boudry, M. (2011). Why machine-information metaphors are bad for science and science education. *Science and Education, 20,* 453–471.

Pinsker, H. M., Hening, W. A., Carew, T. J., & Kandel, E. R. (1973). Long-term sensitization of a defensive withdrawal reflex in Aplysia. *Science, 182,* 1039–1042.

Pirone, J. R., & Elston, T. C. (2004). Fluctuations in transcription factor binding can explain the graded and binary responses observed in inducible gene expression. *Journal of Theoretical Biology, 226,* 111–121.

Popova, B. C., Tada, T., Takagi, N., Brockdorff, N., & Nesterova, T. B. (2006). Attenuated spread of X-inactivation in an X;autosome translocation. *Proceedings of the National Academy of Sciences USA, 103,* 7706–7711.

Poulter, M. O., Du, L., Weaver, I. C. G., Palkovits, M., Faludi, G., Merali, Z., ... Anisman, H. (2008). GABA$_A$ receptor promoter hypermethylation in suicide brain: Implications for the involvement of epigenetic processes. *Biological Psychiatry, 64,* 645–652.

Powledge, T. M. (2011). Behavioral epigenetics: How nurture shapes nature. *BioScience, 61,* 588–592.

Provençal, N., Suderman, M. J., Caramaschi, D., Wang, D., Hallett, M., Vitaro, F., ... Szyf, M. (2013). Differential DNA methylation regions in cytokine and transcription factor genomic loci associate with childhood physical aggression. *PLoS ONE, 8*(8), e71691. doi:10.1371/journal.pone.0071691

Provençal, N., Suderman, M. J., Guillemin, C., Massart, R., Ruggiero, A., Wang, D., ... Szyf, M. (2012). The signature of maternal rearing in the methylome in rhesus macaque prefrontal cortex and T cells. *Journal of Neuroscience, 32,* 15626–15642.

Provençal, N., Suderman, M. J., Guillemin, C., Vitaro, F., Côte, S. M., Hallett, M., ... Szyf, M. (2014). Association of childhood chronic physical aggression with a DNA methylation signature in adult human T cells. *PLoS ONE, 9*(4), e89839. doi:10.1371/journal.pone.0089839

Ptashne, M. (2010). Questions over the scientific basis of epigenome project. *Nature, 464,* 487.

Radiolab (Producer). (2012a, November 19). *Leaving your Lamarck* [Audio podcast]. Retrieved from http://www.radiolab.org/2012/nov/19/leaving-lamarck/

Radiolab (Producer). (2012b, November 19). *You are what your grandpa eats* [Audio podcast]. Retrieved from http://www.radiolab.org/2012/nov/19/you-are-what-your-grandpa-eats/

Radtke, K. M., Ruf, M., Gunter, H. M., Dohrmann, K., Schauer, M., Meyer, A., & Elbert, T. (2011). Transgenerational impact of intimate partner violence on methylation in the promoter of the glucocorticoid receptor. *Translational Psychiatry, 1,* e21. doi:10.1038/tp.2011.21

Rakyan, V. K., & Beck, S. (2006). Epigenetic variation and inheritance in mammals. *Current Opinion in Genetics and Development, 16,* 573–577.

Rakyan, V. K., Chong, S., Champ, M. E., Cuthbert, P. C., Morgan, H. D., Luu, K. V. K., & Whitelaw, E. (2003). Transgenerational inheritance of epigenetic states at the murine *Axin^{Fu}* allele occurs after maternal and paternal transmission. *Proceedings of the National Academy of Sciences USA, 100,* 2538–2543.

Rakyan, V. K., Down, T. A., Maslau, S., Andrew, T., Yang, T.-P., Beyan, H., . . . Spector, T. D. (2010). Human aging-associated DNA hypermethylation occurs preferentially at bivalent chromatin domains. *Genome Research, 20,* 434–439.

Rastan, S., & Robertson, E. J. (1985). X-chromosome deletions in embryo-derived (EK) cell lines associated with lack of X-chromosome inactivation. *Journal of Embryology and Experimental Morphology, 90,* 379–388.

Ravelli, G. P., Stein, Z. A., & Susser, M. W. (1976). Obesity in young men after famine exposure *in utero* and early pregnancy. *New England Journal of Medicine, 295,* 349–353.

Razin, A. (1998). CpG methylation, chromatin structure, and gene silencing—a three-way connection. *The EMBO Journal, 17,* 4905–4908.

Reddy, T. E., Pauli, F., Sprouse, R. O., Neff, N. F., Newberry, K. M., Garabedian, M. J., & Myers, R. M. (2009). Genomic determination of the glucocorticoid response reveals unexpected mechanisms of gene regulation. *Genome Research, 19,* 2163–2171.

Redon, C., Pilch, D., Rogakou, E., Sedelnikova, O., Newrock, K., & Bonner, W. (2002). Histone H2A variants H2AX and H2AZ. *Current Opinion in Genetics and Development, 12,* 162–169.

Reik, W., Dean, W., & Walter, J. (2001). Epigenetic reprogramming in mammalian development. *Science, 293,* 1089–1093.

Reppert, S. M., & Weaver, D. R. (2002). Coordination of circadian timing in mammals. *Nature, 418,* 935–941.

Richards, E. J. (2006). Inherited epigenetic variation—Revisiting soft inheritance. *Nature Reviews: Genetics, 7,* 395–401.

Rice, W. R., Friberg, U., & Gavrilets, S. (2012). Homosexuality as a consequence of epigenetically canalized sexual development. *Quarterly Review of Biology, 87,* 343–368.

Robert, J. S. (2002). How developmental is evolutionary developmental biology? *Biology and Philosophy, 17,* 591–611.

Robert, J. S. (2004). *Embryology, epigenesis, and evolution: Taking development seriously.* New York: Cambridge University Press.

Robert, J. S. (2008). Taking old ideas seriously: Evolution, development and human behavior. *New Ideas in Psychology, 26,* 387–404.

Roemer, I., Reik, W., Dean, W., & Klose, J. (1997). Epigenetic inheritance in the mouse. *Current Biology, 7,* 277–280.

Roth, T. L. (2012). Epigenetics of neurobiology and behavior during development and adulthood. *Developmental Psychobiology, 54,* 590–597.

Roth, T. L., Lubin, F. D., Funk, A. J., & Sweatt, J. D. (2009). Lasting epigenetic influence of early-life adversity on the BDNF gene. *Biological Psychiatry, 65,* 760–769.

Rothstein, M. A., Cai, Y., & Marchant, G. E. (2009). The ghost in our genes: Legal and ethical implications of epigenetics. *Health Matrix, 19,* 1–62.

Rudenko, A., & Tsai, L.-H. (2014). Epigenetic regulation in memory and cognitive disorders. *Neuroscience, 264,* 51–63.

Rusak, B., Robertson, H. A., Wisden, W., & Hunt, S. P. (1990). Light pulses that shift rhythms induce gene expression in the suprachiasmatic nucleus. *Science, 248,* 1237–1240.

Russell, L. B. (1963). Mammalian X-chromosome action: Inactivation limited in spread and in region of origin. *Science, 140,* 976–978.

Rutten, B. P. F., & Mill, J. (2009). Epigenetic mediation of environmental influences in major psychotic disorders. *Schizophrenia Bulletin, 35,* 1045–1056.

Sahoo, T., del Gaudio, D., German, J. R., Shinawi, M., Peters, S. U., Person, R. E., . . . Beaudet, A. L. (2008). Prader-Willi phenotype caused by paternal deficiency for the HBII-85 C/D/ box small nucleolar RNA cluster. *Nature Genetics, 40*, 719–721.

Santos, K. F., Mazzola, T. N., & Carvalho, H.F. (2005). The prima donna of epigenetics: The regulation of gene expression by DNA methylation. *Brazilian Journal of Medical and Biological Research, 38*, 1531–1541.

Sapienza, C., Peterson, A. C., Rossant, J., & Balling, R. (1987). Degree of methylation of transgenes is dependent on gamete of origin. *Nature, 328*, 251–254.

Sapolsky, R. M. (2005). The influence of social hierarchy on primate health. *Science, 308*, 648–652.

Scafidi, F. A., Field, T. M., Schanberg, S. M., Bauer, C. R., Tucci, K., Roberts, J., . . . Kuhn, C.M. (1990). Massage stimulates growth in preterm infants: A replication. *Infant Behavior and Development, 13*, 167–188.

Schneider, S. M. (2012). *The science of consequences: How they affect genes, change the brain, and impact our world.* Amherst, NY: Prometheus Books.

Scoville, W. B., & Milner, B. (1957). Loss of recent memory after bilateral hippocampal lesions. *Journal of Neurology, Neurosurgery, and Psychiatry, 20*, 11–21.

Shen, L., & Zhang, Y. (2012). Enzymatic analysis of Tet proteins: Key enzymes in the metabolism of DNA methylation. *Methods in Enzymology, 512*, 93–105.

Shoguchi, E., Hamaguchi, M., & Satoh, N. (2008). Genomewide network of regulatory genes for construction of a chordate embryo. *Developmental Biology, 316*, 498–509.

Shuel, R. W., & Dixon, S. E. (1960). The early establishment of dimorphism in the female honeybee, *Apis mellifera*, L. *Insectes Sociaux, 7*, 265–282.

Shulevitz, J. (2012, September 8). Why fathers really matter. *New York Times.* Retrieved from http://www.nytimes.com/2012/09/09/opinion/sunday/why-fathers-really-matter.html?pagewanted=all&_r=0

Sinclair, K. D., Allegrucci, C., Singh, R., Gardner, D. S., Sebastian, S., Bispham, J., . . . Young, L. E. (2007). DNA methylation, insulin resistance, and blood pressure in offspring determined by maternal periconceptional B vitamin and methionine status. *Proceedings of the National Academy of Sciences USA, 104*, 19351–19356.

Singh, S. M., Murphy, B., & O'Reilly, R. L. (2003). Involvement of gene–diet/drug interaction in DNA methylation and its contribution to complex diseases: From cancer to schizophrenia. *Clinical Genetics, 64*, 451–460.

Skinner, M. K. (2011). Role of epigenetics in developmental biology and transgenerational inheritance. *Birth Defects Research (Part C), 93*, 51–55.

Skinner, M. K., Savenkova, M. I., Zhang, B., Gore, A. C., & Crews, D. (2014). Gene bionetworks involved in the epigenetic transgenerational inheritance of altered mate preference: Environmental epigenetics and evolutionary biology. *BMC Genomics, 15*, 377. doi:10.1186/1471-2164-15-377

Smith, L. B. (1999). Do infants possess innate knowledge structures? The con side. *Developmental Science, 2*, 133–144.

Spencer, J. P., Blumberg, M. S., McMurray, B., Robinson, S. R., Samuelson, L. K., & Tomblin, J. B. (2009). Short arms and talking eggs: Why we should no longer abide the nativist–empiricist debate. *Child Development Perspectives, 3*, 79–87.

Spiegelman, A. (1986). *Maus: A survivor's tale.* New York: Pantheon.

Spilianakis, C. G., Lalioti, M. D., Town, T., Lee, G. R., & Flavell, R. A. (2005). Interchromosomal associations between alternatively expressed loci. *Nature, 435*, 637–645.

Stahle, D. W., Cleaveland, M. K., Blanton, D. B., Therrell, M. D., & Gay, D. A. (1998). The Lost Colony and Jamestown droughts. *Science, 280*, 564–567.

Stensmyr, M. C., Stieber, R., & Hansson, B. S. (2008). The Cayman crab fly revisited—Phylogeny and biology of *Drosophila endobranchia*. *PLoS ONE, 3*(4), e1942. doi:10.1371/journal.pone.0001942

Strahl, B. D., & Allis, D. (2000). The language of covalent histone modifications. *Nature, 403,* 41–45.

Sturm, R. A., & Frudakis, T. N. (2004). Eye colour: Portals into pigmentation genes and ancestry. *Trends in Genetics 20,* 327–332.

Suderman, M., Borghol, N., Pappas, J. J., Pereira, S. M. P., Pembrey, M., Hertzman, C., . . . Szyf, M. (2014). Childhood abuse is associated with methylation of multiple loci in adult DNA. *BMC Medical Genomics, 7,* 13. doi:10.1186/1755-8794-7-13

Sun, J.-M., Chen, H. Y., Espino, P. S., & Davie, J. R. (2007). Phosphorylated serine 28 of histone H3 is associated with destabilized nucleosomes in transcribed chromatin. *Nucleic Acids Research, 35,* 6640–6647.

Surani, M. A. H., Barton, S. C., & Norris, M. L. (1987). Influence of parental chromosomes on spatial specificity in androgenetic ←→ parthenogenetic chimaeras in the mouse. *Nature, 326,* 395–397.

Susser, E. S., & Lin, S. P. (1992). Schizophrenia after prenatal exposure to the Dutch Hunger Winter of 1944-1945. *Archives of General Psychiatry, 49,* 983–988.

Susser, M., & Stein, Z. (1994). Timing in prenatal nutrition: A reprise of the Dutch famine study. *Nutrition Reviews, 52,* 84–94.

Sweatt, J. D. (2009). Experience-dependent epigenetic modifications in the central nervous system. *Biological Psychiatry, 65,* 191–197.

Szyf, M., & Bick, J. (2013). DNA methylation: A mechanism for embedding early life experiences in the genome. *Child Development, 84,* 49–57.

Szyf, M., McGowan, P., & Meaney, M. J. (2008). The social environment and the epigenome. *Environmental and Molecular Mutagenesis, 49,* 46–60.

Takahashi, K., & Yamanaka, S. (2006). Induction of pluripotent stem cells from mouse embryonic and adult fibroblast cultures by defined factors. *Cell, 126,* 663–676.

Tanaka, Y., Naruse, I., Maekawa, T., Masuya, H., Shiroishi, T., & Ishii, S. (1997). Abnormal skeletal patterning in embryos lacking a single *Cbp* allele: A partial similarity with Rubinstein-Taybi syndrome. *Proceedings of the National Academy of Sciences USA, 94,* 10215–10220.

Taverna, S. D., Li, H., Ruthenburg, A. J., Allis, C. D., & Patel, D. J. (2007). How chromatin-binding modules interpret histone modifications: Lessons from professional pocket pickers. *Nature Structural and Molecular Biology, 14,* 1025–1040.

Terry, M. B., Ferris, J. S., Pilsner, R., Flom, J. D., Tehranifar, P., Santella, R. M., . . . Susser, E. (2008). Genomic DNA methylation among women in a multiethnic New York City birth cohort. *Cancer Epidemiology, Biomarkers and Prevention, 17,* 2306–2310.

Tobi, E. W., Lumey, L. H., Talens, R. P., Kremer, D., Putter, H., Stein, A. D., . . . Heijmans, B. T. (2009). DNA methylation differences after exposure to prenatal famine are common and timing- and sex-specific. *Human Molecular Genetics, 18,* 4046–4053.

Trafton, A. (2008). Human genes sing different tunes in different tissues. *MIT TechTalk, 53*(8), 6.

Travis, J. (2000). Silence of the Xs: Does junk DNA help women muffle one X chromosome? *Science News, 158,* 92–94.

Tsankova, N. M., Berton, O., Renthal, W., Kumar, A., Neve, R. L., & Nestler, E. J. (2006). Sustained hippocampal chromatin regulation in a mouse model of depression and antidepressant action. *Nature Neuroscience, 9,* 519–525.

Tsankova, N., Renthal, W., Kumar, A., & Nestler, E. J. (2007). Epigenetic regulation in psychiatric disorders. *Nature Reviews: Neuroscience, 8,* 355–367.

Tung, J., Barreiro, L. B., Johnson, Z. P., Hansen, K. D., Michopoulos, V., Toufexis, D., . . . Gilad, Y. (2012). Social environment is associated with gene regulatory variation in the rhesus macaque immune system. *Proceedings of the National Academy of Sciences USA, 109,* 6490–495.

Turnbaugh, P. J., Ley, R. E., Hamady, M., Fraser-Liggett, C. M., Knight, R., & Gordon, J. I. (2007). The human microbiome project. *Nature, 449,* 804–810.

Tylee, D. S., Kawaguchi, D. M., & Glatt, S. J. (2013). On the outside, looking in: A review and evaluation of the comparability of blood and brain "-omes." *American Journal of Medical Genetics Part B: Neuropsychiatric Genetics, 162B,* 595–603.

Uchida, S., Hara, K., Kobayashi, A., Otsuki, K., Yamagata, H., Hobara, T., . . . Watanabe, Y. (2011). Epigenetic status of *Gdnf* in the ventral striatum determines susceptibility and adaptation to daily stressful events. *Neuron, 69,* 359–372.

Vale, W., Spiess, J., Rivier, C., & Rivier, J. (1981). Characterization of a 41-residue ovine hypothalamic peptide that stimulates secretion of corticotropin and β-endorphin. *Science 213,* 1394–1397.

van den Berg, I. M., Laven, J. S. E., Stevens, M., Jonkers, I., Galjaard, R., Gribnau, J., & van Doorninck, J. H. (2009). X chromosome inactivation is initiated in human preimplantation embryos. *American Journal of Human Genetics, 84,* 771–779.

van Gorp, S., Leerink, M., Kakinohana, O., Platoshyn, O., Santucci, C., Galik, J., . . . Marsala, M. (2013). Amelioration of motor/sensory dysfunction and spasticity in a rat model of acute lumbar spinal cord injury by human neural stem cell transplantation. *Stem Cell Research and Therapy, 4*(3), 57.

Van IJzendoorn, M. H., Bakermans-Kranenburg, M. J., & Ebstein, R. P. (2011). Methylation matters in child development: Toward developmental behavioral epigenetics. *Child Development Perspectives, 5,* 305–310.

Van Speybroeck, L. (2002). From epigenesis to epigenetics: The case of C. H. Waddington. *Annals of the New York Academy of Science, 981,* 61–81.

Varmuza, S. (2003). Epigenetics and the renaissance of heresy. *Genome, 46,* 963–967.

Vassoler, F. M., White, S. L., Schmidt, H. D., Sadri-Vakili, G., & Pierce, R. C. (2013). Epigenetic inheritance of a cocaine-resistance phenotype. *Nature Neuroscience, 16,* 42–47.

Veldic, M., Guidotti, A., Maloku, E., Davis, J. M., & Costa, E. (2005). In psychosis, cortical interneurons overexpress DNA-methyltransferase 1. *Proceedings of the National Academy of Sciences USA, 102,* 2152–2157.

Vickers, M. H., Gluckman, P. D., Coveny, A. H., Hofman, P. L., Cutfield, W. S., Gertler, A., . . . Harris, M. (2005). Neonatal leptin treatment reverses developmental programming. *Endocrinology, 146,* 4211–4216.

Voineagu, I., Wang, X., Johnston, P., Lowe, J. K., Tian, Y., Horvath, S., . . . Geschwind, D. H. (2011). Transcriptomic analysis of autistic brain reveals convergent molecular pathology. *Nature, 474,* 380–384.

Waddington, C. H. (1968). The basic ideas of biology. In C. H. Waddington (Ed.), *Towards a Theoretical Biology* (Vol. 1: Prolegomena, pp. 1–32). Edinburgh: Edinburgh University Press.

Wadsworth, J. S., McBrien, D. M., & Harper, D. C. (2003). Vocational guidance and employment of persons with a diagnosis of Prader-Willi syndrome. *Journal of Rehabilitation, 69,* 15–21.

Wang, E. T., Sandberg, R., Luo, S., Khrebtukova, I., Zhang, L., Mayr, C., . . . Burge, C. B. (2008). Alternative isoform regulation in human tissue transcriptomes. *Nature, 456,* 470–476.

Wang, Z., Zang, C., Rosenfeld, J. A., Schones, D. E., Barski, A., Cuddapah, S., . . . Zhao, K. (2008). Combinatorial patterns of histone acetylations and methylations in the human genome. *Nature Genetics, 40,* 897–903.

Waterland, R. A., & Jirtle, R. L. (2003). Transposable elements: Targets for early nutritional effects on epigenetic gene regulation. *Molecular and Cellular Biology, 23,* 5293–5300.

Waterland, R. A., Travisano, M., & Tahiliani, K. G. (2007). Diet-induced hypermethylation at *agouti viable yellow* is not inherited transgenerationally through the female. *FASEB Journal, 21,* 3380–3385.

Watson, J. D., & Crick, F. H. C. (1953). Molecular structure of nucleic acids: A structure for deoxyribose nucleic acid. *Nature, 171,* 737–738.

Weaver, I. C. G. (2007). Epigenetic programming by maternal behavior and pharmacological intervention: Nature versus nurture: Let's call the whole thing off. *Epigenetics, 2*, 22–28.

Weaver, I. C. G., Cervoni, N., Champagne, F. A., D'Alessio, A. C., Sharma, S., Seckl, J. R., . . . Meaney, M. J. (2004a). Epigenetic programming by maternal behavior. *Nature Neuroscience, 7*, 847–854.

Weaver, I. C. G., Champagne, F. A., Brown, S. E., Dymov, S., Sharma, S., Meaney, M. J., & Szyf, M. (2005). Reversal of maternal programming of stress responses in adult offspring through methyl supplementation: Altering epigenetic marking later in life. *Journal of Neuroscience, 25*, 11045–11054.

Weaver, I. C. G., D'Alessio, A. C., Brown, S. E., Hellstron, I. C., Dymov, S., Sharma, S., . . . Meaney, M. J. (2007). The transcription factor nerve growth factor-inducible protein A mediates epigenetic programming: Altering epigenetic marks by immediate-early genes. *Journal of Neuroscience, 27*, 1756–1768.

Weaver, I. C. G., Diorio, J., Seckl, J. R., Szyf, M., & Meaney, M. J. (2004b). Early environmental regulation of hippocampal glucocorticoid receptor gene expression: Characterization of intracellular mediators and potential genomic target sites. *Annals of the New York Academy of Science, 1024*, 182–212.

Weaver, I. C. G., Meaney, M. J., & Szyf, M. (2006). Maternal care effects on the hippocampal transcriptome and anxiety-mediated behaviors in the offspring that are reversible in adulthood. *Proceedings of the National Academy of Sciences USA, 103*, 3480–3485.

Wei, G., & Mahowald, A. P. (1994). The germline: Familiar and newly uncovered properties. *Annual Review of Genetics, 28*, 309–324.

Weismann, A. (1889). *Essays upon heredity and kindred biological problems.* London: Frowde.

West, M. J., & King, A. P. (1987). Settling nature and nurture into an ontogenetic niche. *Developmental Psychobiology, 20*, 549–562.

Wilkinson, L. S. (2010). Which parental gene gets the upper hand? *Science, 329*, 636–637.

Williams, C. A., Beaudet, A. L., Clayton-Smith, J., Knoll, J. H., Kyllerman, M., Laan, L. A., . . . Wagstaff, J. (2006). Angelman syndrome 2005: Updated consensus for diagnostic criteria. *American Journal of Medical Genetics, 140A*, 413–418.

Wilmut, I., Schnieke, A. E., McWhir, J., Kind, A. J., & Campbell, K. H. S. (1997). Viable offspring derived from fetal and adult mammalian cells. *Nature, 385*, 810–813.

Wilson, R. S., Mendes de Leon, C. F., Barnes, L. L., Schneider, J. A., Bienias, J. L., Evans, D. A., & Bennett, D. A. (2002). Participation in cognitively stimulating activities and risk of incident Alzheimer disease. *Journal of the American Medical Association, 287*, 742–748.

Wolff, G. L. (1978). Influence of maternal phenotype on metabolic differentiation of agouti locus mutants in the mouse. *Genetics, 88*, 529–539.

Wong, C. C. Y., Caspi, A., Williams, B., Craig, I. W., Houts, R., Ambler, A., . . . Mill, J. (2010). A longitudinal study of epigenetic variation in twins. *Epigenetics, 5*, 516–526.

Wong, C. C. Y., Mill, J., & Fernandes, C. (2011). Drugs and addiction: An introduction to epigenetics. *Addiction, 106*, 480–489.

Woodward, T. E., & Gills, J. P. (2012). *The mysterious epigenome: What lies beyond DNA.* Grand Rapids, MI: Kregel Publications.

World Health Organization, International Agency for Research on Cancer (2004). Betel-quid and areca-nut chewing and some areca-nut-derived nitrosamines. *IARC Monographs on the Evaluation of Carcinogenic Risks to Humans, 85*.

Wu, C. -t., & Morris, J. R. (2001). Genes, genetics, and epigenetics: A correspondence. *Science, 293*, 1103–1105.

Xu, J., & Gordon, J. I. (2003). Honor thy symbionts. *Proceedings of the National Academy of Sciences USA, 100*, 10452–10459.

Yaffe, K., Barnes, D., Nevitt, M., Lui, L.-Y., & Covinsky, K. (2001). A prospective study of physical activity and cognitive decline in elderly women: Women who walk. *Archives of Internal Medicine, 161*, 1703–1708.

Yehuda, R., & Bierer, L. M. (2009). The relevance of epigenetics to PTSD: Implications for the DSM-V. *Journal of Traumatic Stress, 22*, 427–434.

Yokota, S., Hori, H., Umezawa, M., Kubota, N., Niki, R., Yanagita, S., & Takeda, K. (2013). Gene expression changes in the olfactory bulb of mice induced by exposure to diesel exhaust are dependent on animal rearing environment. *PLoS ONE, 8*(8), e70145. doi:10.1371/journal.pone.0070145

Zeisel, S. H. (2009). Importance of methyl donors during reproduction. *American Journal of Clinical Nutrition, 89*, 673S–677S.

Zhang, Q., Andersen, M. E., & Conolly, R. B. (2006). Binary gene induction and protein expression in individual cells. *Theoretical Biology and Medical Modelling, 3*(18). doi:10.1186/1742-4682-3-18

Zhang, T.-Y., Bagot, R., Parent, C., Nesbitt, C., Bredy, T. W., Caldji, C., . . . Meaney, M. J. (2006). Maternal programming of defensive responses through sustained effects on gene expression. *Biological Psychology, 73*, 72–89.

Zhang, T.-Y., & Meaney, M. J. (2010). Epigenetics and the environmental regulation of the genome and its function. *Annual Review of Psychology, 61*, 439–466.

Zovkic, I. B., & Sweatt, J. D. (2012). Epigenetic mechanisms in learned fear: Implications for PTSD. *Neuropsychopharmacology Reviews*. Advance online publication. doi:10.1038/npp.2012.79

INDEX